HOT TOPICS

Infectious Diseases

Vincent Lo Re III, MD
Clinical and Research Fellow
Division of Infectious Diseases
Center for Clinical Epidemiology and Biostatistics
University of Pennsylvania School of Medicine
Philadelphia, Pennsylvania

HANLEY & BELFUS
An Affiliate of Elsevier

HANLEY & BELFUS, INC.
An Affiliate of Elsevier

The Curtis Center
Independence Square West
Philadelphia, Pennsylvania 19106

Note to the reader: Although the information in this book has been carefully reviewed for correctness of dosage and indications, neither the editor, nor the authors, nor the publisher can accept any legal responsibility for any errors or omissions that may be made. No warranty is expressed or implied with respect to the material contained herein. Before prescribing any drug, the reader must review the manufacturer's current product information (package inserts) for accepted indications, absolute dosage recommendations, and other information pertinent to the safe and effective use of the product described.

Library of Congress Control Number: 2003107382

INFECTIOUS DISEASES: HOT TOPICS   ISBN 1-56053-580-6

Printed in the United States of America

Last digit is the print number: 9 8 7 6 5 4 3 2 1

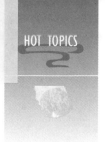

Infectious
Diseases

Contents

HOT TOPICS

Contributors

Valerianna Amorosa, MD
Clinical and Research Fellow, Department of Medicine, Division of Infectious Diseases, University of Pennsylvania School of Medicine, Philadelphia, Pennsylvania

Todd Daniel Barton, MD
Instructor, Division of Infectious Diseases, University of Pennsylvania School of Medicine, and Associate Program Director, Internal Medicine Residency Program, Hospital of the University of Pennsylvania, Philadelphia, Pennsylvania

Leanne Beers, MD
Clinical and Research Fellow, Division of Infectious Diseases, University of Pennsylvania School of Medicine, Philadelphia, Pennsylvania

Emily A. Blumberg, MD
Associate Professor, Department of Medicine, Division of Infectious Diseases, University of Pennsylvania School of Medicine, Philadelphia, Pennsylvania

Serena Cardillo, MD
Medical Resident, Department of Internal Medicine, University of Pennsylvania School of Medicine, Philadelphia, Pennsylvania

Maureen Cassin, MD
Medical Resident, Department of Internal Medicine, University of Pennsylvania School of Medicine, Philadelphia, Pennsylvania

Stephen J. Gluckman, MD, FACP
Chief, Infectious Diseases Clinical Services, Hospital of the University of Pennsylvania, Philadelphia; Professor of Medicine, Division of Infectious Diseases, University of Pennsylvania School of Medicine, Philadelphia, Pennsylvania

Carolyn V. Gould, MD
Clinical and Research Fellow, Department of Medicine, Division of Infectious Diseases, University of Pennsylvania School of Medicine, Philadelphia, Pennsylvania

Kelly J. Henning, MD
Director of Epidemiology, Division of Epidemiology, New York City Department of Health and Mental Hygiene, New York, New York; Adjunct Associate Professor, University of Pennsylvania School of Medicine, Philadelphia, Pennsylvania

Janet M. Hines, MD
Assistant Professor, Department of Medicine, Division of Infectious Diseases, University of Pennsylvania School of Medicine, and Associate Director, Immunodeficiency Program, Hospital of the University of Pennsylvania, Philadelphia, Pennsylvania

Barry E. Kenneally, MD
Adjunct Professor, Department of Family Practice and Community Medicine, University of Pennsylvania School of Medicine, Philadelphia, Pennsylvania

Paul A. Kinniry, MD
Clinical and Research Fellow, Division of Pulmonary and Critical Care, Hospital of the University of Pennsylvania, Philadelphia, Pennsylvania

Jay R. Kostman, MD
Chief, Division of Infectious Diseases, Presbyterian Hospital, Philadelphia; Associate Professor, Department of Medicine, Division of Infectious Diseases, University of Pennsylvania School of Medicine, Philadelphia, Pennsylvania

Vincent Lo Re III, MD
Clinical and Research Fellow, Division of Infectious Diseases, Center for Clinical Epidemiology and Biostatistics, University of Pennsylvania School of Medicine, Philadelphia, Pennsylvania

Kathryn A. Novello, MD
Medical Resident, Department of Medicine, Hospital of the University of Pennsylvania, Philadelphia, Pennsylvania

Harvey Rubin, MD
Associate Dean of Student Affairs; Director, Institute for Strategic Threat Analysis and Response; Professor of Medicine, Division of Infectious Diseases, University of Pennsylvania School of Medicine, Philadelphia, Pennsylvania

Henry M. Wu, MD, DTM&H
Clinical and Research Fellow, Department of Internal Medicine, Division of Infectious Diseases, University of Pennsylvania School of Medicine, Philadelphia, Pennsylvania

Preface

The field of infectious diseases changes rapidly. Almost yearly, new infectious agents are identified, while other known entities increase in incidence and expand their geographic locations. The emergence and spread of West Nile virus in the United States in 1999, the anthrax bioterrorist attacks of 2001, and the recognition of the global systemic acute respiratory syndrome (SARS) outbreak in 2003 are just a few recent examples of the constant evolution of infectious diseases and their subsequent impact on humanity.

Infectious Diseases Hot Topics was created to summarize key information on the clinical presentation, diagnosis, management, and prevention of many important and emerging infectious diseases. As you review the table of contents, you will see that a number of the chapters review subjects that are currently considered to be truly hot topics in infectious diseases, such as West Nile virus and other causes of viral encephalitis (Chapter 3), management of chronic hepatitis C (Chapter 12), travel medicine (Chapters 27–29), and agents of bioterrorism (Chapter 30). Other chapters cover subjects that may not appear to be hot but are so commonly encountered and discussed in clinical settings as to necessitate their inclusion in any list of hot topics.

This book is intended for physicians and other primary care providers who manage patients with infectious diseases. In particular, house officers, medical students, and other trainees will find that each chapter presents an overall approach to the management of a particular infectious illness, facilitating bedside care and aiding in preparation for rounds and clinical conferences. Internists, family physicians, emergency medicine physicians, nurse practitioners, and various specialists will also appreciate this book as a quick reference to assist in the management of many infections. It is designed in a concise, readable format that is easy to use in any practice setting. Numerous figures and tables emphasize key diagnostic and treatment information. All of the contributing authors have incorporated current advances up to the time of publication.

I hope that you enjoy reading it as much as we enjoyed writing it!

Vincent Lo Re III, MD
EDITOR

ACKNOWLEDGMENTS

I wish to thank Dr. Harvey Rubin for giving me the opportunity to bring my vision of this book into reality. I also want to thank my superb contributing authors for their time and hard work. The editors of Hanley & Belfus, particularly Jacqueline M. Mahon, provided me with valuable assistance and support. Most importantly, I thank my incredible wife, Serena, for her constant patience with me during our first year of marriage as I spent it tied to the computer, writing and editing these chapters.

Dedication

For my wife, Serena, who was so supportive of my efforts on this book. She is the light of my life. Vivo per lei, bella.

And for my parents, who helped me achieve my dream of becoming a doctor. I love and admire you both dearly.

V.L.R. III

Acute Bacterial Meningitis

Valerianna Amorosa, M.D.

chapter

1

The suspicion of acute bacterial meningitis is a medical emergency and always a "hot topic" among clinical practitioners. Although fewer than 25,000 cases occur per year in the United States,[1] acute bacterial meningitis carries an overall mortality rate of 25% and accounts for significant morbidity despite advances in therapy. Based on initial clinical suspicion, the clinician must move swiftly toward timely diagnosis and institution of therapy. In these situations, treatment should not be postponed for more than 30 minutes beyond the initial presentation and should not await the results of diagnostic procedures.

This chapter reviews the common pathogens implicated in acute bacterial meningitis, provides an overview of the key clinical findings, presents the critical diagnostic findings on lumbar puncture, and discusses the indications for neuroimaging. Choices for empiric and definitive therapy, including relevant therapeutic adjuncts, are also reviewed. Finally, the role of isolation and chemoprophylaxis in cases of *Neisseria meningitidis* infection are also addressed.

Causes of Acute Bacterial Meningitis

Streptococcus pneumoniae. In North American series, infection with *S. pneumoniae* is overall the most common cause of acute bacterial meningitis, occurring in more than 50% of community-acquired cases.[3,4] Pneumoccocal meningitis occurs with the highest incidence in patients 6 to 24 months of age and those over 65 years of age, but it can be seen across all age groups. It can be associated with significant neurologic complications, particularly deafness. A number of conditions can allow more severe disease, and these include asplenism, multiple myeloma, alcoholism, malnutrition, cirrhosis, and renal disease. The organisms may be identified in the cerebrospinal fluid (CSF) as lancet-shaped gram-positive cocci in pairs. The mortality rate associated with pneumococcal meningitis is 19% overall, although this is much higher in elderly and debilitated people.[12] Beta-lactam-resistant pneumococcus has emerged over the last decade, leading to revised recommendations for empiric therapy that now include vancomycin.

Neisseria meningitidis. Infection with *N. meningitidis* occurs most commonly in children and young adults and carries a mortality rate of 3% to 13%.[1] Most people acquire the disease from an asymptomatic carrier through face-to-face contact . Certain host factors can predispose individuals to disease, and these include age, level of immunity, and the presence of alcoholism.[13] The incubation period of *N. meningitidis* is typically 2 to 10 days, with an initial presentation of fever and malaise followed by headache, nausea, vomiting, stiff neck, and a maculopapular, purpuric, or petecheal rash.[13] The rash is evident with concomitant meningococcemia and evolves rapidly. The organisms appear as gram-negative diplococci on Gram stain of the CSF.

Listeria monocytogenes. Infection with *L. monocytogenes* is the second most common cause of meningitis in people older than 60 years.[1] The incidence of listeriosis varies from year to year in different regions and is occasionally associated with outbreaks related to contaminated deli meats and dairy products.[14] Since cell-mediated immunity is involved in *Listeria* defense, patients with depressed cellular immunity are at particular risk for infection with this agent. In addition to those with comorbidities, *Listeria* meningitis can occur sporadically in healthy adults, although most commonly in elderly people. While the disease is associated with a high mortality rate (exceeding 20%), when it occurs in otherwise healthy people, the mortality rate is low.[3,4] *Listeria* appears as a gram-positive rod on Gram stain of the CSF, but it is rarely visualized.[6]

Group B Streptococci. Group B streptoccal infection accounts for up to 4% of cases of meningitis in adults and is most often a consideration in peripartum and neonatal patients. However, group B streptococcal meningitis can also be seen in non-pregnant patients, particularly the elderly and those with underlying diabetes mellitus or cirrhosis. Often a distant infectious site, such as endometritis or endocarditis, is present.[15] The organisms appear as gram-positive cocci in pairs and chains.

Gram-Negative Bacilli. Gram-negative rods can be associated with acute bacterial meningitis in neonates, neurosurgical patients, immunosuppressed hosts, and elderly people. *Escherichia coli* and *Klebsiella pneumoniae* are the most common gram-negative pathogens isolated.[6] Meningitis can also occur in the context of gram-negative sepsis.[5]

Haemophilus influenzae. Since the use of the conjugated *Haemophilus influenzae B* vaccine, *Haemophilus influenzae* is no longer a major pathogen in infant and childhood meningitis. Fewer than 1200 cases per year are now reported to the Centers for Disease Control and Prevention, with fewer than 300 cases occurring in children.[1] *Haemophilus* meningitis in anyone older than 6 years is uncommon and suggests other underlying conditions such as sinusitis, otitis media, pneumonia, diabetes, alcoholism, asplenism, a CSF leak, or an immune deficiency.[6,17] The organisms can be identified as small gram-negative coccobacilli on Gram stain of the CSF.

Staphylococci. *Staphylococcus aureus* meningitis is most commonly associated with prior neurosurgery, head trauma, or CSF shunt infections.[4] One sees gram-positive cocci in clusters on Gram stain. *S. aureus* meningitis can also be seen in cases of underlying infective endocarditis, paraspinal infection, sinusitis, osteomyelitis, or pneumonia. *Staphylococcus epidermidis* is the most common pathogen seen in CSF shunt infections.

Miscellaneous Pathogens. *Nocardia* species, long filamentous gram-positive rods, may cause meningitis in patients with underlying immunosuppression. *Capnocytophaga canimorsus*, a gram-negative rod, is a rare cause of meningitis and can be seen in association with dog and cat bites, most fulminantly in asplenic people.[18] It is a fastidious organism that is not grown on standard culture. Thus, it should be considered when gram-negative rods are identified in the CSF and no growth is seen with subsequent cultures.[18] Group A streptococci are a rare cause of meningitis and are seen typically in those with predisposing sinusitis or otitis media.[16]

Clinical Findings

Several case series have looked at signs and symptoms associated with bacterial meningitis.[2–4] The classic clinical triad of fever, headache, and nuchal rigidity was present in 66% of patients in two recent case series.[3,4] In 50% of cases, patients present with an altered level of consciousness. Photophobia, seizures, nausea, vomiting, neurologic deficits, and rashes or other skin lesions may also be present.[3–5] In elderly people, the presentation may be subtle, with an altered mental status (often in the absence of fever) as the only presenting sign.[6]

When symptoms and signs are suggestive of meningitis, the patient's history can be useful in determining possible causes. Key historical features include the following:

- Patient's age
- Recent or prior neurosurgical procedures
- Presence of an intraventricular shunt
- History of head trauma
- History of recent sinusitis, otitis media, or meningitis
- Pregnancy status
- Immunosuppression due to human immunodeficiency virus, organ transplant, malignancy, diabetes, cirrhosis, or alcohol abuse

- History of sick contact
- Animal and insect exposures
- Travel history
- Meningococcal and vaccination history

Certain findings on physical examination can be useful in assessing for meningeal inflammation. Nuchal rigidity typically suggests meningeal inflammation, as do the classic Kernig and Brudzinski signs, although these lack sensitivity and specificity. Kernig's sign is pain elicited behind the patient's knee while the examiner extends the knee from a flexed hip, bent knee position as the patient lies on his or her back.

Brudzinski's sign is present if the patient flexes his or her hips and knees as the examiner flexes the patient's neck. One recent study noted that these physical signs were present in only 5% of patients with meningitis.[2] However, other investigators have noted their presence in up to 50% of cases.[5] A Japanese study found that "jolt accentuation," which is defined as an increasing severity of headache caused by turning the patient's head back and forth horizontally two to three times in 1 minute was more sensitive and specific for meningitis than any other diagnostic maneuver.[7]

Neuroimaging

When a history and physical examination suggest bacterial meningitis, the practitioner should proceed swiftly to lumbar puncture to establish a diagnosis. However, the clinician is faced with the question of whether the procedure will put the patient at risk for herniation and subsequent neurologic deterioration. To assess this risk, physicians often order head computed tomography (CT) scans prior to performing the procedure. In certain populations, provided there is no delay in delivery of empiric antibiotics, this approach may be appropriate.

It is generally accepted that patients with coma, papilledema, or other focal neurologic deficits should undergo neuroimaging prior to lumbar puncture for suspected acute bacterial meningitis.[5] Hasbrun et al[8] have determined that in such patients, head CT scanning should be used in making the decision to perform lumbar puncture.

A recent prospective study has confirmed, however, that clinical features can be used to determine which patients are unlikely to have an abnormal CT scan and can thus undergo lumbar puncture without delay.[9] In this study of 235 patients who underwent a head CT scan prior to lumbar puncture, abnormalities were more often associated with certain historical features and neurologic findings. Patients older than 60 years with known immune deficiency (due to human immunodeficiency virus, immunosuppression, or transplantation), central nervous system disease, or a history of seizure 1 week prior to presentation were more likely to have abnormal head CT scans. Patients with focal neurologic findings were also more likely to have abnormal scans. In the patients with none of these features, only 3% of the CT scans were abnormal, and there was no evidence of mass lesion or herniation risk that precluded subsequent lumbar puncture.[8] Kastenbauer et al[9] retrospectively studied the records of 75 adults with pneumococcal meningitis and similarly determined that patients with focal neurologic deficits, seizures, and reduced level of consciousness (Glasgow coma score ≤12) were more likely to have head CT abnormalities.

Diagnosis

The lumbar puncture is critical to the diagnosis of acute bacterial meningitis. Several case series have looked at the presence of various CSF abnormalities of the lumbar puncture in cases of acute bacterial meningitis.[3,4] Opening pressure is typically greater than 18 cm H_2O and can be very high when cerebral edema is present.[4] Generally, 80% of the time, the fluid is turbid. Gram stain is positive in 50% to 60% of cases. CSF cultures are positive in 65% to 75% of cases, although less often if antibiotics precede the lumbar puncture. The CSF cell count often exceeds 1000 cells/mm³. Neutrophilic predominance, with more than 80% neutrophils, is present in 80% of cases, although there are cases of lymphocyte predominance, seen most commonly with *Listeria* infection. The total protein usually exceeds 45 mg/dL in more than 95% of cases and is greater than 200 mg/dL in more than 50% of cases. The CSF glucose level is less than 50 mg/dL in approximately 70% of cases. However, these initial indices can be relatively normal in immunocompromised and neutropenic patients, and excluding the diagnosis of acute bacterial menigitis may necessitate a follow-up lumbar puncture.[5] Partial antibiotic treatment, which is defined as the administration of intravenous antibiotics within 6 hours, oral antibiotics within 12 hours, or a prior recent course of antibiotics, does not usually not have a significant effect on CSF indices.[3] Bacterial antigen tests in the CSF have been shown to have sensitivities of less than 75% and cannot be used to rule out disease.[11] CSF analysis, combined with blood culture data, determines the diagnosis of acute bacterial meningitis.

Gram stain and culture of the CSF results should be performed immediately after the lumbar puncture and can direct antibiotic therapy. Since blood cultures are positive in more than 50% of cases of acute bacterial meningitis, two sets of blood cultures should be drawn prior to the administration of any antibiotic therapy.[10]

Treatment

Empiric Treatment

As has been mentioned, antibiotic selection in cases of acute bacterial meningitis is of paramount importance. Since antibodies and complement are lacking in the CSF, allowing for rapid bacterial multiplication, bactericidal antibiotics are needed to sterilize the CSF. Due to the inflammation at the blood-brain barrier, antibiotics can more readily enter the CSF. The chosen antibiotics must have adequate CSF penetration, reach bactericidal concentrations in the CSF, and retain activity in the low pH and high protein environment of infected spinal fluid.[12] To facilitate this, antibiotic dosages used to treat acute bacterial meningitis are generally higher than those used for other infections.

The latest data from the Centers for Disease Control and Prevention indicate that almost 20% of clinical isolates of pneumococcus are resistant to penicillin and another 10% display intermediate susceptibility.[7] Moreover, 7.5% of isolates are noted to be resistant to third-generation cephalosporins and another 10% have intermediate resistance.[1] Recommendations have thus evolved to include vancomycin in addition to ceftriaxone or cefotaxime as part of initial empiric therapy.

Additionally, given the high prevalence of *Listeria* infection in people older than 50 years and those with significant comorbidities or immune dysfunction, clinicians should also add ampicillin to their initial empiric coverage. For the population aged 18 to 50 years, both a third-generation cephalosporin and vancomycin should be part of the initial empiric regimen (Table 1). For patients with a prior neurosurgical procedure, broad empiric coverage is initially recommended with vancomycin and an antipseudomonal cephalosporin such as cefepime.

There are cases in which the clinical presentation and CSF indices are consistent with acute bacterial meningitis but Gram stain, CSF cultures, and blood cultures fail to reveal a pathogen. This occurs most often in cases of partial antibiotic treatment. Empiric therapy with a third-generation cephalosporin, vancomycin, and, if indicated, ampicillin, is warranted in these situations as well.

Quite frequently, patients are noted to have a true penicillin allergy, which necessitates alterations in first-line therapy. In these situations, empiric therapy should include chloramphenicol with the addition of vancomycin (see Table 1). Combination vancomycin and rifampin may be the best definitive regimen for pneumococcal disease when penicillin is contraindicated.[16] When *Listeria* is a consideration, trimethoprim-sulfamethoxazole should be added. The necessarily high doses of intravenous antibiotic comes with a high fluid load, which may necessitates close attention to volume status in a patient with potential cardiac disease.

TABLE 1. Empiric Therapy for Bacterial Meningitis (Delayed Lumbar Puncture or Negative Cerebrospinal Fluid Gram Stain)

Host	Potential Pathogens	Empiric Antibiotic
Normal immunity, >3 months to <18 years old	Neisseria meningitidis, Streptococcus pneumoniae	Third-generation cephalosporin and vancomycin
Age >50 years or pregnant	S. pneumoniae, Listeria monocytogenes, gram-negative bacilli	Third-generation cephalosporin, vancomycin, and ampicillin
Impaired cellular immunity*	L. monocytogenes, gram-negative bacilli, S. pneumoniae	Antipseudomonal cephalosporin, ampicillin, vancomycin
Head trauma, neurosurgery, cerebrospinal fluid shunt	Staphylococcus aureus, Staphylococcus epidermidis, gram-negative bacilli, S. pneumoniae	Vancomycin, antipseudomonal cephalosporin

*For discussion of those with impaired cellular immunity, see text.
Adapted from Tunkel AR, Scheld WM: Acute meningitis. In Mandell GL, Bennett JE, Dolin R (eds): Mandell, Douglas and Bennett's Principles and Practice of Infectious Diseases, 5th ed. Philadelphia, Churchill Livingstone, 2000, 959–997; and Quagliarello VJ, Scheld WM: Treatment of bacterial meningitis. N Engl J Med 336:708–716, 1997.

Once a pathogen is identified, definitive therapy should use the best agents possible. In many cases, desensitization to penicillin may be necessary given the known clinical failures of chloramphenicol for pneumococcus and fears about poor penetration of vancomycin into the CSF.

Definitive Treatment

Streptococcus pneumoniae. If pneumococcus is isolated, the patient should be given both vancomycin and a third-generation cephalosporin. Vancomycin has been shown in vitro to be synergistic with ceftriaxone against ceftriaxone-resistant pneumococcal strains.[12] If the organism is found to be resistant to penicillin and to ceftriaxone, this synergistic regimen should be continued. Given the concern that steroid use can decrease the ability of vancomycin to penetrate the CSF, one should consider the addition of rifampin to promote sterilization of the CSF when using steroids.[12] If the strain is susceptible to penicillin, this antibiotic is the ideal therapy (Tables 2 and 3).

Neisseria meningitidis. If gram-negative diplococci are seen on Gram stain or N. meningitidis is isolated, ceftriaxone is the recommended initial therapy. Since resistant strains have been isolated in the United States, penicillin use is not recommended until the susceptibilities are known.[1]

Listeria monocytogenes. If Listeria is isolated, treatment with ampicillin is appropriate. Since the beta-lactams may not be bactericidal against L.

TABLE 2. Antibiotic Recommendations Based on Gram Stain	
Finding	Antibiotic
Gram-positive cocci	Vancomycin plus broad-spectrum cephalosporin
Gram-positive rods	Ampicillin +/− aminoglycocide
Gram-negative rods	Antipseudomonal cephalosporin plus aminoglycocide
Gram-negative diplococci or small gram-negative coccobacilli	Broad-spectrum cephalosporin

Adapted from Tunkel AR, Scheld WM: Acute meningitis. In Mandell G, Bennett JE, Dolin R (eds): Mandell, Douglas and Bennett's Principles and Practice of Infectious Diseases, 5th ed. Philadelphia, Churchill Livingstone, 2000, 959–997; and Quagliarello VJ, Scheld WM: Treatment of bacterial meningitis. N Engl J Med 336:708–716, 1997.

monocytogenes, it is recommended that ampicillin be used in combination with gentamicin. Trimethoprim-sulfamethoxazole is an alternative bactericidal therapy against *Listeria* and has shown clinical success.[12]

Group B Streptococci. For group B streptococcal meningitis, penicillin or ampicillin alone may be used (Table 4). However, in children and those with severe illnesses, the addition of gentamicin should also be considered.

Gram-Negative Bacilli. The development of broad-spectrum cephalosporins has dramatically improved the mortality rate from meningitis due to gram-negative bacilli. First-line therapy for community-acquired gram-negative meningitis includes a third-generation cephalosporin, such as ceftriaxone, with the addition of gentamicin, administered either intraventricularly or intravenously. There is the possibility of the emergence of antibiotic resistance during therapy for gram-negative meningitis, and, in some cases, repeat lumbar puncture may be necessary to guide therapeutic decisions.

Staphylococci. For both *S. aureus* and coagulase-negative staphylococcal infections, vancomycin is appropriate initially, but an antistaphylococ-

TABLE 3. Definitive Therapy of Acute Bacterial Meningitis, by Organism	
Organism	Treatment
Streptococcus pneumoniae	Vancomycin with third-generation cephalosporin
Neisseria meningitidis	Ceftriaxone
Listeria monocytogenes	Ampicillin and gentamicin
Group B streptococcus	Penicillin G
Haemophilus influenzae	Ceftriaxone
Enterobacteriaceae	Third-generation cephalosporin and aminoglycoside
Pseudomonas aeruginosa, Acinetobacter	Antipseudomonal cephalosporin and aminoglycoside

Adapted from Tunkel AR, Scheld WM: Acute meningitis. In Mandell GL, Bennett JE, Dolin R (eds): Mandell, Douglas and Bennett's Principles and Practice of Infectious Diseases, 5th ed. Philadelphia, Churchill Livingstone, 2000, 959–997; and Quagliarello VJ, Scheld WM: Treatment of bacterial meningitis. N Engl J Med 336:708–716, 1997.

TABLE 4. Antimicrobial Susceptibility Data for Common Organisms Causing Acute Bacterial Meningitis

Organism	First-Line Therapy
Streptococcus pneumoniae	
PCN MIC < 0.1 μg/ml	Penicillin G or ampicillin
PCN MIC 0.1–1.0 μg/ml	Ceftriaxone or cefotaxime
PCN MIC ≥ 2.0 μg/ml	Vancomycin plus third-generation cephalosporin (above)
Neisseria meningitidis	
PCN MIC < 0.1 μg/ml	Penicillin G or ampicillin
PCN MIC 0.1–1.0 μg/ml	Third-generation cephalosporin (above)
Listeria monocytogenes	Ampicillin +\− aminoglycoside
Staphylococcus aureus	
Methicillin sensitive	Nafcillin or oxacillin
Methicillin resistant	Vancomycin
Haemophilus influenzae	
Beta-lactamase negative	Ampicillin
Beta-lactamase positive	Third-generation cephalosporin (above)
Enterobacteriaceae	Third-generation cephalosporin plus aminoglycoside*
Pseudomonas aeruginosa	Cefepime plus aminoglycoside
Group B streptococci	Ampicillin or penicillin G (consider addition of aminoglycoside)
Staphylococcus epidermidis	Vancomycin (consider addition of rifampin)

*Unless susceptibility data dictate otherwise or extended-spectrum beta-lactamase producing organism.
Adapted from Tunkel AR, Scheld WM: Acute meningitis. In Mandell G, Bennett JE, Dolin R (eds): Mandell, Douglas and Bennett's Principles and Practice of Infectious Diseases, 5th ed. Philadelphia, Churchill Livingstone, 2000, 959–997; and Quagliarello VJ, Scheld WM: Treatment of bacterial meningitis. N Engl J Med 336:708–716, 1997.

cal penicillin (such as nafcillin) is ideal therapy if the organism is susceptible (see Table 4). In CSF shunt infections, intraventricular antibiotics are often warranted (Table 5), and most often the shunt will need to be removed.

Duration of Therapy

The duration of therapy for various pathogens should be guided by clinical response. No large studies have examined appropriate duration of treatment for the majority of pathogens, although it is known that short therapeutic regimens are adequate for *N. meningitidis* and *H. influenzae*.[12] Recommendations for treatment durations are listed in Table 6.

Adjunctive Therapy

Steroid Use

Given that many of the damaging sequelae of acute bacterial meningitis are due to the host's inflammatory response, several studies have

TABLE 5. Dosages of Antibiotics Used in the Treatment of Acute Bacterial Meningitis*		
Drug	Daily dose (intravenous)	Dosing interval (hours)
Ampicillin	12 g	4
Cefepime	4 g	12
Cefotaxime	8–12 g	4–6
Ceftriaxone	4 g	12–24
Chloramphenicol[†]	4–6 g	6
Gentamicin[‡]	3–5 mg/kg	8
Nafcillin	9–12 g	4
Oxacillin	9–12 g	4
Penicillin G	24 million units	4
Rifampin	600 mg (oral)	24
Trimethaprim-sulfamethoxazole	10–20 mg/kg	6–12
Vancomycin[§]	2–4 g	8–12

*Dosing may need to be modified in cases of renal or hepatic impairment.
[†]Higher doses or alternate regimen recommended for pneumococcus.
[‡]May need to monitor serum levels
[§]May need to monitor serum and CSF levels in critical patients
Adapted from Tunkel AR, Scheld WM: Acute meningitis. In Mandell G, Bennett JE, Dolin R (eds): Mandell, Douglas and Bennett's Principles and Practice of Infectious Diseases, 5th ed. Philadelphia, Churchill Livingstone, 2000, 959–997; and Quagliarello VJ, Scheld WM: Treatment of bacterial meningitis. N Engl J Med 336:708–716, 1997.

looked at the role of steroids as an adjunctive measure. Many of the studies have been done in children, and steroids have been shown to decrease the incidence of hearing loss in cases of *H. influenzae* meningitis in this population.[5] Corroborating retrospective studies, a recent randomized double-blinded study from the Netherlands found significant mortality and morbidity benefit with the use of dexamethasone during the first 4 days of therapy for acute bacterial meningitis, convincingly for pneumococcal meningitis.[19,20] The authors used doses of 10 mg IV every 6 hours for 4 days, commencing before or concomitant with the first dose of antibiotics. While they did not demonstrate better out-

TABLE 6. Duration of Antibiotic Therapy Depending on Organism Isolated	
Organism	Duration (days)
Neisseria meningitidis	7
Streptococcus pneumoniae	10–14
Listeria monocytogenes	14–21
Group B streptococci	14–21
Gram-negative bacilli (*Haemophilus influenzae*)	21

Adapted from Tunkel AR, Scheld WM: Acute meningitis. In Mandell G, Bennett JE, Dolin R (eds): Mandell, Douglas and Bennett's Principles and Practice of Infectious Diseases, 5th ed. Philadelphia, Churchill Livingstone, 2000, 959–997; and Quagliarello VJ, Scheld WM: Treatment of bacterial meningitis. N Engl J Med 336:708–716, 1997.

comes with steroids for nonpneumococcal meningitides, the number of nonpneumococcal cases was too small to reach a conclusion. Early steroid use should strongly be considered when the clinical picture with or without CSF data points to bacterial meningitis.

Supportive Care

Each patient's neurologic status should be monitored closely and vigilantly for clinical deterioration, and, if this occurs, the practitioner should consider prompt reimaging, the use of modalities to lower intracranial pressure, and neurosurgical consultation for placement of a ventricular shunt or other neurosurgical intervention. While debate has surrounded intravenous fluid administration and cerebral edema, it is now generally accepted that fluids are often needed to maintain an adequate mean arterial pressure to provide sufficient cerebral perfusion pressure.[21]

Prevention of Meningococcal Disease

When a patient is diagnosed with meningococcal meningitis, there is often confusion concerning who should receive secondary prophylaxis. Chemoprophylaxis should be given to close contacts, such as household members, day care center contacts, and those exposed to the patient's oral secretions. Prophylaxis should be given in the first 24 hours because the rate of secondary disease is highest in the first days after disease onset in the index patient. Table 7 gives prophylaxis recommendations.

In the United States, the quadrivalent meningococcal vaccine has been used during outbreaks to limit disease spread. In addition, given the higher prevalence of meningococcal disease among college freshmen living in dorms than the general population, the Centers for Disease Control and Prevention has recommended vaccination for this

TABLE 7. Prophylaxis Recommendations for Meningococcal Exposure	
Patient Group	**Regimen**
Children	
< 1 month	Rifampin: 5 mg/kg twice daily × 2 days
> 1 month	Rifampin: 10 mg/kg twice daily × 2 days
Adults	• Ciprofloxacin 500 mg × 1 dose
	or
	Ofloxacin 400 mg × 1 dose
	• Azithromycin 500 mg × 1 dose
	• Rifampin: 600 mg twice daily × 2 days

Adapted from Ziad M: Meningococcal disease and travel. Clin Infect Dis 34:84–90, 2002.

population. Vaccination is also recommended for asplenic individuals and travelers to areas where meningococcal disease is endemic.

References

1. Summary of notifiable diseases, United States 2002. MMWR Morbid Mortal Wkly Rep 49:1–102, 2002.
2. Thomas KE, Hasbun R, Jekel J, Quagliarello VJ: The diagnostic accuracy of Kernig's sign, Brudzinski's sign, and nuchal rigidity in adults with suspected meningitis. Clin Infect Dis 35:46–52, 2002.
3. Hussein AS, Shafran SD: Acute bacterial meningitis in adults: A 12-year review. Medicine (Baltimore) 79:360–368, 2000.
4. Durand ML, Calderwood SB, Weber DJ, et al: Acute bacterial meningitis in adults: A review of 493 episodes. N Engl J Med 328:21–28, 1993.
5. Tunkel AR, Scheld WM: Acute meningitis. In Mandell GL, Bennett JE, Dolin R (eds): Mandell, Douglas, and Bennett's Principles and Practice of Infectious Diseases, 5th ed. Philadelphia, Churchill Livingstone, 2000, 959–997.
6. Choi C: Bacterial meningitis in aging adults. Clin Infect Dis 33:1380–1385, 2001.
7. Uchihara T, Tsukagoshi J: Jolt accentuation of headache: The most sensitive sign of CSF pleocytosis. Headache 31:167–171, 1991.
8. Hasbun R, Abrahams J, Jekel J, Quagliarello VJ: Computed tomography of the head before lumbar puncture in adults with suspected meningitis. N Engl J Med 345: 1727–1733, 2001.
9. Kastenbauer S, Winkler F, Pfister HW: Cranial CT before lumbar puncture in suspected meningitis. N Engl J Med 346:1248–1251, 2002.
10. Jackson LA, Wenger JD: Laboratory surveillance for meningococcal disease in selected areas, U.S., 1989–91. MMWR Morbid Mortal Wkly Rep 42:21–30, 1993.
11. Mein J, Lum G: CSF bacterial antigen detection tests offer no advantage over Gram's stain in the diagnosis of bacterial meningitis. Pathology 31:67–69, 1999.
12. Quagliarello VJ, Scheld WM: Treatment of bacterial meningitis. N Engl J Med 336: 708–716, 1997.
13. Ziad M: Meningococcal disease and travel. Clin Infect Dis 34:84–90, 2002.
14. Update: Foodborne Listeriosis—United States, 1988–1990. MMWR Morbid Mortal Wkly Rep 41:251,257–258, 1992.
15. Domingo P, Barquet N, Alvarez M, et al: Group B streptococcal meningitis in adults: Report of 12 cases and review. Clin Infect Dis 25:1180–1187, 1997.
16. Van de Beek D, de Gans J, Spanjaard L, et al: Group A streptococcal meningitis in adults: Report of 41 cases and a review of the literature. Clin Infect Dis 34:e32–36, 2002.
17. Schuchat A, Robinson K, Wenger JD, et al: Bacterial meningitis in the U.S. in 1995. N Engl J Med 337:970–976, 1997.
18. Pers C, Gahrn-Hansen B, Frederiksen W: *Capnocytophaga canimorsus* septicemia in Denmark, 1982–95: Review of 39 cases. Clin Infect Dis 23:71–75, 1996.
19. Auburtin M, Porcher R, Bruneel F, et al: Pneumococcal meningitis in the intensive care unit: Prognostic factors of clinical outcome in a series of 80 cases. Am J Respir Crit Care Med 165:713–717, 2002.
20. De Gans J, van de Beek D: Dexamethasone in adults with bacterial meningitis. N Engl J Med 347:1549–1556, 2002.
21. Roos KL: Acute bacterial meningitis. Neurology 20:293–306, 2000.

Aseptic Meningitis

Kathryn A. Novello, M.D.

chapter

2

The term *aseptic meningitis* refers to any meningitis for which a cause is not apparent after initial evaluation of the cerebrospinal fluid (CSF) with routine Gram stain and culture.[1] The incidence of aseptic meningitis is difficult to identify, as many cases are likely unreported.[2] The Centers for Disease Control and Prevention estimated that between 1982 and 1988, there were approximately 8300 to 12,700 cases of aseptic meningitis.[3] Although viral causes are the most common, there are numerous causes, ranging from self-limited to life-threatening. Differentiating among these can be challenging.

Aseptic meningitis is most commonly caused by enteroviruses, with estimates ranging from 80% to 95% of cases.[1,2,4] Other infectious causes include arboviruses, herpes simplex virus, partially treated bacterial meningitis, Lyme disease, tuberculosis, and various fungi (Table 1). However, a number of noninfectious causes; notably drugs, autoimmune diseases, and malignancies, have also been implicated. This chapter discusses the common causes of acute aseptic meningitis in immunocompetent adults.

Viral Causes of Aseptic Meningitis

Enteroviruses

Enteroviruses remain the most common cause of aseptic meningitis in those cases in which a diagnosis is made. Approximately two thirds of all culture-negative CSF from patients with aseptic meningitis will be positive for enteroviruses by polymerase chain reaction (PCR).[5,6] The most common enteroviruses causing meningitis include coxsackieviruses A and B, echovirus, and enteroviruses 68 to 71. Poliovirus is also classified as an enterovirus, but its incidence has declined greatly since vaccination.[1] Enteroviruses are transmitted by a fecal-oral route. In temperate climates, disease is most common in the summer and early fall months, although it may occur throughout the year. Symptoms generally include nonspecific flu-like symptoms, along with fever, headache, nausea, vomiting, and

13

TABLE 1. Infectious Origins of Aseptic Meningitis

Origin	Common Pathogens	Less Common/Rare Pathogens
Viruses	Enteroviruses Human immunodeficiency virus Herpes simplex virus type 2 Arboviruses	Mumps virus Lymphocytic choriomeningitis virus Adenovirus Herpes simplex type 1 Varicella-zoster virus Cytomegalovirus Epstein-Barr virus Influenza A and B Parainfluenza Measles Rubella
Bacteria	Partially treated bacterial meningitis Parameningeal infection Subacute bacterial endocarditis *Borrelia burgdorferi* (Lyme disease) *Mycobacterium tuberculosis*	*Treponema pallidum* (syphilis) *Leptospira* sp. *Brucella* sp. *Mycoplasma hominis* *Mycoplasma pneumoniae* *Chlamydia psittaci* *Listeria monocytogenes* *Nocardia* sp. *Actinomyces*
Fungi		*Cryptococcus neoformans* *Coccidioides imimitis* *Histoplasma capsulatum* *Blastomyces dermatitidis* *Candida* sp. *Aspergillus* sp.
Parasites		*Angiostrongylus cantonensis* *Gnathostoma spinigerum* *Baylisascaris procyonis* *Toxoplasma gondii*

Adapted from Connolly KJ, Hammer SM: The acute aseptic meningitis syndrome. Infect Dis Clin North Am 4:599–622, 1990.

meningismus. A maculopapular rash may also be seen. Focal neurologic signs are rare in the adult population.[7]

The CSF leukocyte count is usually less than 500 cells/mm^3 but may be higher. There is classically a predominance of lymphocytes, but early in the illness there may be a predominance of neutrophils (Table 2).[1] The CSF protein level may be mildly elevated, and hypoglycorrhachia, a low CSF glucose, is usually mild if present.[2] Enterovirus may be grown in culture, but PCR can make the diagnosis more rapidly and may shorten hospitalization and courses of empiric antibiotics.[5,6]

Although the clinical course in adults is usually self-limited, morbidity may still be high.[2] In a 1998 study of the clinical course of aseptic meningitis in adults, 82% of patients were hospitalized, with an average

	White Blood	Predominant	Glucose	Protein
Origin	Cell Count	Cell Type	Level	Level
Bacteria	100–1000s	Neutrophils	Decreased	Increased
Viruses	10s–100s	Neutrophils	Normal to	Normal to
Parameningeal infections		(early)	slightly	slightly
		Lymphocytes	decreased	increased
		(after 6–48		
		hours)		
Partially treated	10–100s	Neutrophils and	Normal to	Increased
bacterial meningitis		lymphocytes	slightly	
			decreased	
Leptospira	100–500	Lymphocytes	Normal	Increased
Lyme disease	100–500	Lymphocytes	Normal	Increased
Drugs	100–500	Neutrophils and	Normal	Increased
		lymphocytes		
Mycobacteria	10s–100s	Lymphocytes	Decreased	Increased
		and monocytes		
Fungi	10–100s	Lymphocytes	Decreased	Increased
		and monocytes		
Autoimmune diseases	10s–100s	Neutrophils	Normal to	Normal to
			slightly	slightly
			decreased	increased

TABLE 2. Cerebrospinal Fluid Patterns During Meningitis

Adapted from Rothart HA; Viral meningitis and the aseptic meningitis syndrome. In Scheld M, Whitley R, Durack D, eds: Infections of the Central Nervous System, 2nd ed. New York: Raven, 1997:23–46.

duration of stay of 4 days and 9 days of missed work.[8] The treatment of aseptic meningitis is primarily supportive. However, trials involving the use of antiviral agents are ongoing. One drug, pleconaril, has been shown to be effective for compassionate use and continues to be investigated in ongoing trials.[8,9]

Herpesviruses

Aseptic meningitis has been reported with herpes simplex virus (HSV) types 1 and 2, varicella-zoster virus, Epstein-Barr virus, cytomegalovirus, and human herpesvirus 6.

Aseptic meningitis is more common with HSV-2 (HSV-1 is typically associated with encephalitis) and accounts for approximately 1% to 3% of all cases of aseptic meningitis.[1,2] In one series, 36% of women and 13% of men with primary genital HSV-2 reported a headache, stiff neck, and photophobia.[2,10] Meningeal symptoms usually start 3 to 12 days after the onset of genital lesions and are usually self-limited in immunocompetent persons.[10]

Cerebrospinal fluid leukocyte counts range from 10 to 1000 cells/mm³ and are predominantly lymphocytic.[10] The CSF protein level is usually elevated, and the CSF glucose level is typically normal, although hypoglycorrhachia has been reported.[1] HSV-2 meningitis can be diagnosed by viral culture, but PCR assay is more sensitive.[10]

Intravenous acyclovir is recommended for the treatment of HSV meningitis.[1,10] Isolation of herpesviruses with resistance to acyclovir have occurred, and alternative therapies include vidarabine and foscarnet.[11]

Human Immunodeficiency Virus

Acute human immunodeficiency virus (HIV) infection may cause acute aseptic meningitis, and the patient may present with symptoms of fever, malaise, lymphadenopathy, maculopapular rash, and pharyngitis.[12] Acute meningoencephalitis may occur in 5% to 10% of patients around the time of seroconversion.[4] HIV can infect the meninges early and persist. Aseptic meningitis may occur in a previously infected patient as well.[4]

The CSF typically shows a mildly increased leukocyte count with a lymphocytic predominance (usually less than 200 cells/mm^3), an elevated protein level, and a normal or mildly decreased glucose level.[1,2] A high index of suspicion is necessary for diagnosis, particularly in patients who have risk factors for HIV. Although HIV has been cultured from CSF, this is not routinely performed as a diagnostic test.[13] The diagnosis can be confirmed with the HIV enzyme-linked immunosorbent assay or by PCR.[1] In most patients, the meningitis syndrome itself will resolve without specific treatment, although seizures, alterations in mental status, and other neurologic complications have been reported.[2] Early treatment of HIV with combination antiretroviral-drug therapy should be strongly considered.[12]

Lymphocytic Choriomeningitis Virus

Lymphocytic choriomeningitis (LCM) virus, an arenavirus, was one of the earliest viruses to be reported as a cause of aseptic meningitis. It accounted for a significant number of cases in early studies but is now rarely reported.[2,4] It is transmitted to humans by contact with rodents or their excreta.[1] LCM virus most commonly affects young adults in the late fall and winter. Symptoms include malaise, severe headache, photophobia, lightheadedness, and myalgias.[1] A small subset of patients may experience orchitis, arthritis, myopericarditis, or alopecia as late manifestations, hypothesized to be immunologic complications.[1]

Cerebrospinal fluid findings are not different from other causes of aseptic meningitis, although hypoglycorrhachia is seen in up to one fourth of cases.[1,2] The diagnosis is most often made serologically. Most cases resolve spontaneously, although convalescence may be prolonged. Fatal cases and those with severe neurologic sequelae are rare.[2] Treatment is primarily supportive.

Mumps

Prior to the introduction of mumps vaccine in 1967, mumps virus, a paramyxovirus, was an important cause of aseptic meningitis. It remains an important cause worldwide and in unimmunized populations.[1,4] Mumps is transmitted via a respiratory route, with most infections occurring in winter and spring months. Symptomatic meningitis is estimated to occur in 10% to 30% of mumps patients.[4] When mumps meningitis is associated with parotitis, diagnosis is relatively straightforward. However, meningitis may precede parotitis or occur without it in 40% to 50% of cases.[1,2]

Examination of the CSF typically shows higher leukocyte counts, which occasionally have a neutrophilic predominance.[1] The diagnosis is usually made serologically.[2]

There is no specific treatment for mumps illness.[2] Most often, meningitis due to mumps is a benign illness, and patients recover fully. Uncommonly, patients may develop more severe neurologic sequelae.[1]

Arboviruses

Although encephalitis is the most commonly recognized and clinically significant neurologic manifestation of most arthropod-borne illnesses, some arboviruses may cause aseptic meningitis.[1,2] In the United States, the most common arboviral cause of meningitis is the St. Louis encephalitis virus, a flavivirus.[1,2,4] Aseptic meningitis accounts for about 15% of symptomatic cases of St. Louis encephalitis and is more common in patients younger than 60 years.[4] Other arboviral causes include the California encephalitis group (most importantly the La Crosse virus), and Colorado Tick fever virus. These agents may be difficult to distinguish from enteroviruses clinically. Treatment is supportive. Recently, the West Nile virus has emerged as a major arbovirus causing encephalitis, but it may rarely cause an aseptic meningitis.[14]

Miscellaneous Viruses

Measles and adenoviruses are causes of encephalitis and meningoencephalitis but may cause aseptic meningitis as well.[1,2] Measles may be associated with a pleocytosis in about one third of cases, although most patients are asymptomatic.[2] Adenovirus is commonly associated with a respiratory illness.[1] Parainfluenza virus as well as influenza A and B have also been associated with aseptic meningitis.[2]

Bacterial Causes of Aseptic Meningitis

Partially treated bacterial meningitis may manifest as aseptic meningitis and should be strongly considered in patients who have had prior antibiotic treatment. Subacute bacterial endocarditis is associated with aseptic meningitis. In addition, parameningeal foci of infections, such as an epidural abscess, are also associated with a CSF pleocytosis. Several rickettsial infections may be associated with aseptic meningitis. Aseptic meningitis may be a manifestation of the second phase of Lyme disease, caused by *Borrelia burgdorferi*. This is more often associated with other neurologic findings such as cranial neuropathies.[16] Headache and stiff neck may occur in the first stage, but the CSF is often normal during that stage.[2] The CSF often shows a lymphocytic pleocytosis with slightly elevated protein level and normal glucose level.[16] Prognosis is good with appropriate antibiotic therapy.[2] Secondary syphilis may be associated with meningitis as well.[1,2] Aseptic meningitis may also occur in approximately one half of cases due to leptospirosis, which is acquired by contact with animal body fluids.[1,2]

Although tuberculous meningitis often appears subacutely and with neurologic manifestions other than meningitis, it, too, should be considered in the differential diagnosis of aseptic meningitis.[1,2] Approximately 75% of patients with tuberculous meningitis have evidence of extrameningeal disease, but 25% do not.[2] In addition, the tuberculin skin test may be negative. These patients often have a delay in diagnosis and increased severity of disease. Cranial nerve palsies, the syndrome of inappropriate antidiuretic hormone secretion, and a change in mental status are often present.[1] Diagnosis is often difficult without such signs, as cultures of CSF for *Mycobacterium tuberculosis* are slow and may be insensitive. It can be confused with enteroviral infections, and dual infections with viruses have been reported.[2] CSF in late disease will show a lymphocytic pleocytosis with increased protein and decreased glucose but may differ in early disease.[1] Newer culture techniques and antigen testing are currently ongoing.[15] Prognosis is often progressive and fatal, especially without therapy.[15]

Fungal Causes of Aseptic Meningitis

Fungal meningitis occurs more often in immunocompromised individuals but may rarely affect immunocompetent individuals. The most common cause of fungal meningitis is *Cryptococcus neoformans,* which may be associated with encephalitis as well as abscess or granuloma formation.[1,2] The endemic mycoses, such as *Coccidioides immitis, Histoplasma capsulatum,* and *Blastomyces dermatitidis,* can cause aseptic meningitis as well. Fungal infections of the central nervous system are usually indolent, and CSF findings resemble those of viral meningitis.[2]

Noninfectious Causes of Aseptic Meningitis

Medications

Many drugs can cause aseptic meningitis, but the incidence of this illness remains unknown.[17] Nonsteroidal anti-inflammatory drugs (NSAIDs), antibiotics, intravenous immunoglobulin, and the immune modulating agent OKT3 have all been reported to cause aseptic meningitis.[17,23] The mechanism is unclear, but it appears that a cellular immune hypersensitivity reaction may be involved.

Patients present with symptoms similar to those of viral meningitis, although a few may have findings such as rash, pruritis, and facial edema consistent with a hypersensitivity reaction.[1] Meningitis may occur hours to days after ingestion of the drug and may even be associated with a history of prior exposure.[1,17] CSF findings include a predominantly neutrophilic pleocytosis, normal to low glucose level, and slightly increased protein level.[17]

Originally, drug-induced meningitis was reported more often in patients with underlying autoimmune disorders such as systemic lupus erythematosus, rheumatoid arthritis, and Sjögren's syndrome. However, it has been subsequently found in patients with no known underlying predisposition.[1,2,17] Patients usually improve once the drug is stopped, which helps differentiate drug-induced meningitis from other causes. Table 3 presents a list of drugs reported to cause aseptic meningitis.

Autoimmune Disorders

Aseptic meningitis has also been associated with autoimmune diseases. In particular, approximately 2% to 4% percent of patients with systemic lupus erythematosus may develop aseptic meningitis.[2] In addition to malaise, fever, and headache, aseptic meningitis due to systemic lupus erythematosus may be accompanied by myelopathy, stroke, and decreased serum complement levels.[17,18] The CSF typically has a neutrophilic pleocytosis.[2]

Malignancy

Central nervous system tumors may manifest as acute or recurrent aseptic meningitis. This may result from direct invasion of the meninges with the tumor, and there may be involvement from leukemia, lymphoma, or metastatic tumors. A chemical meningitis, caused by lipid spillage from tumors such as craniopharyngiomas or pituitary adenomas, may also occur.[1] Aseptic meningitis due to a malignancy may cause a very low glucose level. In addition, patients may present with focal neurologic findings. Neuroimaging is warranted.[1] The prognosis is usually poor.[19]

TABLE 3. Medications Implicated in Drug-Induced Aseptic Meningitis	
Drug Group	**Drugs Involved**
Nonsteroidal anti-inflammatory drugs	Ibuprofen
	Tolmetin
	Sulindac
	Naproxen
	Diclofenac sodium
	Ketoprofen
	Rofecoxib[23]
Antibiotics	Sulfamethoxazole
	Trimethoprim
	Trimethoprim-sulfamethoxazole
	Isoniazid
	Ciprofloxacin
	Penicillin
	Metronidazole
	Cephalosporin
	Pyrazinamide
	Sulfisoxazole
Miscellaneous	OKT3
	Azathioprine[1]
	Valacyclovir
	Infliximab
	Intravenous immunoglobulin
	Cytosine arabinoside[1]
	Carbemezapine[1]
	Phenazopyridine[1]
	Cytaribine

Adapted from Moris G, Garcia-Monco JC: The challenge of drug-induced aseptic meningitis. Arch Intern Med 159:1185–1194, 1999.

Mollaret's Meningitis

Mollaret's meningitis is a rare syndrome of recurrent acute meningitis. The symptoms of an individual episode will resolve spontaneously in 2 to 6 days but then recur in weeks to months.[4] The disease is most common in young adults. The CSF demonstrates a mixed lymphocytic and neutrophilic pleocytosis.[4] Early in an attack, large fragile mononuclear cells are seen, which have been demonstrated to be monocytes.[4] Studies have shown links with HSV 1 and 2 as well as Epstein-Barr virus.[4]

Approach to the Patient

The management of patients with aseptic meningitis is complicated by its diverse origins. If there is any suspicion of bacterial meningitis (immunosuppressed, at the extremes of age, previously received antibiotics, indeterminate CSF findings), there should be a low threshold for empiric antibiotics. Algorithms and nomograms have been studied and validated in one report, but practitioners should use their clinical judgment.[20,21] Studies of patients with bacterial meningitis have shown that a delay in antiobiotic therapy is associated with adverse clinical outcome.[22]

A complete history is critical and should focus on symptoms, preceding antibiotic treatment, travel and exposures, HIV risk factors, and recent medication use. Physical examination may show specific findings, such as a rash, neurologic deficits, or changes in cognition. Diagnostic tests, as discussed earlier, should be performed based on the patient's history, physical findings, and, possibly, geographic locations.

References

1. Connolly KJ, Hammer SM: The acute aseptic meningitis syndrome. Infect Dis Clin North Am 4:599–622, 1990.
2. Rotbart HA: Viral meningitis and the aseptic meningitis syndrome. In Scheld M, Whitley R, Durack D, eds: Infections of the Central Nervous System, 2nd ed. New York: Raven, 1997:23–46.
3. Centers for Disease Control and Prevention: Summary of notifiable diseases, United States, 1988. MMWR Morbid Mortal Wkly Rep 37:1–57, 1989.
4. Tunkel AR, Scheld WM: Acute meningitis. In Mandell GL, Bennett JE, Dolin R, eds: Mandell, Douglas, and Bennett's Principles and Practice of Infectious Diseases, 5th ed. Philadelphia: Churchill Livingstone, 2000:959–1006.
5. Rotabart HA: Diagnosis of enteroviral meningitis with the polymerase chain reaction. J Pediatr 117:85–89, 1990.
6. Sawyer MH, Holland D, Aintablian N: Diagnosis of enteroviral central nervous system infection by polymerase chain reaction during a large community outbreak. Pediatr Infect Dis J 13:177–182, 1994.
7. Rotbart HA: Enteroviral infections of the central nervous system. Clin Infect Dis 20:971–981, 1995.
8. Rotbart HA, Brennan PJ, Fife KH, et al: Enterovirus meningitis in adults. Clin Infect Dis 27:896–898, 1998.
9. Rotbart HA, Webster DA: Treatment of potentially life-threatening enterovirus infections with pleconaril. Clin Infect Dis 32:228–235, 2001.
10. Corey L: Herpes simplex virus. In Mandell GL, Bennett JE, Dolin R, eds: Mandell, Douglas, and Bennett's Principles and Practice of Infectious Diseases, 5th ed. Philadelphia: Churchill Livingstone, 1564–1575, 2000.
11. Gateley A, Gander RM, Johnson PC, et al: Herpes simplex virus type 2 meningoencephalitis resistant to acyclovir in a patient with AIDS. J Infect Dis 161:711–715, 1990.
12. Kahn JO, Walker BD: Acute human immunodeficiency virus type 1 infection. N Engl J Med 339:33–39, 1998.
13. Ho DD, Rota TR, Schooley RT, et al: Isolation of HTLV-III from cerebrospinal fluid and neural tissues of patients with neurologic syndromes related to the acquired immunodeficiency syndrome. N Engl J Med 313:1493–1497, 1985.
14. Asnis DS: West Nile virus infection in the United States: A review and update. Infect Med 19:266–278, 2002.

15. Thwaites G, Chau TT, Mai NT, et al: Tuberculous meningitis. J Neurol Neurosurg Psychiatry 68:289–299, 2000.
16. Pachner AR, Steer AC: The triad of neurologic manifestations of Lyme disease: Meningitis, cranial neuritis, and radiculoneuritis. Neurology 35:47–53, 1985.
17. Moris G, Garcia-Monco JC: The challenge of drug-induced aseptic meningitis. Arch Intern Med 159:1185–1194, 1999.
18. Jennekens FG, Kater L: The central nervous system in systemic lupus erythematosis part one: Clinical syndromes a literature investigation. Rheumatology 41:605–618, 2002.
19. Blaney SM, Poplack DG: Neoplastic meningitis: Diagnosis and treatment considerations. Med Oncol 17:151–162, 2000.
20. Spanos A, Harrell FE, Durack DT: Differential diagnosis of acute meningitis: An analysis of the predictive value of initial observations. JAMA 262:2700–2707, 1989.
21. Aronin SI, Peduzzi, P, Quagliarello VJ: Community-acquired bacterial meningitis: Risk stratification for adverse clinical outcome and effect of antibiotic timing. Ann Intern Med 129:862–869, 1998.
22. McKinney WP, Heudebert GR, Harper SA, et al: Validation of a clinical prediction rule for the differential diagnosis of acute meningitis. J Gen Intern Med 9:8–12, 1994.
23. Bonnel RA, Villalba ML, Karwoski CB, et al: Aseptic meningitis associated with rofecoxib. Arch Intern Med 162:713–715, 2002.

Viral Encephalitis

Vincent Lo Re III, M.D., and
Stephen J. Gluckman, M.D., FACP

chapter

3

The emergence of West Nile virus in New York City in 1999 and the subsequent outbreak in Louisiana in 2002 have made encephalitis a "hot topic" and forced clinicians to reevaluate their knowledge on this subject. *Encephalitis* refers to an inflammation of the brain and is distinguished from meningitis by the presence of abnormalities in brain function, which may include altered mental status, motor or sensory deficits (sometimes focal but generally diffuse), or behavioral or speech disturbances. Nearly 100 different agents have been associated with encephalitis, but viral pathogens remain the most common cause.

Encephalitis resulting from viral infection manifests as two distinct disease entities:

- *Acute viral encephalitis*—causes direct infection of neurons with subsequent inflammation and neuronal destruction, mainly in the gray area.
- *Postinfectious encephalomyelitis*—follows a variety of primarily viral infections and is associated with inflammation and demyelination of the white matter.

Clinicians should develop a broad differential diagnosis when assessing a new patient who presents with symptoms and signs of encephalitis. To assist in this endeavor, the unique characteristics of viral encephalitic syndromes of interest in the United States are reviewed.

Acute Viral Encephalitis

The clinical hallmarks of acute viral encephalitis include fever, headache, and an altered level of consciousness. Other common clinical findings include behavioral changes, speech disturbances, and focal or diffuse neurologic signs such as seizure or hemiparesis.

Establishing a diagnosis of viral encephalitis may be difficult, so clinicians should inquire about certain epidemiologic features:

- Season of the year
- Prevalent diseases within the community

23

- History of travel
- Recreational activities
- Occupational exposures
- Animal contacts (insects or animal bites)

The use of neurodiagnostic tests, including electroencephalogram (EEG), computed tomographic scan, and magnetic resonance imaging (MRI), can provide useful information in the evaluation of encephalitis. Although only herpes simplex encephalitis has specific treatment, the confirmation of other viral causes can provide helpful prognostic information and minimize unnecessary and ineffective therapies. Evaluation and management of acute viral encephalitis can be complex, and practitioners should seek consultation with an infectious diseases specialist for assistance. The viral causes of acute encephalitis are summarized in Table 1, and seasonal incidences of key viral pathogens are presented in Table 2.

TABLE 1. Viral Causes of Acute Encephalitis
Arthropod-borne viruses (indigenous to US)
Eastern equine encephalitis virus
Jamestown Canyon virus
La Crosse virus
Powassan virus
Snowshoe hare virus
St. Louis encephalitis virus
Venezuelan equine encephalitis
Western equine encephalitis virus
West Nile virus
Enteroviruses
Coxsackievirus A and B
Echoviruses
Polioviruses
Herpesviruses
Cytomegalovirus
Epstein-Barr virus
Herpes simplex type 1
Herpes simplex type 2
Human herpesvirus 6
Simian herpes B virus
Varicella-zoster virus
Other viruses
Adenovirus
Human immunodeficiency virus
Influenza
JC virus
Lymphocytic choriomeningitis virus
Measles virus
Mumps virus
Rabies

TABLE 2. Seasonal Incidence of Selected Viral Causes of Encephalitis	
Time of Year	**Virus**
Summer/Fall	Eastern equine encephalitis virus
	La Crosse virus
	St. Louis encephalitis virus
	Western equine encephalitis virus
	West Nile virus
Winter/Spring	Measles virus
	Mumps virus
	Varicella-zoster virus
Any Season	Herpes simplex virus type 1
	Human immunodeficiency virus
	Rabies

Herpes Simplex Virus

Herpes simplex virus (HSV) encephalitis due to HSV type 2 occurs in babies infected perinatally. However, HSV type 1 is the most common cause of acute nonepidemic viral encephalitis among healthy children (older than 6 months of age) and adults.[1] The estimated frequency of HSV type 1 encephalitis in the United States is 1 in 250,000 to 1 in 500,00 persons per year.[2] This encephalitis has no seasonal preference and can occur at any time of the year. In the absence of therapy, the mortality rate exceeds 70%, and only 2.5% of patients overall (11% of survivors) regain normal function.[2,3] Early treatment is the most important factor in ameliorating the morbidity and mortality of this infection.

Pathogenesis. Encephalitis with HSV type 1 can be due either to reactivation of virus or to primary infection. Approximately one third of patients develop HSV type 1 encephalitis during primary infection, and approximately two thirds acquire the disease through reactivation.[5] Reactivation of latent HSV type 1 in the trigeminal ganglion leads to active replication of virus with subsequent spread directly to the temporal cortex. Primary HSV type 1 encephalitis results from either intranasal inoculation with direct invasion of the olfactory tract or from oral inoculation with spread along the trigeminal nerve.[4] Whether primary infection or reactivation, the clinical syndromes are identical, producing inflammation and necrotizing lesions in the inferior and medial temporal lobes and orbital-frontal cortex.[4,5]

Clinical Presentation. HSV type 1 encephalitis typically has an abrupt onset, although an insidious, subacute presentation has been reported. Fever is almost always present, and headaches are prominent early in the disease course. More than 90% of patients have signs that suggest a localized lesion in one or both temporal lobes, and this localization often takes the form of intense personality changes.[5] Seizures, hemiparesis, visual field defects, and paresthesias may also be present. Symptoms often take 2 to 3 weeks to reach maximal severity, and some patients can progress rapidly to coma and death. Coexistent oral herpetic lesions are rare in HSV type 1 encephalitis.

Diagnosis. Routine diagnostic tests are of limited utility in HSV type 1 encephalitis. Examination of cerebrospinal fluid (CSF) often shows a mononuclear cell pleocytosis (10 to 1000 cells/mm^3), an elevated protein concentration, and a normal or slightly low glucose level.[1] The most helpful CSF finding, if present, is red blood cells in the absence of a traumatic lumbar puncture. This suggests necrotizing HSV type 1 encephalitis in the appropriate clinical setting. MRI with enhancement demonstrates lesions earlier than computed tomographic scan and is superior in localizing lesions to the orbital-frontal and temporal lobes. The EEG pattern in HSV type 1 encephalitis is distinctive and consists of periodic sharp-and-slow wave complexes emanating from the temporal lobe that occur at regular intervals of 2 to 3 seconds.[2,4,5] These discharges can be unilateral or bilateral and are seen in two thirds of pathologically proven cases of HSV encephalitis. Although clinical and imaging studies can suggest HSV type 1 encephalitis, the diagnosis is correct only approximately 50% of the time when based on these criteria.[7] Therefore, laboratory confirmation of the diagnosis is required. Polymerase chain reaction (PCR) on CSF for HSV type 1 is the procedure of choice, and results can be obtained in 1 hour. In one series, PCR was shown to be 98% sensitive and 100% specific.[6] Serum antibodies are unhelpful, and CSF viral culture has low sensitivity. Cerebral biopsy with virus isolation has been the gold standard for diagnosis. It is rarely indicated unless CSF abnormalities are atypical, a CSF PCR study is negative, MRI and EEG are nonspecific, or clinical course is progressive despite acyclovir therapy. If CSF PCR is not available, early stereotactic brain biopsy is favored over empiric antiviral treatment, since the clinical diagnosis is only 50% accurate and alternative treatable diagnoses are found in as many as 15% of cases when biopsy is peformed.[7]

Therapy. Acyclovir is the treatment of choice for herpes encephalitis and should be instituted upon suspicion of the disease. The effects of the illness can be significantly reduced if acyclovir is begun before there is a major alteration in the patient's level of consciousness. Therapy has reduced the mortality rate to 19% (versus 70% in untreated control subjects), with 38% of patients returning to normal function.[5] The recommended dose is 10 mg/kg intravenously every 8 hours for 10 to 14 days.[1] The dose should be adjusted in patients with renal failure. Patients with a Glasgow Coma Score below 6 at the beginning of therapy, age older than 30 years, or the presence of encephalitis for more than 4 days before the initiation of treatment have a very poor outcome.[1,8]

Patients who survive herpes encephalitis may have severe, debilitating sequelae, including motor and sensory deficits, aphasia, and problems with cognitive function.[1-3,5] Relapse of encephalitis is occasionally seen 1 week to 3 months after completion of acyclovir therapy and initial improvement. Retreatment with acyclovir or acyclovir and vidarabine is indicated in these cases.[5]

Arboviruses

Arthropod-borne viruses (arboviruses) are a common cause of sporadic and epidemic encephalitis in the United States. They are a heterogeneous group of organisms that are transmitted by arthropod vectors (mosquitoes and ticks).[9] West Nile virus is an arbovirus.

Pathogenesis. Arboviruses are inoculated into a host by a mosquito or tick bite and undergo local replication at the skin site.[4] If there is a large enough inoculum, viremia occurs, with subsequent invasion and infection of the central nervous system. Arboviral encephalitis is predominantly a disease of the cortical gray matter, brainstem, and thalamic nuclei.[4]

Epidemiologic Factors. Arboviruses have different epidemiologic features, but their clinical manifestations are indistinguishable. Arboviral encephalitis is seen mainly in the summer, when the vectors are present. Clinicians can narrow the list of arboviral pathogens causing encephalitis based on (1) location where the infection was acquired, (2) incidences of other cases caused by a specific arbovirus, and (3) age of the patient. Specific features of the main arboviruses causing encephalitis in the United States are discussed below and presented in Table 3.

- *West Nile virus*—In August 1999, an epidemic of encephalitis occurred in and around New York City.[10] The outbreak was initially attributed to St. Louis encephalitis virus. However, the simultaneous deaths of numerous birds in the area suggested that St. Louis encephalitis virus, which typically spares its avian host, was not the culprit. Ultimately, the causative agent was identified as West Nile virus. West Nile virus was well described in Africa and the Middle East but had not been previously encountered in the western hemisphere.[12] West Nile virus has continued to appear each summer in the United States with a rapidly expanding geographic distribution, and the epizootic has spread to 42 states and the District of Columbia as of October 2002.[11] Most human infections are subclinical, but febrile illnesses ranging from a nonspecific viral syndrome to fatal encephalitis have been reported. Profound muscle weakness, occasionally suggesting Guillain-Barré syndrome, is a relatively unique feature of this viral encephalitis.[10,12,13] Severe neurologic involvement occurs primarily in elderly patients.[10,12,13] A maculopapular rash occurs in approximately 20% of patients and may last

TABLE 3. Characteristics of Selected Mosquito-Borne Encephalitides in the United States

Virus	Geographic Distribution	Age-Group Affected	Case-Fatality Rate	Symptoms
West Nile	East coast USA	Adults (esp. elderly)	4–12%	Altered mental status, seizures, myelitis
La Crosse	Central, eastern USA	Children	<1%	Altered mental status, seizures, paralysis, focal weakness
St. Louis	Central, western, southern USA	Adults (esp. elderly)	10–20%	Headache, nausea, vomiting, irritability, altered mental status
Western equine encephalitis	West, Midwest USA	Infants and adults	3%	Headache, altered mental status, seizures
Eastern equine encephalitis	East, Gulf Coast, southern USA	Children and adults	>30%	Headache, altered mental status, seizures

Adapted from Whitley RJ, Gnann JW: Viral encephalitis: Familiar infections and emerging pathogens. Lancet 359:507–514, 2002.

up to 1 week.[10] Case-fatality rates range from 4% to 12%.[10,13] There is currently no vaccine to prevent West Nile virus infection. Prevention includes vector avoidance and mosquito control.

- *La Crosse virus*—This arbovirus, a member of the California encephalitis group, causes aseptic meningitis and encephalitis in primarily school-age children. The largest numbers of cases occur in wooded areas of the Midwestern and mid-Atlantic states.[4] The majority of cases improve after a 1-week period.
- *St. Louis encephalitis virus*—Found throughout the United States, this arbovirus causes epidemics of encephalitis primarily in the Midwestern and Southern states. Clinical infection frequently affects adults above the age of 50 years. The case-fatality rate is approximately 10% (but may be higher in the elderly), and approximately 10% of survivors experience residual cognitive or motor deficits.[4]
- *Western equine encephalitis virus*—Seen primarily in very young children, this arbovirus is found only in the western United States. The case-fatality rate is 3% to 4%.[9]
- *Eastern equine encephalitis virus*—The most virulent of the arboviral encephalitides, eastern equine encephalitis virus has a case-fatality rate exceeding 30% and leaves severe neurologic sequelae in survivors.[9] The disease is limited to the Atlantic and Gulf coast regions.

- *Powassan virus*—Powassan virus is a flavivirus that is transmitted by ticks and is very uncommon in the United States. However, between September 1999 and July 2001, four Maine and Vermont residents with encephalitis were found to be infected with Powassan virus.[14] Powassan virus has been isolated from four tick species in North America, including *Ixodes cookei, Ixodes marxi, Ixodes spinipalpus,* and *Dermacentor andersoni.*[14] Encephalitis is associated with significant long-term morbidity and has a case-fatality rate of 10% to 15%.[14] There is no specific therapy for Powassan encephalitis, and the best means of prevention is protection from tick bites.
- *Venezuelan equine encephalitis*—Endemic in South America, this alphavirus is a rare cause of encephalitis in Central America and the southern United States, particularly Texas and Florida.[4,9] The virus most commonly produces subclinical disease or a mild illness characterized by fever, headaches, or gastrointestinal symptoms. Encephalitis is quite uncommon. The case-fatality rate is less than 1%.[9]

Clinical Presentation. The onset of arboviral encephalitis may be acute or subacute, and symptoms caused by these agents are typically nonspecific, including fever, headache, nausea, and vomiting. Virtually any central nervous system abnormality can occur, and clinical manifestations vary from minimal alterations in mental status to hemiparesis, seizure, and coma.

Diagnosis. CSF generally reveals a mild lymphocytic or mononuclear pleocytosis, a moderately elevated protein level, and a normal glucose level.[5] Arboviral infections are generally diagnosed by serologic testing of acute and convalescent (obtained 4 weeks later) sera. Specimens should be sent during the acute illness to detect virus-specific IgM antibodies in the serum and CSF.[4] Viral cultures of the CSF are generally negative.

Therapy. Treatment of arboviral encephalitis is primarily supportive, with fluids, anticonvulsants (if seizures occur), and mechanical ventilation (if necessary). No antiviral agents against these organisms are available.

Other Viral Origins

In addition to the arboviruses and herpes simplex virus type 1, many other viruses can cause encephalitis (see Table 1).

Enteroviruses. Certain types of enteroviruses, particularly polio and enterovirus 71, have potential to cause severe encephalitis.[2] The clinical features are fever, macular or maculopapular rash, and seizures. Examination of the CSF may reveal a lymphocytic pleocytosis with a mildly elevated protein level.[4] The enteroviruses can be isolated in viral culture of the CSF and can be detected by the use of PCR.[4] There is no specific antiviral therapy for enteroviral encephalitis.

Varicella-zoster virus. Encephalitis can be a complication of varicella-zoster virus infection. Acute cerebellar ataxia is the most common neurologic complication of varicella (chickenpox) and generally develops toward the end of the first week of the exanthem. Approximately 1 in 4000 patients who have varicella virus infection and who are younger than 15 years of age develop this complication.[4] Encephalitis may also complicate a herpes zoster eruption within days to months of the rash and usually occurs in the setting of dissemination. The diagnosis is suspected on clinical grounds. Evidence of ischemic or hemorrhagic infarctions as well as demyelinating lesions may be seen on MRI scan.[4] Analysis of CSF shows a mild lymphocytic pleocytosis, slight increase in protein level, and a normal glucose level. PCR can be used to detect varicella-zoster virus DNA in the CSF, and virus can be grown in culture. There is no proven treatment once encephalitis develops, although acyclovir is often given.

Measles Virus. Encephalitis is an infrequent complication of measles virus and is of three distinct types:

1. *Postinfectious encephalomyelitis*—manifests as sudden recurrence of fever, altered mental status, and multifocal neurologic signs approximately 4 to 8 days after the measles rash. The mortality rate is 10% to 20%, and the majority of survivors are left with permanent neurologic sequelae.[15]

2. *Subacute sclerosing panencephalitis*—manifests as the insidious onset of neurologic dysfunction with myoclonus and seizure activity 6 or more years after an acute measles infection. Progression to coma and death occurs in 1 to 2 years.[4]

3. *Subacute measles*—manifests with a decline in mentition, focal seizures (epilepsia partialis continua), or focal neurologic deficits in an immunocompromised individual 1 to 2 months after a measles infection.

Diagnosis can be confirmed by brain biopsy. Therapy is supportive. A live attenuated vaccine is very effective in preventing measles.

Mumps Virus. Encephalitis due to mumps virus is a rare sequela of infection. Encephalitis can precede, occur with, or develop up to 2 weeks after the parotitis caused by the virus. It can also occur in the absence of parotitis. Other associated findings include orchitis, oophoritis, and pancreatitis. Examination of the CSF may demonstrate two important findings. The CSF leukocyte count is often elevated above 1000 cells/mm³ in cases of central nervous system mumps infection, and there is a modest decrease in the glucose concentration.[16] The diagnosis can be confirmed either with viral culture or by serology. Most patients with mumps encephalitis make a complete recovery, although neurologic sequelae such as deafness, a seizure disorder, or decline in cognitive function can occur. A live virus vaccine can prevent mumps and is indicated for all people born after 1963 who have not had mumps.

Human Immunodeficiency Virus (HIV). Acute self-limited encephalitis symptoms have been reported at the time of primary HIV disease and seroconversion to HIV infection.[5]

Rabies. In cases of encephalitis due to rabies virus infection, patients demonstrate agitation, hyperactivity, hydrophobia, and spasms of the larynx and pharynx.[17] The symptoms wax and wane but ultimately progress to coma and death. The disease carries a 100% mortality rate.[17] The incubation period can be as long as a year. Because of the public health implications, this diagnosis must be considered in every patient with undiagnosed encephalitis. In the United States, most human rabies infections are due to the bat variant, although a history of a bat bite is unusual. In addition to bats, other mammals that have a relatively high prevalence of carrying rabies include raccoons, foxes, and skunks. There has never been a documented case of rabies acquired from the bite of a rodent or lagamorph (rabbit).

Postinfectious Encephalomyelitis

Postinfectious encephalomyelitis is an acute inflammatory demyelinating disease of the brain and spinal cord that, as its name implies, occurs after the onset of a viral illness. It has also been called *acute disseminated encephalomyelitis, acute demyelinating encephalomyelitis,* and *postviral encephalomyelitis.* This disorder generally develops after a respiratory tract infection, a viral exanthem (particularly measles or varicella), or an immunization (historically, smallpox immunization with vaccinia virus).[5] It is more common in children than in adults. Worldwide, measles remains the most important cause of postinfectious encephalomyelitis. In the United States, postinfectious encephalomyelitis is most commonly associated with varicella infection and infections of the respiratory tract, especially influenza.[4] The incidence of this diseases is unknown but probably accounts for 10% to 15% of cases of acute encephalitis in the United States.[5]

Pathogenesis. Postinfectious encephalomyelitis is likely an autoimmune disease triggered by a viral infection. Investigators have suggested that the viral infection activates peripheral blood lymphocytes to migrate into the central nervous system and react against the myelin of neurons.[18] Perivascular inflammation and demyelination of brain tissue are prominent pathologic findings.

Clinical Presentation. Many symptoms and signs of postinfectious encephalomyelitis resemble those of acute viral encephalitis. Patients present with abrupt onset of fever, confusion, and multifocal neurologic signs. There is usually a history of nonspecific respiratory or gastrointestinal illness for about 5 days to 3 weeks prior to the onset of the encephalomyelitis.

Diagnosis. This disorder should be considered if encephalomyelitis occurs days to weeks after an infection or immunization. Examination of the CSF typically demonstrates a mononuclear or lymphocytic pleocytosis, elevated protein level, and normal glucose level, but the results of this analysis are normal in one third of patients.[4,5] An EEG usually reveals diffuse slowing of brain waves. MRI may show enhancement of multifocal white matter lesions. Abnormalities resemble multiple sclerosis, but the lesions of postinfectious encephalomyelitis are all of the same age, whereas those of multiple sclerosis are of varying age.[4]

Therapy. Treatment of postinfectious encephalomyelitis is supportive and includes the following:

- Lowering patient's temperature with antipyretic agents
- Administering adequate fluids
- Treating seizures, if they develop
- Reducing intracranial pressure
- Initiating mechanical ventilation, if necessary

Treatment with high-dose intravenous methylprednisolone has been suggested, but well-controlled clinical trials detailing its benefit have not been performed. Aggressive supportive therapy is needed, because patients with postinfectious encephalomyelitis can make remarkable recoveries after prolonged period of coma.

References

1. Whitley RJ, Lakeman F: Herpes simplex virus infections of the central nervous system: Therapeutic and diagnostic considerations. Clin Infect Dis 20:414–420, 1995.
2. Whitley RJ, Gnann JW: Viral encephalitis: Familiar infections and emerging pathogens. Lancet 359:507–514, 2002.
3. Whitley RJ: Viral encephalitis. N Engl J Med 323:242–250, 1990.
4. Roos KL: Encephalitis. Neurol Clin 17:813–833, 1999.
5. Johnson RT: Acute encephalitis. Clin Infect Dis 23:219–226, 1996.
6. Lakeman FD, Whitley RJ, et al: Diagnosis of herpes simplex encephalitis: Application of polymerase chain reaction to cerebrospinal fluid from brain-biopsied patients and correlation with disease. J Infect Dis 171:857–863, 1995.
7. Barza M, Pauker SG: The decision to biopsy, treat, or wait in suspected herpes encephalitis. Ann Intern Med 92:641–649, 1980.
8. Gutierrez KM, Prober CG: Encephalitis: Identifying the specific cause is key to effective management. Postgrad Med 103:123–143, 1998.
9. Tsai TF: Arboviral infections in the United States. Infect Dis Clin North Am 5:73–102, 1991.
10. Nash D, Farzad M, Fine A, et al: The outbreak of West Nile virus infection in the New York City area in 1999. N Engl J Med 344:1807–1814, 2001.
11. Centers for Disease Control and Prevention: West Nile Virus Activity—United States, October 24–30, 2002. MMWR Morbid Mortal Wkly Rep 51:974–975, 2002.
12. Marfin AA, Gubler DJ: West Nile encephalitis: An emerging disease in the United States. Clin Infect Dis 33:1713–1719, 2001.

13. Petersen LR, Marfin AA: West Nile virus: A primer for the clinician. Ann Intern Med 137:173–179, 2002.
14. Centers for Disease Control and Prevention: Outbreak of Powassan Encephalitis—Maine and Vermont, 1999–2001. MMWR Morbid Mortal Wkly Rep 50:761–764, 2001.
15. Johnson RT, Griffin DE, Hirsch RL, et al: Measles encephalomyelitis—clinical and immunologic studies. N Engl J Med 310:137–141, 1984
16. Wilfert CM: Mumps meningoencephalitis with low cerebrospinal-fluid glucose, prolonged pleocytosis, and elevation of protein. N Engl J Med 280:855–859, 1969.
17. Fishbein DB, Robinson LE: Rabies. N Engl J Med 329:1632–1638, 1993.
18. Johnson RT: The pathogenesis of acute viral encephalitis and postinfectious encephalomyelitis. J Infect Dis 155:359–364, 1987.

Approach to the Patient With Acute Conjunctivitis

chapter

4

Vincent Lo Re III, M.D.

A red eye is the most common presenting complaint seen by primary care physicians.[1] The clinical term *red eye* is applied to a variety of distinct infectious or inflammatory ocular disorders that involve one or more tissue layers of the eye (Table 1). In some cases, a red eye signals a vision-threatening condition that requires urgent referral to an ophthalmologist (Table 2).[2] The majority of cases, however, are benign and can be treated by primary care physicians. Conjunctivitis is the most common cause of the red eye in the community setting.[1] This chapter reviews the main causes of conjunctivitis, highlights key elements of the history and ocular examination, and reviews essential principles of management.

Definitions

The conjunctiva is a thin mucous membrane with both bulbar and palpebral portions. The palpebral portion of the conjunctiva covers the inside surface of the eyelids, while the bulbar portion covers the surface of the globe up to the limbus (the junction of the sclera and cornea). Underneath the conjunctiva lie the episclera, sclera, and uveal tissue layers. The conjunctiva is generally transparent, but when it is inflamed, as in conjunctivitis, it appears pink or red at a distance. The superficial blood vessels within the conjunctiva become engorged (termed *injection*), and edema of the conjunctiva may become apparent.

Causes of Conjunctivitis

Conjunctivitis encompasses a broad group of conditions manifesting as inflammation of the conjunctiva. It is useful to characterize conjunctivitis into four main categories: bacterial, viral, allergic, and nonspecific.

Bacterial Conjunctivitis

Hyperacute Bacterial Conjunctivitis. Hyperacute bacterial conjunctivitis is a severe sight-threatening ocular infection primarily caused by *Neisse-*

TABLE 1.   Causes of Red Eye
Angle closure glaucoma
Anterior uveitis
Blepharitis
Chalazion (internal hordeolum)
Conjunctivitis
Contact lens overuse
Corneal abrasion/ulcer
Dry eye syndrome
Episcleritis/scleritis
Foreign body
Keratitis
Orbital cellulitis
Pterygium
Sty (external hordeolum)
Subconjunctival hemorrhage
Trauma

ria gonorrhoeae. Gonococcal ocular infection may present in neonates (a cause of *ophthalmia neonatorum*) or in sexually active young adults. Transmission of the organism to infants occurs during vaginal delivery, and affected infants develop ocular discharge 3 to 5 days after birth.[3] In adults, the organism is usually transmitted from the genitalia to the hands and then the eyes.

Hyperacute bacterial conjunctivitis has an abrupt onset and is characterized by purulent discharge that reaccumulates rapidly after being wiped away.[4] The discharge often accumulates in the lashes and runs down the patient's cheek. The conjunctiva is bright red, tender, and edematous (called *chemosis*), and an inflammatory membrane of leukocytes and fibrin may develop on the palpebral conjunctival surface. Preauricular lymphadenopathy is often present. One eye is usually involved first, but within several days, the second eye becomes involved through autoinoculation. As the conjunctival swelling and reaction increases, a peripheral corneal ring ulcer can develop because of compression of the corneal vessels.[5]

Gram-negative intracellular diplococci can be identified on Gram stain of the discharge. Patients with hyperacute bacterial conjunctivitis require

TABLE 2.   Causes of Red Eye that Require Urgent Referral to an Ophthalmologist
Angle closure glaucoma
Anterior uveitis
Episcleritis/scleritis
Infectious keratitis
Orbital cellulitis

immediate ophthalmologic referral. If a gonococcal ocular infection is left untreated, rapid progression to corneal perforation and permanent loss of vision can occur.[4] Since gonococcal conjunctivitis is a sexually transmitted disease, clinicians should inquire about concomitant urethritis or vaginitis and ask about sexual partners who might be infected.

Acute Bacterial Conjunctivitis. This is caused by a wide range of gram-positive and gram-negative organisms but is most often due to *Staphylococcus aureus, Streptococcus pneumoniae,* and *Haemophilus influenzae.*[6] *S. aureus* conjunctivitis is common in adults, whereas the other pathogens are more likely in children. Contact lens wearers are at greater risk for *Pseudomonas aeruginosa* conjunctivitis.[6] Acute bacterial conjunctivitis is highly contagious and can be spread by direct contact with the patient or with contaminated fomites.

The symptoms and signs of acute bacterial conjunctivitis are far less severe and less rapid in onset than those of hyperacute bacterial conjunctivitis.[3] There typically is redness and continuous purulent discharge from one eye, although both eyes can be involved. Patients may complain that the affected eyelids are "matted together" or "stuck shut," but this is not useful in distinguishing this type of conjunctivitis from others. More purulent discharge appears within minutes after wiping the lids.

Acute bacterial conjunctivitis is usually self-limited, lasting approximately 1 to 2 weeks, and does not cause any serious harm. In most cases, the diagnosis is based on clinical evaluation. Laboratory studies to identify an organism and determine its sensitivity are usually performed in severe cases or in those that are unresponsive to initial therapy.[1]

Chlamydial Conjunctivitis. Ocular *Chlamydia trachomatis* infection can occur in two distinct forms: trachoma (associated with serotypes A through C) and inclusion conjunctivitis (associated with serotypes D through H).[6]

Trachoma, one of the leading causes of blindness worldwide, is uncommon in North America. It is characterized by a chronic inflammation of both the cornea and conjunctiva (*keratoconjunctivitis*) that ultimately leads to scarring and blindness.

Inclusion conjunctivitis occurs in both newborns (the other cause of *ophthalmia neonatorum*) and adults. Infants exposed to *C. trachomatis* during vaginal delivery develop conjunctival inflammation, discharge, and eyelid edema 5 to 12 days after birth. In adults, transmission occurs by conjunctival contact with infected genital tract secretions. The usual presentation is a subacute or chronic infection characterized by unilateral or bilateral eye redness, mucopurulent discharge, foreign body sensation, and preauricular lymphadenopthy.[3] Scarring of the conjunctiva, which is characteristic of trachoma, is rarely present in cases of inclusion conjunctivitis. At least half of affected adults have concurrent, and possibly asymptomatic, urethritis or cervicitis.[7] Coinfection with other sexually transmitted diseases is common and should be evaluated in patients with chlamydial conjunctivitis. Sexual partners should be referred for treatment.

Viral Conjunctivitis

Conjunctivitis due to viral infection is the leading cause of a red eye.[1] Patients typically present with an acutely red eye, watery discharge, and conjunctival and eyelid swelling. The disorder usually affects one eye first and the other several days later. A tender preauricular lymph node supports the diagnosis but is not present in the majority of cases.[1] Viral conjunctivitis may develop during or after an upper respiratory tract infection and is usually self-limited.

Adenovirus is the most common cause of viral conjunctivitis and is often involved in community epidemics in schools or in the workplace. There are three common presentations of adenoviral conjunctivitis:

- *Follicular conjunctivitis*—This is the most common type of ocular adenoviral infection (typically due to serotypes 1, 2, 4, 5, and 6), and it affects children more frequently than adults. It is characterized by the presence of follicles—tiny, round, gray-white patches present on the palpebral conjunctiva. In severe cases, follicles may enlarge into papules and resemble cobblestones.[8] The infection is self-limiting and generally resolves within 2 weeks.
- *Pharyngoconjunctival fever*—This adenoviral conjunctivitis (usually caused by serotypes 3 and 7) is characterized by the abrupt onset of high fever, pharyngitis, and bilateral follicular conjunctivitis.[8] Small petechial hemorrhages can occur on the bulbar conjunctiva. The disease runs a course of 10 to 14 days.
- *Epidemic keratoconjunctivitis*—A particularly fulminant adenoviral infection (commonly associated with serotype 8), epidemic keratoconjunctivitis involves both the conjunctival and corneal epithelia.[8] It is characterized by prominent conjunctival injection, a severe follicular response, and chemosis. Corneal infiltrates then occur, producing a foreign body sensation and photophobia that can prevent spontaneous opening of the eyes.[6] Affected patients often drop several lines of visual acuity on a Snellen chart. The disease is usually self-limited but may take months to completely resolve.

Herpesviruses, particularly herpes simplex virus, may also cause conjunctivitis, although they typically involve the cornea. Herpes simplex virus can produce vesicular lid lesions, preauricular lymphadenopathy, and transient keratitis. Fluorescein staining of the cornea may reveal the dendritic pattern that is pathognomonic for herpetic keratitis.[2]

Allergic Conjunctivitis

Allergic conjunctivitis is an IgE-mediated hypersensitivity reaction to small airborne allergens (usually pollens, animal dander, or dusts). The personal or family history is significant for other atopic conditions such as asthma, allergic rhinitis, or eczema. There is often bilateral eye redness, watery discharge, and chemosis. However, the hallmark of allergic conjunctivitis is itching. It is this complaint as well as the history of allergy that allows the distinction between allergic and viral conjunctivitis.

Nonspecific Conjunctivitis

Nonspecific conjunctivitis should be considered in patients whose presentation does not suggest an infectious or allergic origin. This condition is usually caused by a transient mechanical or chemical insult, including the following:
- Dry eye syndrome[9]
- Contact lens use
- Ocular foreign body[9]
- Ambient chemical exposure (gas or liquid)

Principles of Management

History

Certain historical features can help narrow the diagnostic etiology of a red eye and rapidly determine the need for patient referral. The medical history should include questions regarding the following:
- Change of vision ("Can you read ordinary print with the affected eye?")
- Eye pain
- Photophobia
- History of eye trauma
- Contact lens use
- Time course of illness
- Environmental or work-related exposures
- Eye itching
- Eye discharge
- History of upper respiratory tract infection
- Sexual history/history of sexually transmitted diseases
- Medication history
- Allergies
- History of eye disease

Ocular Examination

The patient with a red eye should be examined in a well-lit room. The physician should carefully observe and examine the face and eyelids and search for regional lymphadenopathy. The ocular examination should focus on the following:

- *Measurement of visual acuity*—If acuity is diminished, the physician should suspect a more worrisome diagnosis (angle closure glaucoma, infectious keratitis, uveitis) and immediately refer the patient to an ophthalmologist.
- *Examination of the pupils*—The size and reactivity of the pupils should be closely observed. A fixed or nonreactive pupil should prompt immediate referral to an ophthalmologist.
- *Examination of the anterior segment*—The clinician should note the presence of any discharge, appearance of the cornea, and pattern of redness. If either ciliary flush (circumcorneal injection) or hypopyon (a layer of leukocytes in the anterior chamber) are seen, urgent referral to an ophthalmologist is required.
- *Fundoscopic examination*—This is usually not helpful in the differential diagnosis of the red eye.

Therapy

The management of conjunctivitis is summarized below and in Table 3.

Hyperacute Bacterial Conjunctivitis. Because of the rising prevalence of penicillin-resistant *N. gonorrhoeae* in the United States, ceftriaxone (Rocephin), a third-generation cephalosporin, is currently the systemic drug of choice.[10] Ciprofloxacin can be used in patients who are allergic to penicillin. The eyes should be lavaged with saline as well. Concurrent treatment for presumed infection with *C. trachomatis* should also be performed. Physicians should ask about partners who might be infected.

Acute Bacterial Conjunctivitis. Acute bacterial conjunctivitis is likely to be self-limited in most cases, but treatment can shorten the clinical course and reduce person-to-person spread.[11] Erythromycin ophthalmic ointment or sulfacetamide ophthalmic drops are effective initial choices. Ophthalmic fluoroquinolones are not first-line therapy because of bacterial resistance and cost.[11] Aminoglycoside drops or ointments are not recommended because they are toxic to the corneal epithelium and can cause a reactive keratoconjunctivitis after several days of use.

Chlamydial Conjunctivitis. Adult inclusion conjunctivitis is treated orally with erythromycin or doxycycline for 7 to 14 days.[1,6] Tetracyclines should not be administered to pregnant women. Adjunctive topical erythromycin ointment may be of benefit. The treatment of sexual partners helps to prevent reinfection.

Viral Conjunctivitis. There is no specific antiviral agent for the treatment of viral conjunctivitis. Contact lens use should be avoided until the

TABLE 3. Management of Conjunctivitis		
Type of Conjunctivitis	Therapy	Comments
Hyperacute bacterial conjunctivitis	• Ceftriaxone (Rocephin) 1 gm IM × 1 or Ciprofloxacin 500 mg PO bid for 7 d • Erythromycin ophthalmic ointment 1/2 inch qid for 5–7 d • Saline irrigation	• Isolate from school or work for 1 to 2 weeks • Requires immediate ophthalmologic referral • Treat sexual partners • Test for concomitant sexually transmitted diseases
Acute bacterial conjunctivitis	• Erythromycin ophthalmic ointment 1/2 inch qid for 5–7 d or Sulfacetamide 1- 2 drops qid for 5–7 d or Ciprofloxacin (Ciloxan) 1–2 drops qid for 5–7 d	• Isolate from school or work for 1 to 2 weeks • Refer to ophthalmology if no improvement occurs
Chlamydial conjunctivitis	• Doxycycline 100 mg PO bid for 7–14 d or Erythromycin 500 mg PO qid for 7–14 d • Erythromycin ophthalmic ointment 1/2 qid for 5–7 d	• Isolate from school or work for 1 to 2 weeks • Doxycycline contra- indicated in pregnancy • Treat sexual partners • Test for concomitant sexually transmitted diseases
Viral conjunctivitis	• Visine AC 1–2 drops qid as needed for ~3 wks • Naphcon-A 1–2 drops qid as needed for ~3 wks	• Isolate from school or work for 1 to 2 weeks • Warm/cool compresses • Refer to ophthalmology if no improvement occurs
Allergic conjunctivitis	• Visine AC 1–2 drops qid as needed for ~3 wks • Naphcon-A 1–2 drops qid as needed for ~3 wks • Patanol 1–2 drops bid as needed	• Avoid systemic antihistamines
Nonspecific conjunctivitis	• Hypotears (artificial tears) 1–2 drops q 1 hr to qid as needed • Lacrilube ointment 1/2 inch at bedtime as needed	• Avoid topical corticosteroids

IM = intramuscular, PO = oral, bid = twice daily, tid = three times daily, qid = four times daily

eyes are without discharge and no longer red. The use of warm or cool compresses may provide additional symptomatic relief. Some patients feel improvement with topical antihistamines and decongestants, which are available in over-the-counter formulations. Physicians should explain that these agents treat the symptoms but not the disease. Patients should further be told that irritation and discharge may get worse for 3 to 5 days before improving and that symptoms can persist for up to 3 weeks.

Allergic Conjunctivitis. Over-the-counter topical antihistamines or decongestants are reasonable first-line therapies for symptomatic relief. Systemic antihistamines and decongestants are of little benefit in allergic conjunctivitis, since they tend to dry the ocular surface, exacerbating the sense of irritation.

Nonspecific Conjunctivitis. Symptomatic relief of nonspecific conjunctivitis may be achieved with over-the-counter topical lubricants (artificial tears or ointments). Topical ocular ointments provide long-lasting relief but can blur vision, so they should be used at bedtime.

Return to Work or School

Bacterial and viral conjunctivitis are both highly contagious. Infected individuals should not share towels, handkerchiefs, or other linens and should carefully wash their hands with soap and water after any contact with their eyes. Patients should be isolated from school or work for 1 to 2 weeks after the onset of symptoms.

References

1. Leibowitz H: The red eye. N Engl J Med 343:345–351, 2000.
2. Hara JH: The red eye: Diagnosis and treatment. Am Fam Phys 54:2423–2430, 1996.
3. Morrow GL, Abbott RL: Conjunctivitis. Am Fam Phys 57:735–746, 1998.
4. Wan WL, Farkas GC, May WN, Robin JB: The clinical characteristics and course of adult gonococcal conjunctivitis. Am J Ophthalmol 102:575–583, 1986.
5. Schachat AP: The red eye. In Barker LR, Burton JR, Zieve PD, eds: Principles of Ambulatory Medicine, 5th ed. Philadelphia, Lippincott Williams & Wilkins, 1999, 1488–1495.
6. O'Brien TP: Conjunctivitis. In Mandell GL, Bennett JE, Dolin R, eds: Mandell, Douglas, and Bennett's Principles and Practice of Infectious Diseases, 5th ed. Philadelphia: Churchill Livingstone, 2000:1251–1256.
7. Postema EJ, Remeijer L, van der Meijden WI: Epidemiology of genital chlamydial infection in patients with chlamydial conjunctivitis: A retrospective study. Genitourin Med 72:203–205, 1996.
8. Weber CM, Eichenbaum JW: Acute red eye: Differentiating viral conjunctivitis from other less common causes. Postgrad Med 101:185–196, 1997.
9. Shields SR: Managing eye disease in primary care. Part 2: How to recognize and treat common eye problems. Postgrad Med 108:83–96, 2000.
10. Haimovici R, Roussel TJ: Treatment of gonococcal conjunctivitis with single-dose intramuscular ceftriaxone. Am J Ophthalmol 107:511–514, 1989.
11. Chung CW, Cohen EJ: Eye disorders: Bacterial conjunctivitis. West J Med 173:202–205, 2000.

Upper Respiratory Tract Infections

Paul A. Kinniry, M.D.

chapter

5

Upper respiratory tract infections are among the most common diagnoses seen in the primary care physician's office. These include viral rhinosinusitis (the common cold), acute sinusitis, and acute pharyngitis. Other, more serious upper respiratory tract infections include epiglottitis and croup. Most upper respiratory tract infections are self-limited and do not require treatment with antibiotics. In some instances, antibiotics are crucial in the management. However, upper respiratory tract infections are associated with widespread misappropriate use of antibiotics.[1] This chapter reviews the different clinical presentations of upper respiratory tract infections, appropriate diagnostic testing, and indications for the use of antibiotics.

Viral Rhinosinusitis

Viral rhinosinusitis, otherwise known as the common cold, is a viral infection of the sinuses and nasal mucosa. It is the most common acute illness in the United States. Most adults have, on average, two to four infections each year, and children average six to eight of these infections annually.[2] The typical causes of viral rhinosinusitis are outlined in Table 1.[3] Transmission may occur through direct contact or by aerosol spread. The viral incubation time is typically 24 hours to 72 hours.[3]

Clinical features include nasal congestion and discharge, cough, headache, sneezing, and sore throat. General malaise is common, but more severe systemic symptoms are often minimal. High-grade fevers are rare and should raise suspicion of an alternative diagnosis. Symptoms typically last less than 7 days; however, up to 25% of patients may continue to be symptomatic at 14 days.[4] Examination of the nasal mucosa reveals erythema and edema, often with prominent watery discharge. Other physical examination findings are scarce. When symptoms persist beyond 7 days, the clinician should begin to consider complications such as bronchitis, secondary bacterial sinusitis, or otitis media.

43

TABLE 1. Common Cold Viruses
Common Causes
Rhinoviruses
Adenoviruses
Coronaviruses
Parainfluenza viruses
Respiratory syncytial virus (RSV)
Influenza A, B
Less common causes
Enteroviruses
Epstein-Barr virus
Adapted from Neiderman MS, Sarosi GA: Respiratory tract infections. Chest Medicine, 4th ed. Philadelphia, Lippincott Williams & Wilkins, 2000; 381–384.

Treatment of viral rhinosinusitis is supportive. There is no role for the use of antibiotics in this setting.[5] Oral decongestants may be used (pseudoephedrine, 30 mg to 60 mg every 6 hours) to alleviate rhinorrhea and nasal congestion in otherwise healthy adults, and acetaminophen may be used to reduce fever, headache, and other systemic symptoms.[6] Children should not be treated with aspirin, owing to concerns for the development of Reye's syndrome. The oral decongestant phenylpropanolamine should not be used because of recent concerns of a small risk of hemorrhagic stroke associated with its use.[7] Intranasal ipratropium bromide (0.06% ipratropium, two 42 μg sprays per nostril three or four times daily for 4 days) has been shown to reduce the severity of rhinorrhea.[8]

Many therapies for the common cold have been studied, with conflicting or confusing results. Zinc lozenges, vitamin C, and echinacea have all been studied for the treatment of the common cold. Data on the utility of these therapies are currently inconclusive. One study found that zinc was useful in reducing the length of symptoms, but side effects including bad taste and nausea, were common.[9] A recent meta-analysis showed conflicting results.[10] Based on available evidence, the use of zinc and echinacea is not recommended for the treatment of the common cold.[11–13] Vitamin C may produce a little benefit in reducing cold symptoms but is not effective in preventing the onset of cold if taken daily.[14]

Acute Sinusitis

Sinusitis is perhaps the most misunderstood infection of the upper respiratory tract. Sinusitis is defined as inflammation of the paranasal sinuses and contiguous nasal mucosa, regardless of the cause.[15] Acute sinusitis is a among the most common conditions treated by primary care physicians and is a common reason for the administration of antibiotics.[15] Many clinicians consider sinusitis to be primarily of bacterial origin, but this is untrue. Although acute bacterial sinusitis does occur, acute sinusitis is often viral and therefore does not necessitate treatment with antibiotics. Distinguishing viral from acute bacterial sinusitis is difficult, and this has led to the widespread overuse of antibiotics for the treatment of sinusitis.[15]

The clinical features of sinusitis include purulent nasal discharge, nasal congestion, facial pain, maxillary toothache, and occasionally fever or cough. The clinical features of viral rhinosinusitis and acute bacterial sinusitis are similar. However, acute bacterial sinusitis typically develops secondarily to viral rhinosinusitis.[16] During a viral upper respiratory tract infection, thick nasal secretions accumulate in the sinuses. Bacterial superinfection can subsequently result. Some authors have suggested that the high intranasal pressures generated during nose blowing may be a contributing factor for the introduction of bacterial pathogens into the sinus cavities.[17] Other causes of acute bacterial sinusitis are less common and include seasonal allergies, mechanical obstruction of sinus drainage, swimming, prolonged nasal intubation, and extension from a dental infection into the sinus cavity.[16]

No diagnostic test easily distinguishes between viral rhinosinusitis and acute bacterial sinusitis.[18] Sinus aspiration, although performed in some research studies, is not practical for routine diagnosis of acute bacterial sinusitis. The value of radiologic studies, including computed tomographic scans of the sinuses, is also limited because radiographic studies are unable to distinguish changes due to viral rhinosinusitis from those caused by acute bacterial sinusitis.[18]

The decision to treat patients with antibiotics most often must be made on clinical grounds alone. Acute bacterial sinusitis is unlikely in patients whose symptoms are less than 7 days in duration.[18] Patients whose symptoms have lasted more than 7 days are more likely to have bacterial sinusitis. However, the duration of illness alone is insufficient to suggest bacterial sinusitis. As discussed earlier, up to 25% of patients with viral rhinosinusitis will still have symptoms at 14 days.[4] Other clinical predictors that suggest acute bacterial sinusitis include maxillary tooth or facial pain (especially unilateral), unilateral sinus tenderness, and mucopurulent nasal discharge.[19] Worsening of symptoms after initial improvement is another clue to acute bacterial sinusitis.[20]

Even if a patient is suspected of having an acute bacterial sinusitis based upon these clinical predictors, it is often not necessary to prescribe antibiotics.[15,18] A recent meta-analysis showed that although there is some benefit to treating patients with acute bacterial sinusitis, the benefit is small, and resolution of symptoms typically occurs without antibiotics.[21] Patients with mild or moderate symptoms can be treated with nasal decongestants and analgesics, as discussed in the previous section. Current recommendations suggest the use of antibiotics in patients with severe symptoms of acute bacterial sinusitis, as outlined earlier.[15,18] Even if antibiotics are used, decongestants should be administered to maintain sinus drainage.

The choice of initial antibiotic therapy is empiric and based on knowledge of the organisms likely to cause acute bacterial sinusitis (Table 2). Current recommendations and dosages are outlined in Table 3. Failure of treatment should result in a broadening of the antibiotic spectrum and prompt consideration of diagnostic sinus aspiration.

Complications of bacterial sinusitis are rare but can be serious. These complications include meningitis, brain abscess, and periorbital cellulitis. Currently, there are no data to suggest that early treatment prevents the development of these complications.[18,21]

The possibility of fungal sinusitis should be strongly considered in the immunocompromised host. Rhinocerebral mucormycosis is an acute invasive fungal sinusitis that typically occurs in patients with organ transplants, diabetes mellitus, or neutropenia (due to hematologic malignancy or immunosuppressive medications). It rarely affects hosts with a normal immune system. A black necrotic palatal or nasal eschar may be seen and is a clue to the diagnosis. When an invasive fungal sinusitis is suspected, therapy with intravenous amphotericin B should be initiated, and urgent surgical consultations should be obtained.[22]

TABLE 2. Common Causes of Acute Sinusitis
Viral
Rhinoviruses
Adenoviruses
Coronaviruses
Parainfluenza viruses
Respiratory syncytial virus (RSV)
Influenza A, B
Bacterial
Streptococcus pneumoniae
Haemophilus influenzae
Moraxella catarrhalis
Staphylococococcus aureus
Anaerobic bacteria
Fungal
Rhizopus species
Mucor species
Aspergillus species
Adapted from Gwaltney JM Jr: Acute sinusitis. Up to Date (11.1). Accessed Dec 2, 2002 at www.uptodateonline. com.

TABLE 3. Suggested Antibiotic Therapy for Acute Bacterial Sinusitis	
Antibiotic Choice	**Adult Dosage**
Amoxicillin	500 mg orally three times daily
Clarithromycin	500 mg orally twice daily
Cefdinir	300 mg orally every 12 hours
Cefuroxime axetil	250 mg orally twice daily
If the patient has received antibiotics within the last month, treatment with the above choices may lead to clinical failure (prevalence of drug-resistant *Streptococcus pneumoniae* exceeds 30% in this situation). Antibiotic treatment should be broadened and include:	
Amoxicillin-clavulante	875/125 mg orally every 12 hours
Levofloxacin	500 mg orally daily
Gatifloxacin	400 mg orally daily
Moxifloxacin	400 mg orally daily

Acute Pharyngitis

Acute pharyngitis is another common infection of the upper respiratory tract seen commonly by primary care physicians, accounting for 10% of primary care visits and 50% of the outpatient antibiotic usage.[23] Most cases of acute pharyngitis are viral in origin and do not require antibiotics. As with sinusitis, one of the key principles in the management of acute pharyngitis is to distinguish between bacterial and viral causes. The organisms commonly responsible for causing acute pharyngitis in adults are listed in Table 4 and reviewed in the following sections.

TABLE 4. Causes of Acute Pharyngitis
Viral
Rhinoviruses
Coronaviruses
Adenovirus
Herpes simplex virus
Parainfluenza virus
Influenza virus
Epstein-Barr virus
Human immunodeficiency virus
Bacterial
Streptococcus pyogenes (group A streptococci)
Neisseria gonorrhoeae
Corynebacterium diphtheriae
Mycoplasma pneumoniae
Chlamydia pneumoniae
Arcanobacterium Haemolyticum
Adapted from Bisno AL: Acute pharyngitis. N Engl J Med 344:205–211, 2001.

Acute Group A Streptococcal Pharyngitis

By far the most common bacterial cause of acute pharyngitis is group A streptococci (*Streptococcus pyogenes*), commonly called "strep throat." Treatment is important to decrease the risk of rheumatic fever, reduce the incidence of suppurative complications, and decrease spread of infection.[24] Several clinical predictors for the diagnosis of group A streptococcal pharyngitis exist. The presence of tonsilar exudates, fever exceeding 101°F, anterior cervical lymphadenopathy, and a history of recent exposure all increase the likelihood that group A streptococcal pharyngitis is present.[25,26] If three or four of these elements are present, the likelihood of group A streptococcal pharyngitis is high, with a positive predictive value of 40% to 60%. If two or fewer are present, group A streptococcal pharyngitis is less likely.[27] Children under the age of 3 years or those who have had prior tonsillectomy may not present with many of these elements.

A throat culture or group A streptococcal rapid antigen detection test can confirm the diagnosis of pharyngitis due to *S. pyogenes*. In children and adolescents, the rapid antigen test can be used as an initial screen; however, current recommendations suggest that if the rapid antigen test result is negative, it should be followed up by a throat culture.[24] Because of the low incidence of *S. pyogenes* infection in children and adolescents presenting with pharyngitis, some investigators have suggested that rapid antigen testing may not be cost effective in this population.[28] It is reasonable to initiate therapy on an acutely ill child with clinical features suggestive of group A streptococcal pharyngitis while awaiting results of the throat culture. Antibiotics should be discontinued if the cultures do not reveal evidence of *S. pyogenes*.[24]

In adults older than 20 years of age, the incidence of group A streptococcal pharyngitis is even lower, as is the risk for subsequent development of rheumatic fever. Thus, less rigorous evaluation is necessary. A reasonable management strategy for adults with pharyngitis is outlined below.[27,29]

1. Empirically treat all patients with four clinical predictors (Table 5).

2. Withhold treatment and testing in patients with one or no clinical predictors.

3. Perform rapid antigen testing for patients with two or three clinical predictors and prescribe antibiotics only if the test result is positive.

TABLE 5.   Clinical Criteria Suggestive of Group A Streptococcal Pharyngitis[25,29]
Tonsillar exudate
Anterior cervical lymphadenopathy
Absence of cough
Fever exceeding 101°F

An accepted alternative approach is to test patients with two or more clinical criteria empirically and reserve treatment for patients with positive group A streptococcal rapid antigen.[27,29] Antibiotics are given to patients with two clinical criteria if they have a positive rapid antigen test result. These recommendations hold only for adults and do not apply to patients with history of rheumatic fever, valvular heart disease, immunosuppression, or chronic pharyngitis. They also do not apply during an epidemic of group A streptococcal pharyngitis or rheumatic fever.[27]

Once the decision to treat the patient for group A streptococcal pharyngitis has been made, an appropriate antibiotic regimen must be decided upon. Penicillin is considered to be the first choice. Adult dosage is penicillin V 500 mg PO bid or 250 mg PO qid for 10 days. If poor patient compliance is suspected, a one-time intramuscular dose of benzathine penicillin 1.2 million units can be given, but pain at the injection site may occur. Erythromycin, azithromycin, clindamycin, or a second-generation oral cephalosporin are acceptable alternatives if the patient is allergic to or intolerant of penicillin.[24] Table 6 lists appropriate antibiotic regimens for the treatment of group A streptococcal pharyngitis. A shorter duration of therapy (4 to 6 days) is likely to be effective with use of a second-generation cephalosporin.

Patients with either viral or bacterial pharyngitis should be offered supportive care. Oral fluid intake should be encouraged, and inability to swallow due to severe pain should trigger immediate evaluation. Antipyretics and analgesics should be recommended. Patients may have some symptomatic relief with warm salt-water gargles or over-the-counter throat lozenges that contain a mild topical anesthetic.

Other Bacterial Causes of Acute Pharyngitis

Mycoplasma pneumoniae and *Chlamydia pneumoniae* are rare causes of acute pharyngitis that can affect primarily young healthy adults. Their

TABLE 6. Suggested Antibiotic Therapy for Acute Bacterial Pharyngitis		
Agent	Dose	Duration of Therapy
First Choice		
Penicillin V	500 mg PO twice daily	10 days
	250 mg PO qid	
Benzathine penicillin	1.2 million units IM	1 dose
Alternative Choice		
Erythromycin	500 mg PO 4 times daily	10 days
Clarithromycin	250 mg PO twice daily	10 days
Azithromycin	500 mg PO x 1 dose then 250 mg PO daily	5 days
Cefdinir	300 mg PO every 12 hours	10 days
Cefuroxime axetil	250 mg PO twice daily	10 days
Cefprozil	500 mg PO daily	10 days
Cefditoren	200 mg PO twice daily	10 days

clinical characteristics are similar. Both are often associated with lower tract symptoms, such as acute bronchitis or even pneumonia, but can cause pharyngitis in the absence of lower tract symptoms. Both respond to erythromycin.[24,29]

Neisseria gonorrhoeae is another rare cause of acute bacterial pharyngitis that occurs in sexually active adults as the result of oral-genital contact. If suspected, the diagnosis can be confirmed with culture on a Thayer-Martin medium. Antibiotic therapy should be initiated for gonorrhea as well as for possible coexisting genital infection with *Chlamydia trachomatis*.[24] Testing for other sexually transmitted disease should be strongly considered, including human immunodeficiency virus (HIV).

Group C and group G streptococci are rare causes of acute bacterial pharyngitis that manifest similar to group A streptococcal pharyngitis. However, the symptoms and signs are often less severe with these organisms. The benefits of treatment of group C and group G streptococci are unknown, and they should be susceptible to the antibiotics used to treat group A streptococcal pharyngitis.[24]

Diphtheria is caused by *Corynebacterium diphtheriae*. This disease has become rare in the United States, occurring mainly in incompletely immunized patients. Diphtheria usually manifests more gradually, with mild constitutional symptoms, low-grade fevers, and pharyngitis. The most distinct physical finding is a gray pseudomembrane that typically covers both tonsils and may extend throughout the oropharynx, nasopharynx, larynx, and tracheobronchial tree.[24] If there is extensive involvement of the upper airway, airway compromise can occur. *C. diphtheriae* can produce a toxin that causes myocarditis and neurologic sequelae (primarily cranial neuropathies and peripheral neuritis). In addition to antibiotics, equine hyperimmune antitoxin should be administered in patients with confirmed cases of diphtheria.[24]

Viral Pharyngitis

Most community-acquired cases of acute pharyngitis are viral (see Table 4). In general, viral pharyngitis is a self-limited illness isolated to the upper respiratory tract. Treatment is generally supportive with antipyretics, analgesics, and adequate oral intake. Some viral causes of pharyngitis have more systemic consequences, and these will be discussed in more detail below.

Infectious Mononucleosis. Infectious mononucleosis is a clinical syndrome consisting of fever, lymphadenopathy, and pharyngitis, caused by the Ebstein-Barr virus. Lymphadenopathy may be present in the anterior cervical and posterior cervical regions, but axillary and inguinal nodes may also be involved.[29] There may be a prodome consisting of fever and malaise that precedes this classic triad. In addition to these features, splenomegaly is common, and hepatitis can occur. Pharyngitis and fatigue may persist for longer than is usually suspected with other forms of pharyngitis. Clues to the diagnosis include lymphocytosis, often with more than 10% lymphs. Testing for heterophil antibodies can confirm the diagnosis.[24] Treatment is generally supportive. Patients should be instructed not to participate in sports or other vigorous activities because of the risk of splenic rupture. Corticosteroids may be needed for patients with severe thrombocytopenia, hemolytic anemia, or upper airway edema that threatens airway obstruction.[24]

Acute Human Immunodeficiency Virus Infection. Acute HIV infection may cause a syndrome of fatigue, weight loss, fevers, rash, and pharyngitis. It should be considered in any young adult with these symptoms. Patients should be questioned for risk factors for HIV. Lymphadenopathy, splenomegaly, and transaminitis are also often present. Laboratory testing may show lymphopenia.[30] Chapter 20 reviews the signs and symptoms associated with acute HIV infection and discusses HIV testing.

Influenza. Influenza may also manifest with pharyngitis but tends to manifest with more severe constitutional symptoms than most viral upper respiratory tract infection. The presence of an epidemic in the community may provide a clue to the diagnosis. Treatment options for influenza are reviewed in Chapter 6.

Epiglottitis

Epiglottitis occurs mainly in children and is a rare form of upper respiratory tract infection in adults. Epiglottitis refers to acute inflammation and edema of the epiglottis and aryepiglottic folds.[4] It can cause airway compromise and death, especially in children over the age of 2 years. *Haemophilus influenzae* type B is the most common bacterial cause. In adults, *Streptococcus pneumoniae, Staphylococcus aureus,* and *Klebsiella* species may also cause epiglottitis.

Epiglottitis classically manifests with acute onset of dyspnea, dysphagia, dysphonia, and drooling.[31] Cough is usually not a prominent feature. High fever may also be present. Adults and young children (<10 years) may have less severe symptoms. Physical examination may reveal an erythematous epiglottis. A tongue blade should not be used because it can precipitate total airway obstruction.[4] A lateral neck radiograph may show an enlarged epiglottis (the "thumb sign"). However, even a patient with severe epiglottitis can be present with a normal appearing radiograph.[4] An emergency consultation with an otorhinolaryngologist should be requested, and the diagnosis can be confirmed with laryngoscopy.

The most important issue in the treatment of epiglottitis is to secure the airway. In children, it is recommended that intubation be performed

TABLE 7. Common Causes of Croup
Viruses
Parainfluenza viruses (especially types 1 and 3)
Influenza A, B
Respiratory syncytial virus
Adenovirus
Enteroviruses
Rhinoviruses
Measles virus (rubeola)
Bacteria
Mycoplasma pneumoniae

Adapted from Neiderman MS, Sarosi GA: Respiratory tract infections. Chest Medicine, 4th ed. Philadelphia, Lippincott Williams & Wilkins, 2000, 381–384.

to ensure airway patency. Intubation for adults must be decided on an individual basis, and careful observation during the first day is crucial.[4]

Antibiotics are required for the treatment of epiglottitis. Antibiotics should cover *H. influenzae, S. pneumoniae, S. aureus* and *Klebsiella* species. Appropriate choices of antibiotics include ceftriaxone, cefuroxime, cefotaxime, or ampicillin/sulbactam. Consultation with an infectious diseases physician is recommended.

Croup

Croup describes infection of the larynx, trachea, and bronchi and affects young children between 3 months and 3 years of age. Patients typically present with acute onset of dyspnea, a barking cough, and stridor. Hoarseness may be present. Symptoms often follow the onset of upper respiratory tract infections.[4] Table 7 presents the most common agents responsible for causing croup. Since most cases of croup are viral, antibiotics are not routinely required. Racemic epinephrine has been used to treat airway symptoms. The role of steroids is controversial, but they probably have benefit in cases of severe croup. Heliox has been used as a bridge therapy until epinephrine and steroids have reduced laryngeal edema.

Key Points: Upper Respiratory Tract Infection

- ☞ Most upper respiratory tract infections are viral and not bacterial and therefore do not require antibiotics; however, these infections are associated with widespread antibiotic misuse.
- ☞ Distinguishing viral causes from bacterial causes in adults requires key information from the history and physical examination.

Key Points (Continued)

↩ Attention to these details is important for decisions regarding appropriate therapy.

↩ This general rule does not apply to patients with epiglotitis, which should be treated as a medical emergency, requiring close observation, antibiotics, and possible intubation.

References

1. Gonzales R, Steiner JF, Sande MA: Antibiotic prescribing for adults with colds, upper respiratory tract infections, and bronchitis by ambulatory care physicians. JAMA 273:214–219, 1997.
2. Turner RB: Epidemiology, pathogenesis, and treatment of the common cold. Ann Allergy Asthma Immunol 78:531–539, 1997.
3. Neiderman MS, Sarosi GA: Respiratory tract infections. In Chest Medicine, 4th ed Philadelphia, Lippincott Williams & Wilkins, 2000, 381–384.
4. Gwaltney JM Jr, Hendley JO, Simon G, Jordan WS Jr: Rhinovirus infections in an industrial population. JAMA 202:494–500, 1967.
5. Hickner JM, Barlett JG, Besser RE, et al: Principles of appropriate antibiotic use for acute rhinosinusitis in adults: Background. Ann Intern Med 134:498–505, 2001.
6. Sperber SJ, Turner RB, Sorrentino JV, et al: Effectiveness of pseudoephedrine plus acetaminophen for the treatment of symptoms attributed to the paranasal sinuses associated with the common cold. Arch Fam Med 9:978–985, 2000.
7. Kernan WN, Viscoli CM, Brass LM, et al: Phenylpropanolamine and the risk of hemorrhagic stroke. N Engl J Med 343:1826–1832, 2000.
8. Hayden FG, Diamond L, Wood PB, et al: Effectiveness and safety of intranasal ipratropium bromide in common colds: A randomized, double-blinded placebo-controlled trial. Ann Intern Med 125:89–97, 1996.
9. Mossad SB, Macknin ML, Medendorp SV, Mason P: Zinc gluconate lozenges for treating the common cold: A randomized, double-blind, placebo-controlled study. Ann Intern Med 125:81–88, 1996.
10. Jackson JL, Peterson C, Lesho E: A meta-analysis of zinc salts lozenges and the common cold. Arch Intern Med 157:2373–2376, 1997.
11. Marshall I: Zinc for the common cold. Cochrane Database of Systemic Reviews, 2000, CD001364.
12. Turner RB, Riker DK, Gangemi JD: Ineffectiveness of Echinacea for prevention of experimental rhinovirus colds. Antimicrob Agents Chemother 44:1708, 2000.
13. Grimm W, Muller HH: A randomized controlled trial of the effect of fluid extract of Echinacea purpurea on the incidence and severity of colds and respiratory infections. Am J Med 106:138–143, 1999.
14. Douglas RM, Chalker EB, Treacy B: Vitamin C for preventing and treating the common cold. Cochrane Database of Systematic Reviews, 2000, CD000980.
15. Snow V, Mottur-Pilson, C, Hickner JM: Principles of appropriate antibiotic use for acute sinusitis in adults. Ann Intern Med 134:495–497, 2001.
16. Gwaltney JM Jr: Acute Sinusitis. Up to Date (11.1). www.uptodateonline.com Accessed Dec 2, 2002.
17. Gwaltney JM Jr, Hendley JO, Phillips CD, et al: Nose blowing propels nasal fluid into the paranasal sinus. Clin Infect Dis 30:387–391, 2000.

18. Hickner JM, Barlett JG, Resser RE, et al: Principles of appropriate antibiotic use for acute sinusitis in adults: Background. Ann Intern Med 134:498–505, 2001.
19. Hanse JG, Schmidt H, Rosborg J, Lund E: Predicting acute maxillary sinusitis in a general practice population. BMJ 311:233–236, 1995.
20. Lindbaek M, Hjortdahl P, Johhnsen UL: Use of symptoms, signs, and blood tests to diagnose acute sinus infections in primary care: Comparison with computed tomography. Fam Med 28:183–188, 1996.
21. Zucher DR, Balk E, Engels E, et al: Diagnosis and treatment of acute bacterial rhinosinusitis. Agency for Health Care Policy and Research Publication No. 99-E016: Evidence Report/Technology Assessment Number 9.
22. DeShazo RD, Chapin K, Swain RE: Fungal sinusitis. N Engl J Med 337:254–259, 1997.
23. Jackler RK, Kaplan MJ: Ears, nose, and throat. In Tierney LM Jr, McPhee SJ, Papadkis MA (eds): Current Medical Diagnosis and Treatment: Adult Ambulatory and Inpatient Management, 41st ed. New York, Lange Medical Books/McGraw-Hill, 2002, pp 253–255.
24. Bisno AL: Acute pharyngitis. N Engl J Med 344:205–211, 2001.
25. Center RM, Witherspoon JM, Dalton HP, et al: The diagnosis of strep throat in adults in the emergency room. Med Decis Making 1:239–246, 1981.
26. Ebell MH, Smith MA, Barry HC, et al: Does this patient have strep throat? JAMA 284:2912–2918, 2000.
27. Cooper RJ, Hoffman JR, Barlett JG, et al: Principles of appropriate antibiotic use for acute pharyngitis in adults: Background. Ann Intern Med 134:509–517, 2001.
28. Tsevat J, Kotagal UR: Management of sore throats in children: A cost-effectiveness analysis. Arch Pediatr Adolesc Med 153:681–688, 1999.
29. Bartlett JG: Approach to acute pharyngitis in adults. UpToDate 2002(11.1). www.uptodateonline.com Accessed Dec 2, 2002.
30. Kahn JO, Walker BD: Acute human immunodeficiency virus type 1 infection. N Engl J Med 339:33–39, 1998.
31. Loos GD: Pharyngitis, croup and epiglottitis. Primary Care 17:335–345, 1990.
32. Rosekrans JA: Viral croup: Current diagnosis and treatment. Mayo Clin Proc 73: 1102–1107, 1998.

Acute Bronchitis

Paul A. Kinniry, M.D.

chapter

6

Acute bronchitis is an acute, self-limited respiratory tract illness in healthy adults. The most significant clinical feature recognized by clini- cians is a cough that typically lasts 1 to 3 weeks, with other causes of acute cough such as pneumonia being excluded.[1,2] Acute bronchitis is one of the most common reasons for patient visits to ambulatory care physicians in the United States and one of the diagnoses most frequently associated with inappropriate use of antibiotics.[3]

In contrast, chronic bronchitis is defined as persistent productive cough for 3 or more months in two successive years in the absence of any other disease that might cause chronic cough and sputum produc- tion. It is most often associated with cigarette smoking. This condition typically occurs in patients with underlying pulmonary disease, such as chronic obstructive pulmonary disease. Acute cough in patients with lung disease is considered a flare of their disease, after pneumonia and other causes are excluded.

This chapter first reviews the pathophysiology, microbiology, and clinical features of acute bronchitis. An overall approach to the diagno- sis is then presented, and the differential diagnosis is discussed. Finally, key treatment strategies are addressed.

Pathophysiology

Acute bronchitis can occur after inoculation of the tracheobronchial mucosa with an infectious agent.[2] The infection elicits an airway inflam- matory response. This initial phase of illness may be accompanied by fevers, myalgias, and malaise or may be relatively asymptomatic. As a re- sult of the inflammatory response, the airways become hyperreactive.[1] The hyperreactivity results in the clinical features of cough, wheezing, and dyspnea and usually lasts 1 to 3 weeks. Airway hyperreactivity may be demonstrated on pulmonary function tests by showing reduction in the forced expiratory volume at 1 second (FEV_1) and an obstructive pattern on

55

spirometry. A reduced FEV_1 has been shown in 40% of healthy adults without prior lung disease who present with acute bronchitis.[4,5] In most patients, the airway hyperreactivity resolves over time.

Microbiology

The identification of a specific microbiologic pathogen occurs in only a minority of cases of acute bronchitis. Respiratory viruses cause the majority of cases of uncomplicated acute bronchitis.[1-3] The viruses that are most commonly implicated include influenza A, influenza B, and respiratory syncytial virus. Viruses that typically cause acute rhinosinusitis may also cause acute bronchitis, and these include coronaviruses, rhinoviruses, and adenovirus.[1]

Less than 10% of patients with uncomplicated acute bronchitis have evidence of a bacterial infection. *Bordetella pertussis, Mycoplasma pneumoniae,* and *Chlamydia pneumoniae* are the most common bacterial pathogens proven to cause acute bronchitis in healthy adults.[1] *Streptococcus pneumoniae, Haemophilus influenzae,* and *Moraxella catarrhalis* may also cause exacerbations of chronic bronchitis in patients with chronic obstructive pulmonary disease. In adults without preexisting lung disease, however, there is no evidence that these organism cause acute bronchitis.[3]

Acute bronchitis may also have noninfectious origins. In particular, inhalational exposures to allergic triggers, either at home or in the workplace, may provoke acute bronchitis. Triggers include tobacco and marijuana smoke, ammonia, and air pollutants. Finally, cough variant asthma should also be considered.[2]

Clinical Features

Cough is a prominent feature of acute bronchitis. The cough may be productive of sputum or may be nonproductive and typically lasts 1 to 3 weeks. Wheezing is often another common feature of acute bronchitis but may also be the result of previously undiagnosed asthma.[2] The distinction between acute bronchitis and an asthma flare is impossible to make at the initial presentation, unless a history of recurrent asthma attacks has been documented. Many of the clinical features common to asthma may be present with acute bronchitis, including reduced peaked flows, or obstructive spirometry results and responsiveness to bronchodilators.[4,5]

Other symptoms of acute bronchitis that may be present in various degrees of severity include dyspnea, chest pain, and shortness of breath. Prominent constitutional symptoms, in addition to other findings suggestive of acute bronchitis, should prompt consideration of influenza or parainfluenza virus as causative agents.[1] Fever is an uncommon finding in patients with acute bronchitis and suggests the possibility of pneumonia or influenza.

Differential Diagnosis

There are many causes of acute cough that prompt patients to present to their primary care physician. Table 1 outlines some of the most common causes of acute cough. Among these are upper respiratory infections, such as viral rhinosinusitis (the common cold) and acute bacterial sinusitis.[6] Noninfectious causes, such as allergic rhinitis and rhinitis due to environmental irritants, are also frequent causes of acute cough.[2,6] Pneumonia, asthma, and congestive heart failure are among the more serious conditions that should be considered.[6] Aspiration of a foreign body is a common cause among young children and among people with swallowing dysfunction.[6]

Approach to the Diagnosis

The diagnosis of acute bronchitis is made on clinical grounds. At the outset, it is critically important to distinguish acute bronchitis from pneumonia. Wheezing, dyspnea, or sputum production may suggest acute bronchitis or pneumonia. Abnormalities of vital signs (pulse >100 beats/min, temperature >38°C, respirations >24 breaths/min) or signs of focal consolidation on physical examination of the chest should alert the clinician to the possibility of pneumonia and prompt a chest radiograph.[7] In the absence of these signs and symptoms, a chest radiograph is usually not necessary in most patients presenting with acute cough, and acute bronchitis is likely. Among the elderly, immunosuppressed, or patients with chronic diseases, however, a high suspicion for pneumonia should always be maintained despite the lack of clinical predictors.[8,9]

TABLE 1.   Common Causes of Acute Cough
Viral rhinosinusitis (viral upper respiratory tract infection)
Bacterial sinusitis
Allergic rhinitis
Acute bronchitis
Asthma
Pneumonia
Congestive heart failure
Chronic obstructive pulmonary disease with flare
Aspiration of foreign body
Adapted from Irwin RS, Madison JM: The diagnosis and treatment of cough. N Engl J Med 343:1715–1721, 2000.

Studies that have used sputum Gram stains, nasopharyngeal swabs, and viral serologies have failed to determine the cause of acute bronchitis in more than two thirds of patients.[1,3] Since acute bronchitis in the majority of patients has a viral origin, sputum Gram staining is not considered useful in the evaluation of otherwise healthy patients. Rapid viral respiratory panels can be obtained by swabbing the nasopharynx and have been used to attempt to determine a viral origin. The utility of viral respiratory panels in clinical practice is limited.

Treatment

The treatment of acute bronchitis is primarily supportive and includes the use of antitussive agents and bronchodilators. Bronchodilators have been use to reduce the incidence of cough and should be considered in patients with acute bronchitis.[10] Patients with prominent cough or wheezing should be prescribed a beta-agonist agent via a meter-dosed inhaler. Inhaled beta-agonists work by relaxing bronchial smooth muscles that are hyperreactive. Albuterol, a common beta-agonist, is typically used at a dose of two puffs four times a day. However, a recent meta-analysis calls into question the use of beta-agonists for the treatment acute bronchitis, noting that they were no better than placebo in reducing symptoms of acute bronchitis and were associated with a higher incidence of adverse events (primarily tremor and nervousness).[11] Patients with an abnormal lung examination finding (mainly wheezing) were not distinguished from those with a normal lung examination findings in this analysis, and patient selection could have led to this result. Thus, patients with wheezing may benefit symptomatically from albuterol, but in the absence of any abnormalities on lung examination, albuterol may not be indicated.

If the cough of acute bronchitis is disturbing sleep or is causing discomfort, an antitussive agent may be used. Dextromethorphan or codeine are common agents used to reduce the severity of a cough. Acetaminophen or nonsteroidal anti-inflammatory drugs can also be used for patients with continued constitutional symptoms or fevers.[1,2]

Based on an extensive amount of available evidence, current clinical practice guidelines strongly recommend that antibiotics not be routinely prescribed in patients with acute bronchitis.[3] In fact, the use of antibiotics for the treatment of acute bronchitis may be the single largest cause of inappropriate antibiotic use in the United States. Purulence of sputum is not useful in distinguishing a bacterial from a viral cause of acute bronchitis and should not be an indication for the use of antibiotics. An overall approach to the management of acute bronchitis is presented in Figure 1.

Bordetella pertussis, the causative agent of "whooping cough," is one

Figure 1. Algorithm for the management of suspected acute bronchitis. (Adapted from Gonzales R, Sande MA: Uncomplicated acute bronchitis. Ann Intern Med 133:981–990, 2000.)

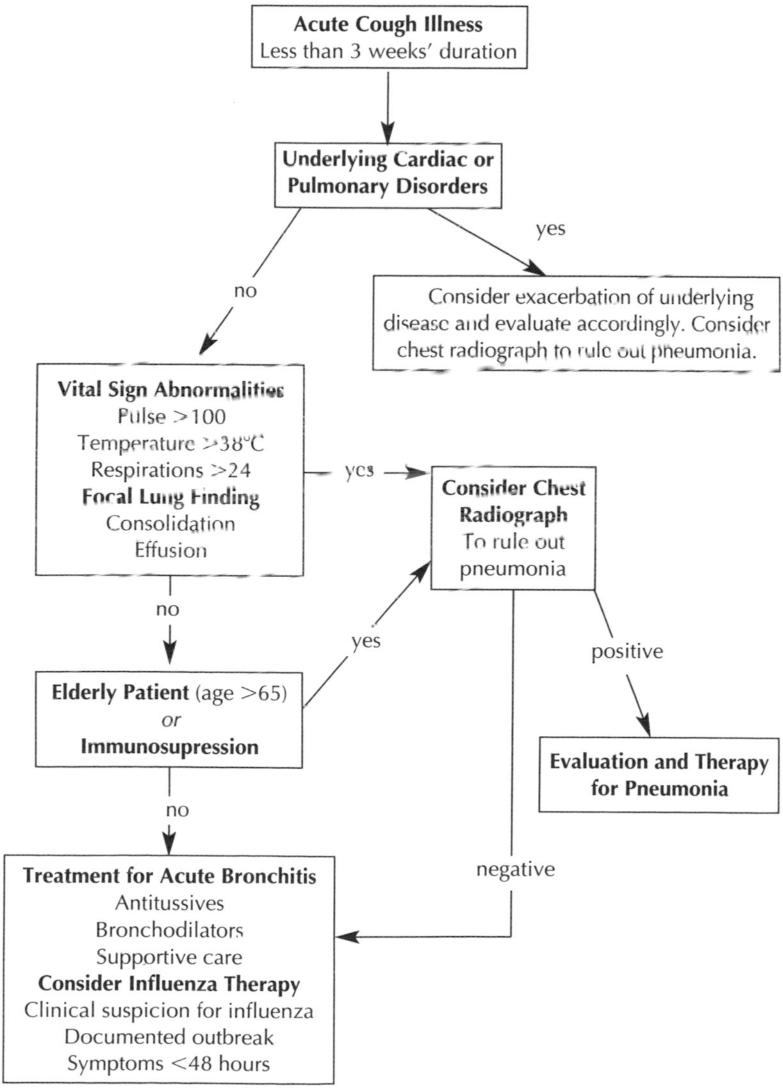

Acute Cough Illness
Less than 3 weeks' duration

↓

Underlying Cardiac or Pulmonary Disorders

yes →

Consider exacerbation of underlying disease and evaluate accordingly. Consider chest radiograph to rule out pneumonia.

no ↓

Vital Sign Abnormalities
Pulse >100
Temperature >38°C
Respirations >24
Focal Lung Finding
Consolidation
Effusion

— yes →

Consider Chest Radiograph
To rule out pneumonia

no ↓

yes ↑

Elderly Patient (age >65)
or
Immunosupression

positive ↓

Evaluation and Therapy for Pneumonia

no ↓

Treatment for Acute Bronchitis
Antitussives
Bronchodilators
Supportive care
Consider Influenza Therapy
Clinical suspicion for influenza
Documented outbreak
Symptoms <48 hours

← negative

bacterial cause of acute bronchitis for which the use of antibiotics may be appropriate.[1–3] If *B. pertussis* is suspected because of a known close contact or during an outbreak, empiric antibiotic treatment should be initiated while awaiting appropriate confirmatory testing. Adults with pertussis often present late in the course of illness, and antibiotics are more important to reduce the spread of the disease than to treat the illness in the presenting patient.

If influenza is suspected, therapy with a neuraminidase inhibitor, such as zanamavir or oseltamivir, or an antiviral agent, such as amantadine or rimantadine, should be considered. These agents have been shown to shorten the course of illness by approximately 1 day if given within 48 hours of the onset of symptoms.[1,12] Side effects of the therapy are common, with central nervous system side effects common with rimantadine and gastrointestinal complaints common with the neuraminidase inhibitors. A 5-day course for both classes of agents is typical. Neuraminidase inhibitors are preferred, given the lower side effect profile[1,12] and since they are effective against both influenza A and influenza B. During documented influenza outbreaks, these agents should be considered in patients presenting with usual symptoms of influenza. Given the need to initiate the treatment within the first 48 hours, the clinician should not wait for confirmatory diagnostic testing. These agents should be especially considered in patients with underlying cardiac or pulmonary disease or other medical comordidities.

Complications of Acute Bronchitis

Bacterial superinfection after viral upper respiratory tract infection is an uncommon complication. The clinician should be alerted to this possibility when patients diagnosed with an uncomplicated case of acute bronchitis subsequently develop fevers and other signs suggestive of pneumonia. Chest radiographs should be obtained in this scenario to evaluate for possible pneumonia.

Severe pain or sudden onset of shortness of breath after coughing may be indicative of a serious complication such as pneumothorax or rib fracture. Cough lasting beyond 3 weeks is unlikely to be from acute bronchitis, and if a cough persists for this duration, another diagnosis should be sought out. The exception to this is acute bronchitis due to *B. pertusis,* which may persist for 4 to 6 weeks.

Key Points: Acute Bronchitis

☞ Acute bronchitis is an acute respiratory tract infection that results in variable degrees of cough (with or without sputum production), wheezing, and dyspnea in otherwise healthy adults, in whom pneumonia has been excluded clinically or by chest radiograph.

Key Points (*Continued*)

- ↪ Acute bronchitis is most often the result of respiratory viral infections.
- ↪ Airway hyperreactivity is responsible for many of the clinical features of acute bronchitis.
- ↪ Treatment of acute bronchitis is supportive and primarily consists of bronchodilators and antitussive agents.
- ↪ The role of antibiotics is *extremely limited,* and they should not be used routinely in the treatment of acute bronchitis.

Reference

1. Gonzales R, Sande MA: Uncomplicated acute bronchitis. Ann Intern Med 133: 981–990, 2000.
2. Knutson D, Braun C: Diagnosis and management of acute bronchitis. Am Fam Phys 65:2039 2044, 2002.
3. Snow V, Mottur-Pilson C, Gonzales R: Principles of appropriate antibiotic use for treatment of acute bronchitis in adults. Ann Intern Med 134:518–520, 2001.
4. Boldy DA, Skidmore SJ, Ayres JF: Acute bronchitis in the community: Clinical features, infective factors, changes in pulmonary function and bronchial reactivity to histamine. Respir Med 84:377–385, 1990.
5. Williamson HA Jr: Pulmonary function tests in acute bronchitis: Evidence for reversible airway obstruction. J Fam Pract 3:251–256, 1987.
6. Irwin RS, Madison JM: The diagnosis and treatment of cough. N Engl J Med 343:1715–1721, 2000.
7. Metlay JP, Kapoor WN, Fine MJ: Does this patient have community-acquired pneumonia? JAMA 278:1440–1445, 1997.
8. Feldman C: Pneumonia in the elderly. Clin Chest Med 20:563–573, 1999.
9. Metlay JP, Schulz R, Li Y-H, et al: Influence of age on symptoms at presentation in patients with community-acquired pneumonia. Arch Intern Med 157:1453–1459, 1997.
10. Hueston W: Albuterol delivered via meter-dosed inhaler to treat acute bronchitis: A placebo controlled double blinded study. J Family Pract 39:437–440, 1994.
11. Smucny JJ, Flynn CA, Becker LA, Glazier RH: Are beta-2 agonists effective treatment for acute bronchitis or acute cough in patients without underlying lung disease? A systematic review. J Fam Pract 50:945 951, 2001.
12. Couch RB: Pevention and treatment of influenza. N Engl J Med 343:1778–1787, 2000.

Community-Acquired Pneumonia

Paul A. Kinniry, M.D.

chapter

7

There are approximately 3 million cases of community-acquired pneumonia annually in the United States, resulting in 500,000 hospitalizations and 45,000 deaths.[1] Community-acquired pneumonia is the sixth leading cause of death in this country and the most common infectious cause.[1] Thus, it is always a "hot topic" in the field of infectious diseases.

Pneumonia may manifest with a wide spectrum of severity. Outpatient mortality rates are reported to be approximately 1%, but the mortality rate is as high as 25% when hospital admission is necessary. The initial severity and ultimate need for hospitalization may not be immediately apparent to the clinician, prompting a fearful respect of this potentially fatal disease.

This chapter first reviews the causes of community-acquired pneumonia and key clinical features of the disease. An approach to the diagnosis is presented, including a discussion of the criteria for hospital admission. Finally, common treatment regimens and important aspects to follow-up care are addressed.

Microbiology

A number of organisms are known to cause pneumonia in the adult (Table 1). The most common agent recovered is *Streptococcus pneumoniae,* and this also accounts for many cases in which no organisms are identified.[2] Other causes of community-acquired pneumonia include the "atypical agents" (*Chlamydia pneumoniae, Legionella* species, *Mycoplasma pneumoniae*), *Haemophilus influenzae,* respiratory viruses, and *Staphylococcus aureus* should also be considered. Gram-negative rods (particularly *Pseudomonas aeruginosa*), *Mycobacterium tuberculosis,* and endemic fungi are less common causes of community-acquired pneumonia. In particular, gram-negative rods and *S. aureus* should be considered for patients admitted to the intensive care unit. For patients who reside in a long-term care facility, *M. tuberculosis,* gram-negative rods, *S. aureus,* and respiratory viruses should be also be considered.[2]

TABLE 1.   Organisms that Commonly Cause Community-Acquired Pneumonia

Bacteria
  Streptococcus pneumoniae
  Mycoplasma pneumoniae
  Chlamydia pneumoniae
  Haemophilus influenzae
  Legionella species
  Staphylococcus aureus
  Pseudomonas aeruginosa
  Klebsiella species
  Anaerobes
  Mycobacterium tuberculosis (rarely)
Respiratory viruses
  Influenza A, B
  Adenovirus
Aspiration (polymicrobial)
Fungi (rarely)
  Histoplasma capsulatum
  Coccidioides immitis
  Cryptococcus neoformans

Adapted from American Thoracic Society: Guidelines for the management of adults with community-acquired pneumonia: Diagnosis, assessment of severity, antimicrobial therapy, and prevention. Am J Respir Crit Care Med 163:1730–1754, 2001.

The possibility of *P. aeruginosa* infection should be considered in certain patient populations. Risk factors for pseudomonal infection include structural lung disease such as cystic fibrosis or bronchiectasis, previous broad-spectrum antibiotic use for more than 1 week in the past month, malnutrition, and corticosteriod use (more than 10 mg of prednisone daily).[2]

One of the most important recent events in the area of community-acquired pneumonia has been the development of drug-resistant *S. pneumoniae,* and resistance to beta-lactam antibiotics, such as penicillins and cephalosporins, may be as high as 35% in some areas. Drug-resistant S. *pneunomiae* does not need to be considered in every patient but should be thought of when specific risk factors exists. These risk factors include. (1) age greater than 65 years, (2) beta-lactam use within the last 3 months, (3) multiple medical comorbidities, (4) exposure to children in day care, and (5) immunosuppressive conditions, including corticosteriod use and HIV infection (Table 2).[2] There appears to be no difference in mortality among patients infected with *S. pneumoniae* with low or intermediate levels of beta-lactam resistance (<4.0 μmg/ml) and beta-lactam sensitive *S. pneumoniae.* In the absence of meningitis, failure of high-dose beta-lactam treatment is unlikely. At higher levels of resistance (>4.0 μmg/ml), however, there is evidence of increased mortality.[3]

TABLE 2. Risk Factors for Developing Penicillin-Resistant Pneumococcal Pneumonia
Age older than 65 years
Beta-lactam therapy in the past 3 months
Alcoholism
Exposure to children in day care
Immunosuppression (including corticosteriod therapy)
Multiple medical comorbidities
Adapted from American Thoracic Society: Guidelines for the management of adults with community-acquired pneumonia: Diagnosis, assessment of severity, antimicrobial therapy, and prevention. Am J Respir Crit Care Med 163:1730–1754, 2001.

Fluoroquinolone-resistant *S. pneumoniae* has also been recently described.[4] Infection with this organism remains rare in the United States but may be increasing in patients with community-acquired pneumonia who were recently treated with flouroquinolones.[4] The increasing development of flouroquinolone-resistant *S. pneumoniae* will most certainly have an impact on empiric antibiotic recommendations in the near future.

Clinical Features

The usual clinical features of community-acquired pneumonia are very familiar. Symptoms include fever, cough (usually productive of purulent sputum), shortness of breath, and chest pain (often described as pleuritic). Symptoms are typically rapid in onset, with most patients presenting within the first few days of symptoms. Patients may experience chills or rigors. Nonspecific symptoms are also common, such as headache, fatigue, myalgias, and occasionally abdominal pain.

Clinical signs of pneumonia include fever, tachycardia, tachypnea, and abnormal breath sounds. Focal crackles, egophony, increased tactile fremitus, and wheezes are the most common physical examination findings associated with pneumonia.[5,6]

Although these signs and symptoms are identified in most patients, atypical presentations occur, especially in elderly or immunosuppressed patients.[7,8] Among these patients, pneumonia may occur without signs or symptoms localizing to the chest and without fever. Elderly patients may be found with mental status changes, failure to thrive, abdominal pain, or exacerbation of underlying chronic diseases.[7,8] Tachypnea (respiratory rate exceeding 26 breaths/minute) may suggest pneumonia in the elderly patient without other obvious clinical features of pneumonia,[9] and this may be the only clinical clue to the diagnosis.

Diagnosis

Leukocytosis is common in patients with community-acquired pneumonia, with white blood cell counts usually between 15,000 and 30,000, and bandemia is typically prominent. Leukopenia, if present, indicates a poor prognosis.[2]

Blood chemistry test findings may suggest volume depletion. Hyponatremia has been suggested to occur with more frequency in patients with *Legionella* pneumonia,[10] but this finding is nonspecific in distinguishing *Legionella* from other forms of pneumonia.

All patients who are clinically suspected of having community-acquired pneumonia should undergo chest radiography. The chest radiograph is important for confirming the diagnosis and may also suggest an alternative diagnosis, such as congestive heart failure or malignancy.[2] Pulmonary complications of pneumonia may also be evident, such as a parapneumonic effusion or lung abscess. Chest radiographs also offer some prognostic information.[11] Patients with multilobar disease tend to have worse outcomes. The chest radiograph has not proved to be reliable in distinguishing "routine" bacterial pneumonia from "atypical" bacterial or viral pneumonia and should not be used in deciding initial antibiotic therapy.[2,12]

Infrequently, a patient presents with clinical features that are highly suggestive of pneumonia, but the chest radiograph is normal. Some authors suggest that this may represent early pneumonia, before consolidation has fully developed, or pneumonia in a volume-depleted patient in whom an infiltrate will blossom after volume resuscitation.[2] This condition has been described in elderly and neutropenic patients, and the frequency at which it occurs is unknown.[7] Nevertheless, the routine use of repeat radiographs in patients with an initial negative study is not recommended. Such individuals should have an evaluation for other possible causes of their presenting symptoms, and if the clinical picture continues to suggest pneumonia, a repeat chest radiograph after volume resuscitation may be useful.

The value of sputum examination is controversial. Current guidelines from the American Thoracic Society do not recommend obtaining sputum Gram stain and culture routinely. The guidelines recommend obtaining sputum when drug-resistant pneumococci, other resistant pathogens, or organisms not routinely covered by the usual empiric antibiotics are suspected. The American Thoracic Society suggests that a sputum culture be used to broaden coverage if necessary.[2] In contrast, the Infectious Diseases Society of America recommends more liberal use of sputum examination and argues that sputum Gram stain and culture should be performed for all patients admitted to the hospital for pneumonia. Furthermore, this group believes that the initial Gram stain should be used to help determine initial therapy.[1] If sputum is obtained, it should be collected immediately, before the initiation of antibiotic therapy, and the collection of sputum should not be allowed to delay the prompt initiation of appropriate antibiotic therapy. In addition to sputum, two peripheral blood culture sets should be obtained, along with routine chemistries, liver function testing, and complete blood cell count with differential.

Some practitioners suggest testing for human immunodeficiency virus (HIV) in all young (15–54 years) patients admitted with community-acquired pneumonia.[1] The utility of HIV testing in patients with community-acquired pneumonia may be somewhat dependent on the prevalence of HIV in the local population. Clearly, if other risk factors for HIV are present, the patient should be tested.

Admission Criteria

The decision to admit a patient to the hospital for community-acquired pneumonia is probably the most important decision made in the care of an adult with community-acquired pneumonia. Clinicians should use their clinical judgment when contemplating hospital admission. In addition, the patient's ability to take oral medications, support structure in place at home, ongoing substance abuse, or other rare coexisting illnesses that complicate the clinical picture should also be considered when contemplating admission.

To help decide hospital admission, prognostic scoring rules have been developed and validated. The Pneumonia Patient Outcomes Research Team (PORT) was designed to predict patient outcomes and suggest the need for hospitalization.[13] This scoring system groups patients into five classes based on history, vital sign abnormalities, and results of diagnostic testing. The low risk of death in classes I and II has suggested that these patients be considered for outpatient therapy. Class III patients have an intermediate risk of death and may be considered for a brief hospital observation period or outpatient therapy. Class IV and class V patients are at high risk of death and should be admitted for inpatient therapy. One advantage of the PORT study is that it can classify patients into the lowest group on the basis of history and physical findings alone, without the need for extensive diagnostic testing. This is particular useful in treating outpatients with community-acquired pneumonia.

Although full discussion of the PORT scoring system is beyond the scope of this chapter, several prognostic factors have been identified in the development of the scoring system. The clinician should be aware of these in making decisions on where to treat patients with community-acquired pneumonia. Clinical factors associated with poor clinical out-comes are outlined in Table 3. Admission to an intensive care unit is in-dicated for patients with severe disease who are at high risk of poor out-come. If a patient requires mechanical ventilation or is in shock, the need for admission to the intensive care unit is apparent. Other clinical clues that highlight the need for admission to the intensive care unit include acute renal failure, confusion, tachypnea (respiratory rate exceeding 30 breaths/minute), multilobar disease on chest radiograph, or high supple-mental oxygen requirements. Patients with one or more of these features should be considered for admission to the intensive care unit.

Treatment

Antibiotic Selection

Once a diagnosis of community-acquired pneumonia is made, treat-ment with antibiotics should be initiated promptly. In patients who re-

TABLE 3.   Clinical Factors Associated with Poor Clinical Outcome
Age >65 years
Laboratory findings
White blood cell count <4 or >30, neutropenia
Hypoxia PaO_2 <60
Hypercapnia PcO_2 >50
Acute renal failure
Multilobar disease
Progression of infiltrates
Anemia
Metabolic acidosis
Coexisting disease
Chronic obstructive pulmonary disease or bronchiectasis
Diabetes
Chronic renal failure
Congestive heart failure
Malignancy
Alcoholism
Postsplenectomy
Physical findings
Diastolic blood pressure < 60 mm Hg
Systolic blood pressure < 90 mm Hg
Pulse > 125 beats/min
Temperature >40° or <35°C
Confusion or change in mental status
Bacteremia or extrapulmonary infection
Respiratory rate > 30

Adapted from Fine MJ, Auble TE, Yealy DM, et al: A prediction rule to identify low-risk patients with community-acquired pneumonia. N Engl J Med 336:243–250, 1997.

quire admission, intravenous antibiotics should be started after collection of sputum and blood cultures. This should be done without delay. Evidence suggests that appropriately selected, rapidly administered empiric antibiotics is associated with a reduced length of stay.[14]

Initial antibiotic selection is empiric and should be based on the patient's location of therapy (outpatient, inpatient, intensive care unit) and the presence of risk factors for drug-resistant streptococcal pneumonia, and risk factors for gram-negative rod infection (Table 4).[2] In addition, the presence of underlying cardiopulmonary disease should be considered. Atypical pathogens should be considered in all patients being treated for community-acquired pneumonia.[2]

For outpatients without cardiac or pulmonary disease and without risk factors for drug-resistant *S. pneumoniae* or gram-negative rods, therapy with a macrolide antibiotic (azithromycin or clarithromycin) is recommended.[2] Doxycycline is an alternative if the patient is allergic to macrolides.[7] The general use of fluoroquinolones for otherwise healthy outpatients with community-acquired pneumonia is discouraged because of concerns for the development of fluoroquinolone-resistant *S. pneumoniae*.[15] For outpatients with cardiopulmonary disease or with risk factors for drug-resistant streptococcal pneumonia, a fluoroquinolone should be used. Alternatively, an oral beta-lactam plus a macrolide can be substituted.[2]

For patients admitted to the hospital, treatment with intravenous beta-lactam plus intravenous macrolide, or intravenous fluoroquinolone alone is recommended as empiric therapy. Patients admitted to the intensive care unit should not be treated with a single agent alone. Empiric therapy should consist of a beta-lactam plus either a macrolide or a fluoroquinolone.[7] For patients with risk for *Pseudomonas,* an antipseudomonal beta-lactam plus a fluoroquinolone should be used for empiric therapy.[2]

Response to Treatment

Most patients with community-acquired pneumonia should begin to show clinical response within 3 days.[2,16] If the patient is improving clinically (with improvement of the fever curve, decreased dyspnea, and decreasing white blood cell count), a switch to oral therapy should be attempted only if the patient is able to tolerate oral medications. Certain medical conditions are associated with delayed response, including immunosuppression, alcoholism, age greater than 65 years, and multiple medical conditions.[2] Multilobar pneumonia and bacteremia are also associated with delayed resolution. If a patient fails to improve after several days or deteriorates clinically, this may be due to inadequate initial therapy, unusual pathogens not covered by usual empiric therapy, a

TABLE 4. Typical Empiric Antibiotic Regimens for Adults*

Patient Group	Primary Regimen	Alternative Regimen
Outpatients with no cardiac or pulmonary disease or risk factors for DRSP	Oral macrolide Azithromycin 500 mg PO × 1 then 250 mg PO qd Clarithromycin 500 mg PO bid	Doxycycline 100 mg PO bid
Outpatients with cardiac or pulmonary disease, medical comorbidities or age >65	Oral second-generation cephalsporin and oral macrolide Cefdinir 300 mg PO q12h Cefpodoxime proxetil 200 mg PO q12h Cefprozil 500 mg PO q12h and Azithromycin 500 mg PO ×1 then 250 mg PO qd Clarithromycin 500 mg PO bid	Oral fluoroquinolone alone Levofloxacin 500 mg PO qd Gatifloxacin 400 mg PO qd Moxifloxacin 400 mg PO qd
Inpatients with no cardiac or pulmonary disease or risk factors for DRSP	Intravenous fluoroquinolone alone Levofloxacin 500 mg IV qd Gatifloxacin 400 mg IV qd Moxifloxacin 400 mg IV qd	Intravenous macrolide alone Azithromycin 500 mg IV ×1 then 250 mg PO qd
Inpatients with cardiac or pulmonary disease, comorbidities, age >65, risk for DRSP	Intravenous beta-lactam and intravenous macrolide Ceftriaxone 1.0 to 2.0 g IV qd Cefotaxime 2.0 g IV q8h and Azithromycin 500 mg IV qd	Intravenous fluoroquinolone alone Levofloxacin 500 mgIV qd Gatifloxacin 400 mgIV qd Moxifloxacin 400 mg IV qd
Intensive care unit without risk factors for pseudomonas	Intravenous beta-lactam and either intravenous fluoroquinolone or intravenous macrolide Ceftriaxone 1.0 to 2.0 g IV QD Cefotaxime 2.0 g IV q8h and Azithromycin 500 mg IV qd Levofloxacin 500 mg IV qd Gatifloxacin 400 mg IV qd Moxifloxacin 400 mg IV qd	
Intensive care unit with risk factors for pseudomonas	Intravenous antipseudo-monal beta-lactam plus intravenous antipseuo-monal quinolone Cefepime 2.0 g IV q12h Piperacillin/tazobactam 3.375 g IV q4h and Levofloxacin 500 mg PO qd	

*Doses may need to be adjusted for renal insufficiency and other factors
DRSP, drug-resistant *Streptococcus pneumoniae*
Adapted from: American Thoracic Society: Guidelines for the management of adults with community-acquired pneumonia: Diagnosis, assessment of severity, antimicrobial therapy, and prevention. Am J Respir Crit Care Med 163:1730–1754, 2001; and Gilbert DN, Moellering RC, Sande MA: The Sanford Guide to Antimicrobial Therapy, 32nd ed. 2002.

complication of pneumonia, or an incorrect initial diagnosis. The initial diagnosis should be questioned, with repeat history focusing on any possible exposures (primarily HIV risk factors, pets, and recent travel) that may suggest unusual pathogens such as *Pneumocystis carinii*, fungal pneumonia, or psittacosis. Careful repeat physical examination may suggest complications of pneumonia, including empyema, meningitis, septic arthritis, and endocarditis.

Conditions other than pneumonia could account for the clinical presentation. Pulmonary embolism, malignancy, congestive heart failure, hypersensitivity pneumonitis, vasculitis, and sarcoidosis can all mimic pneumonia and should be considered.[2] Bronchoscopy may be considered in patients who failed to improve on initial empiric antibiotics for community-acquired pneumonia. Current evidence suggests that the yield of bronchoscopy is low, except in nonsmoking patients with multilobar disease.[17]

Follow-Up

When the patient has clinically stabilized and is tolerating oral medications, he or she can be discharged without an observation period.[16] Safe hospital discharge is dependent on a number of factors other than clinical stability. The patient's social situation is especially important. Repeat chest radiography at time of discharge is not necessary if the patient is clinically stabilized but should be obtained at a follow-up visit approximately 6 weeks after hospital discharge. This follow-up radiograph is particularly important in smokers, to exclude the possibility of malignancy.

Key Points: Community-Acquired Pneumonia

- Community acquired pneumonia is an acute illness characterized by fever, cough, and pulmonary infiltrates.
- Chest radiographs are required to confirm the diagnosis.
- Perhaps the most important decision made in the treatment of community-acquired pneumonia is whether to treat the patient at home or in the hospital.
- Initial antibiotic selection is empiric and should be initiated immediately after obtaining the appropriate cultures.
- Most patients begin to show improvement and clinical stability within 72 hours of initiation of therapy.
- Follow-up chest radiograph is necessary 6 weeks after treatment, especially in elderly smokers.

References

1. Barlett JG, Dowell SF, Mandell LA, et al: Practice guidelines for the management of community-acquired pneumonia in adults. Clin Infect Dis 31:383–421, 2000.
2. Niederman MS, Mandell LA, Anzueto A, et al: Guidelines for the management of adults with community-acquired pneumonia. Diagnosis, assessment of severity, antimicrobial therapy, and prevention. Am J Respir Crit Care Med 163:1730–1754, 2001.
3. Feikin DR, Schuchat A, Kolczak M, et al: Mortality from invasive pneumococcal pneumonia in the era of antibiotic resistance, 1995–1997. Am J Public Health 90:223–229, 2000.
4. Davidson R, Cavlcanti R, Brunton JL, et al: Resistance to levofloxacin and failure of treatment of pneumococcal pneumonia. N Engl J Med 346:747–750, 2002.
5. Metlay JP, Kapoor WN, Fine MJ: Does this patient have community-acquired pneumonia? Diagnosing pneumonia by history and physical examination. JAMA 278:1440–1445, 1997.
6. Wipf JE, Lipsky BA, Hirschmann JV, et al: Diagnosing pneumonia by physical examination. Arch Intern Med 159:1082–1087, 1999.
7. Feldman C: Pneumonia in the elderly. Clin Chest Med 20:563–573, 1999.
8. Metlay JP, Schulz R, Li YH, et al: Influence of age on symptoms at presentation in patients with community-acquired pneumonia. Arch Intern Med 157:1453–1459, 1997.
9. McFadden JP, Price RC, Eastwood HD, et al: Raised respiratory rate in elderly patients: A valuable physical sign. BMJ 284:626–627, 1982.
10. Stout JE, Yu V: Legionellosis. N Engl J Med 337:682–687, 1997.
11. Hasley PB, Albaum MN, Li YH, et al: Do pulmonary radiographic findings at presentation predict mortality in patients with community-acquired pneumonia? Arch Intern Med 156:2206–2212, 1996.
12. Marie TJ: Community-acquired pneumonia. Clin Infect Dis 18:501–513, 1994.
13. Fine MJ, Auble TE, Yealy DM, et al: A prediction rule to identify low-risk patients with community-acquired pneumonia. N Engl J Med 336:243–250, 1997.
14. Battleman DS, Callahan M, Thaler HT: Rapid antibiotic delivery and appropriate antibiotic selection reduce length of hospital stay of patients with community-acquired pneumonia. Arch Intern Med 162:682–688, 2002.
15. Heffelfinger JD, Dowell SF, Jorgensen JH, et al: Management of community-acquired pneumonia in the era of pneumococcal resistance. Arch Intern Med 160:1399–1408, 2000.
16. Ramirez JA, Vargas S, Ritter GW, et al: Early switch from intravenous to oral antibiotics and early hospital discharge. Arch Intern Med 159:2449–2454, 1999.
17. Feinsilver SH, Fein AM, Niederman MS, et al: Utility of fiberoptic bronchoscopy in nonresolving pneumonia. Chest 98:1322–1326, 1990.

Prevention of Infective Endocarditis

chapter 8

Todd D. Barton, M.D., and
Emily A. Blumberg, M.D.

Infective endocarditis (IE) is a rare disease, with an estimated incidence in the United States of one to five cases per 100,000 patient-years. However, the disease carries an overall mortality rate of 20% to 40%, perhaps as high as 70% in some groups. Efforts to prevent IE have long centered on prevention of transient procedure-related bacteremia. The assumption on which these efforts are based is that procedure-related transient bacteremias cause a significant number of IE cases. This hypothesis has never been directly proven and, in fact, has been questioned on the basis of large case-control and population-based studies. However, consensus expert opinions continue to recommend consideration for antibiotic prophylaxis in moderate-risk and high-risk populations undergoing procedures associated with significant risk of bacteremia.[1] Reasons given for this approach include the high rates of morbidity and mortality associated with IE in high-risk populations, the intuitive logic of the transient bacteremia hypothesis, and the relatively low morbidity rate perceived to be associated with the use of the recommended antibiotics.

Issues pertaining to antibiotic prophylaxis of IE are frequently debated by national consensus groups composed mainly of specialists and researchers. However, it is incumbent upon primary care providers to understand the relevant issues and recommendations, as they are the major decision makers who will consider whether or not to prescribe antibiotic prophylaxis to their patients.

In this chapter, we present a focused review of important issues relating to the prevention of IE. We begin by analyzing factors that place patients at increased risk for IE, then review in detail the available data regarding which procedures are most likely to cause bacteremia with organisms known to cause IE. We then discuss the available data regarding effectiveness of antibiotic prophylaxis and conclude with a review of current recommendations and a few notes on cost-effectiveness and controversies.

Risk Factors for Infective Endocarditis

The first step in considering antibiotic prophylaxis for IE is identification of patients at increased risk for contracting the disease. Both cardiac and noncardiac risk factors should be considered in an overall assessment of risk. These risk factors are summarized in Table 1.

The most commonly considered risk factors for IE are underlying cardiac structural abnormalities associated with turbulent blood flow or damage to endocardial surfaces. Those that place patients at significantly increased risk for IE include prosthetic heart valves, hypertrophic obstructive cardiomyopathy, mitral valve prolapse with regurgitation or thickened leaflets, acquired or congenital aortic stenosis, cyanotic congenital heart malformations, or previous infective endocarditis. Although only some of these risk factors are included in the high-risk category in the consensus American Heart Association recommendations, it is worth noting that recent large surveys have not noted significant differences in risk among patients with these conditions.

TABLE 1. Risk Factors for Infective Endocarditis (IE)		
Risk for IE	**Cardiac Conditions**	**Noncardiac Conditions***
Highest	Prosthetic heart valve Prior infective endocarditis Complex cyanotic heart disease Surgically constructed systemic pulmonary shunts or conduits	

Moderate	Mitral valve prolapse with
	  valvular regurgitation or
	  thickened leaflets
	Other congenital heart disease
	Hypertrophic obstructive
	  cardiomyopathy
	Acquired valvular dysfunction	

Potentially Increased	Mitral valve prolapse without
	  valvular regurgitation, in men or
	  in people older than 40 years
	Heart murmur with a normal
	  echocardiogram
		Diabetes mellitus
		Chronic renal disease
		Indwelling central venous
		  catheter
		Systemic lupus erythematosus
		Antiphospholipid antibody
		  syndrome
		Inflammatory bowel disease
		Poor oral health

*Although these conditions may be associated with infective endocarditis, no specific prevention guidelines exist for patients with these diagnoses in the absence of other predisposing cardiac conditions.
Adapted from Dajani AS, Taubert KA, Wilson W, et al: Prevention of bacterial endocarditis: Recommendations by The American Heart Association. Clin Infect Dis 25:1448–1458, 1997.

Prosthetic Valves

The presence of a prosthetic heart valve is probably the most well-recognized risk factor for the development of IE. Overall, the risk for IE is highest in the first 6 months after implantation, and higher if placed during a period of active infection.[2] Neither of these factors can be affected by systemic antibiotic prophylaxis, and therefore the prevention of early prosthetic valve endocarditis, although critically important, falls largely outside the realm of this review. The available data suggest equal risk in patients with bioprosthetic and mechanical heart valves. These data predate the advent of some of the newer materials and preventive techniques (e.g., antibiotic immersion or silver coating), and thus risk assessments may change in the coming years.[3]

Congenital Heart Disease

Patients with congenital heart disease are probably all at increased risk for IE, although a clear spectrum of risk exists.[4–5] Patients at greatest risk are those with surgically constructed shunts, cyanotic heart disease, or congenital outflow tract stenoses (either left- or right-sided), while patients with repaired isolated atrial septal defects are at minimal to no increased risk.

Since most adult medicine practitioners have few patients with congenital heart disease in their practices, it is of paramount importance to maintain close contact with patients' cardiologists. In this way, the primary care provider can develop a better understanding of the nature of the structural heart disease and its evolution over time, and the two physicians can collaborate in a determination of risk for IE when necessary.

Mitral Valve Prolapse

Mitral valve prolapse (MVP) is the most common risk factor for IE.[2] MVP is present to some degree in approximately 2% of the general population and is an underlying cardiac finding in 10% to 30% of IE cases. Overall, however, IE is a rare development in patients with MVP. Therefore, extensive work has been done in an effort to divide patients with MVP into higher and lower risk subsets, with the goal being to more accurately target a higher risk population for consideration for antibiotic prophylaxis.

The most recent consensus recommendations from the American Heart Association rate MVP with valvular regurgitation and/or thickened leaflets as a moderate-risk condition, while MVP without valvular regurgitation is rated as negligible risk.[1]

In the largest retrospective study of population risk factors for endocarditis to date, mitral valve prolapse was as significant a risk factor as the presence of a prosthetic valve.[6] In this study, patients were not sub-categorized as having or not having valvular regurgitation or thickened leaflets. Experts think that it is not MVP that inherently increases risk, but the jet of mitral regurgitation whose shearing forces damage the atrial surface of the valve.[1] This is problematic, because even patients with MVP without regurgitation at rest can develop regurgitation with exertion or volume depletion, and the risk categorization of this subpopulation has not been adequately addressed. Limited data suggest that men or patients older than 40 years of age may be at increased risk for valve damage associated with MVP, so a reasonable approach may be to use these and other modifying factors (e.g., diabetes, renal disease) to help stratify a patient's risk in the absence of thickened valves or valvular regurgitation.

Miscellaneous Risk Factors

Although structural heart diseases are the most studied risk factors for IE, a few other risk factors are worth noting. It is unclear how to quantify the risks from these risk factors, or how their presence may or may not affect the decision to offer antibiotic prophylaxis.

Previous endocarditis, with or without current structural abnormalities on echocardiography, should be considered a high-risk condition.

Diabetes has been identified as a risk factor for IE in several series. It is not clear whether this increased risk is due to microscopic endocardial damage or the relative immunodeficiency associated with diabetes.

Chronic renal disease is common in patients with advanced diabetes but was shown to be an independent risk factor in a large study.[6]

Nosocomial endocarditis accounts for 10% to 20% of all endocarditis cases in most published series.[7–8] Furthermore, patients who acquire endocarditis on the inpatient wards are more likely to contract IE with *Staphylococcus aureus* or *Enterococcus,* and thus have a significantly higher overall mortality rate than outpatients who contract IE. Careful attention must be paid to inpatients who are going to undergo invasive procedures or who have longstanding indwelling central venous catheters.

Systemic lupus erythematosus and the **antiphospholipid antibody syndrome** are both likely elevate a patient's risk of contracting IE.[9] This is most likely due to the 25% to 75% chance of clinically significant valvular disease in patients with these diseases. Especially in the presence of a heart murmur or any history of symptoms potentially related to valve disease, a cardiac work-up should be undertaken in these patients prior to making a determination regarding antibiotic prophylaxis for IE.

The true effect of **immunodeficiency** on the development of IE is unknown. Other immunodeficiencies (human immunodeficiency virus infection, organ transplants) have not been specifically identified as risks for IE, as patients with these conditions have not been included to any significant degree in the older studies that form the basis for current recommendations.

Procedures Associated with Risk of Bacteremia

After assessing a patient's intrinsic risk for developing IE, the next step in considering the role of antibiotic prophylaxis is to determine whether the planned procedure carries a significant risk of bacteremia with organisms known to cause IE. Although there are dozens of papers in the literature that assess postprocedural bacteremia, the interpretation of their results is difficult because of marked differences in several parameters, including the following:

- Time at which cultures were obtained (from 1 to 20 minutes post procedure)
- Isolates considered significant positives (e.g., inclusion or exclusion of coagulase-negative staphylococci or anaerobic bacteria)
- Definitions of significant bacteremia (by both type of bacteria, quantity recovered, and time from procedure)
- Differences in blood culture methods
- Inability to truly standardize all procedures being performed (e.g., chewing)

Despite these limitations to the available data, it is possible to stratify procedures according to a relatively high or low likelihood of inducing bacteremia with organisms known to cause IE. A complete list of procedures can be found in Table 2.

The *highest risk procedures* include the following:[1–2, 10–12]

- Most dental procedures, generally including any invasive procedure or procedures involving gingival manipulation
- Tonsillectomy
- Esophageal stricture dilation
- Variceal sclerotherapy
- Many genitourinary tract procedures (including transrectal biopsy of the prostate)
- Most open surgical operations involving respiratory, intestinal, or genitourinary tract mucosa

A group of *lower risk procedures* includes the following[1–2, 10–12]:

- Noninvasive dental procedures, including orthodontic band adjustments and fluoride treatments
- Esophagogastroduodenoscopy with or without biopsy
- Colonoscopy with or without biopsy
- Uterine dilatation and curettage
- Spontaneous vaginal delivery or uncomplicated caesarian section

TABLE 2. Recommended Prophylaxis Strategies by Procedure and Risk Group

Class	Procedures Higher Risk for Bacteremia	Procedures Low Risk for Bacteremia[†]	Antibiotic Regimens* Oral	Antibiotic Regimens* Intravenous
Dental	Routine cleaning Tooth extraction Periodontal procedures Dental implant placement Reimplantation of avulsed teeth Endodontic instrumentation (root canal) Initial placement of orthodontic bands Intraligamentary local anesthetic injection	Fluoride treatments Taking of oral impressions or radiographs Orthodontic band adjustment Placement of removable orthodontic or prosthodontic appliances Placement of rubber dams Postoperative suture removal Nonintraligamentary local anesthetic injection	Preferred: Amoxicillin, 2 g PO Alternatives: Clindamycin, 600 mg PO Cephalexin, 2 g PO Cefadroxil, 2 g PO Azithromycin, 500 mg PO Clarithromycin, 500 mg PO	Preferred: Ampicillin, 2 g IV Alternatives: Cefazdin, 1 g IV Clindamycin, 600 mg IV
Gastrointestinal	Esophageal stricture dilation Variceal sclerotherapy Endoscopic retrograde cholangiopancreatography/biliary tract surgery Surgical operations that involve intestinal mucosa Tonsillectomy	Upper or lower endoscopy, with or without biopsy Transesophageal echocardiography	For *upper* GI procedures, refer to dental recommendations above. For *lower* GI procedures: Preferred[‡]: Amoxicillin, 2 g PO	Preferred: Ampicillin 2 g IV Alternative: Vancomycin 1 g IV For high-risk patients, add: Gentamicin 1.5 mg/kg IV (not to exceed 120 mg)

Genitourinary	Prostatic surgery Cystoscopy Urethral dilation Vaginal hysterectomy Other surgical operations that involve genitourinary tract mucosa Transrectal biopsy of the prostate Any genitourinary tract procedure involving infected body fluid or tissue (e.g., insertion of a Foley catheter into an infected bladder)	Uncomplicated vaginal delivery or caesarian section Uterine dilatation and curettage Sterilization procedures Insertion or removal of intrauterine devices	Refer to lower GI recommendations above.
Respiratory	Rigid bronchoscopy Surgical operations that involve respiratory mucosa	Flexible bronchoscopy Endotracheal intubation	Refer to dental recommendations above
Other	No other procedures are generally recognized as high-risk procedures in consensus guidelines	Incision and drainage of cutaneous abscesses Cardiac catheterization Placement or removal of a central venous catheter	

*Oral medications should be taken 60 minutes before the procedure; intravenous medications should be administered 30 minutes before the procedure. Only a single dose is recommended.
†Antibiotic prophylaxis is generally not recommended for low-risk procedures.
‡Because of the desire to cover *Enterococcus* in lower gastrointestinal and genitourinary procedures, there are no alternative oral regimens if the patient cannot take amoxicillin.
GI, gastrointestinal.
Adapted from Dajani AS, Taubert KA, Wilson W, et al: Prevention of bacterial endocarditis: Recommendations by the American Heart Association. Clin Infect Dis 25:1448–1458, 1997.

- Flexible bronchoscopy
- Transesophageal echocardiography

Effectiveness of Prophylaxis

Research in animal models has consistently shown that the administration of antibiotics before (or occasionally shortly after) an induced bacteremia can prevent IE on damaged heart valves.[2] However, proof that this approach is effective in humans is lacking. One major problem with the available literature is that multiple studies repeatedly demonstrate that few high-risk patients take antibiotic prophylaxis.[6,13–15] In the largest retrospective case-control studies to date, less than 25% of high-risk patients (based on preexisting structural heart disease) actually took antibiotic prophylaxis before a procedure for which it was indicated. This has led to very small groups of patients in whom an analysis of efficacy can be performed.

- A large population-based case-control study of patients with IE in the Philadelphia metropolitan area failed to show that dental treatment was a risk factor for IE, thereby calling into question the role of prophylactic antibiotics before such treatments.[6] Patients who took antibiotic prophylaxis were not protected against development of IE, but the number of patients who took prophylaxis was very small, making it difficult to draw a conclusion from this study alone.
- One small (eight cases) case-control study from the Cleveland Clinic showed efficacy of antibiotic prophylaxis but was notable for questionable assignment of causality to distant dental procedures.[16]
- A Dutch national case-control study failed to show significant efficacy of antibiotic prophylaxis prior to medical or dental procedures.[14,17]
- A French case-control study concluded that procedures increase the risk of endocarditis but failed to show protective efficacy of antibiotic prophylaxis.[15]

To date, the available literature does not suggest a protective benefit of antibiotic prophylaxis. However, these studies have been underpowered to detect a protective effect as large as 20% or greater.

Recommended Regimens for Antibiotic Prophylaxis

Choice of Antibiotic

When antibiotic prophylaxis is indicated, practitioners should choose a prophylactic regimen based on several considerations, including the following:

- The microbial flora present at the site of the procedure

- The spectrum of activity, cost, and ease of administration of the antibiotic
- Patient history of allergy or sensitivity to antibiotics

Amoxicillin is the preferred antibiotic for endocarditis prophylaxis before most procedures because of its activity against viridans streptococci, favorable side effect profile, low cost, and reasonable bioavailability.[1] When amoxicillin is contraindicated, other oral agents with activity against oral streptococci are reasonable alternatives before oral procedures, including clindamycin, first-generation cephalosporins, or macrolide antibiotics. However, for lower gastrointestinal or genitourinary procedures, vancomycin is recommended because of the perceived need to include coverage for enterococci. In addition, a single dose of an aminoglycoside antibiotic is recommended before lower gastrointestinal or genitourinary procedures in high-risk patients. Table 2 gives a list of recommended antibiotics commonly used for antibiotic prophylaxis.

Risks of Antibiotics

Anaphylaxis is a complication of antibiotic therapy and will occur approximately 4 to 10 times per 100,000 patient-doses of prophylactic oral amoxicillin.[18] For intravenous ampicillin courses, the rate of anaphylaxis may approach 15 to 20 per 100,000 patient-doses. Although anaphylaxis is the most commonly considered potential harm of antibiotic prophylaxis for IE, approximately 10 times more patients will experience minor allergic reactions to these antibiotics, predominantly rashes. In addition, use of even single-dose regimens of antibiotics could cause *Clostridium difficile* colitis, which has significant associated morbidity.

The impact of short-course antibiotic prophylaxis for IE on the development of antimicrobial resistance is unknown. Population studies have not consistently shown a correlation between total antibiotic exposure and emergence of antimicrobial resistance.[19-21] Although it is logical that increasing antibiotic use drives antimicrobial resistance, data to support this hypothesis have been inconsistent.

Practical Considerations

Ideally, antibiotics should be administered to ensure peak concentrations of the antibiotic at the initiation of the procedure. Prophylactic oral antibiotics should be taken 1 hour prior to the procedure. In patients who are unable to take oral medicine, or who are prescribed intravenous medications for prophylaxis, the intravenous antibiotic should be administered within 30 minutes of the procedure. Some animal data support a protective role for postprocedure antibiotics administered within 30 minutes of the procedure.[2]

Patients who are already taking (or have recently taken) antibiotics for other reasons should be prescribed a different antibiotic for prophylaxis of IE. For example, a patient who has completed a course of amoxicillin for a urinary tract infection within the past week might appropriately be given cephalexin prior to a tooth extraction. This is done with the presumption that the remaining bacterial flora in the patient's mouth are likely to be those that are resistant to or tolerant of amoxicillin.

Miscellaneous Considerations

Cost-Effectiveness

Cost-effectiveness studies have suggested benefit from antibiotic prophylaxis, but the assumptions inherent to these studies were inappropriate, limiting the usefulness of their conclusions. Two recent analyses were performed—one in the general population and one in patients with mitral valve prolapse.[18,22] The study in the general population assumed that antibiotic prophylaxis is 100% effective, which is unlikely, and that 15% of IE cases are related to dental procedures, although this number has been estimated to be closer to 4% to 10% in other studies. The mitral valve prolapse analysis also assumed 80% efficacy. Further study in this area is needed, with application of more accurate estimates of patient and physician adherence to recommendations, effectiveness of prophylaxis, and updated costs of complications of endocarditis and costs of antibiotic use.

Considering Referral

The current recommendations for antibiotic prophylaxis of IE are designed to facilitate widespread application by primary care physicians. Some possible reasons for referral would include the work-up of an undiagnosed murmur, clarification of a congenital heart defect, or suspected penicillin allergy.

Future Directions

In the future, a greater emphasis may be placed on providing early patient education, especially for patients with recently implanted artificial valves or recently treated infective endocarditis. It is possible that the use of a wallet card or other such reminder system may be of use in providing accurate, easily accessible information to the patient and any provider preparing to perform a procedure.

Given that animal data strongly support the efficacy of antibiotic prophylaxis, and that the practice is well-entrenched in modern medical care, it is unlikely that there will ever be a more definitive, randomized, placebo-controlled study to assess the efficacy of antibiotic prophylaxis of IE. Because the disease is rare, even in high-risk populations, it has been estimated that such a study would require more than 6000 high-risk patients undergoing procedures likely to induce bacteremia. However, future research can and should be performed to clarify important remaining questions, including how to improve physician and patient education on this topic, how to measure the effect of antibiotic doses on evolving resistance patterns, and how to measure the significance of postprocedural bacteremias.

References

1. Dajani AS, Taubert KA, Wilson W, et al: Prevention of bacterial endocarditis. Recommendations by the American Heart Association. Clin Infect Dis 25:1448–1458, 1997.
2. Durack DT: Prevention of infective endocarditis. N Engl J Med 332:38–44, 1995.
3. Hyde JA, Darouiche RO, Costerton JW: Strategies for prophylaxis against prosthetic valve endocarditis: A review article. J I leart Valve Dis 7:316–326, 1990.
4. Li W, Somerville J: Infective endocarditis in the grown-up congenital heart (GUCH) population. Eur Heart J 19:166–173, 1998.
5. Morris CD, Reller MD, Menashe VD: Thirty year incidence of infective endocarditis after surgery for congenital heart defect. JAMA 279:599–603, 1998.
6. Strom BL, Abrutyn E, Berlin JA, et al: Dental and cardiac risk factors for infective endocarditis: A population-based, case-control study. Ann Intern Med 129:761–769, 1998.
7. Gilleece A, Fenelon L: Nosocomial infective endocarditis. J Hosp Infect 46:83–88, 2000.
8. Chen SC, Dwyer DE, Sorrell TC: A comparison of hospital and community-acquired infective endocarditis. Am J Cardiol 70:1449–1452, 1992.
9. DeRossi SD, Glick M: Lupus erythematosus: Considerations for dentistry. J Am Dent Assoc 129:330–339, 1998.
10. Lockhart PB: The risk for endocarditis in dental practice. Periodontology 23:127–135, 2000.
11. Hall G, Heimdahl A, Nord CE: Bacteremia after oral surgery and antibiotic prophylaxis for endocarditis. Clin Infect Dis 29:1–8, 1999.
12. Olson ES, Cookson BD: Do antimicrobials have a role in preventing septicaemia following instrumentation of the urinary tract? J Hosp Infect 45:85–97, 2000.
13. Moons P, De Volder E, Budts W, et al: What do adult patients with congenital heart disease know about their disease, treatment, and prevention of complications? A call for structured patient education. Heart 86:74–80, 2001.
14. Van der Meer JT, Van Wijk W, Thompson J, et al: Efficacy of antibiotic prophylaxis for prevention of native-valve endocarditis. Lancet 339:135–139, 1992.
15. Lacassin F, Hoen B, Leport C, et al: Procedures associated with infective endocarditis in adults: A case control study. Eur Heart J 16:1968–1974, 1995.
16. Imperiale TF, Horwitz RI: Does prophylaxis prevent postdental infective endocarditis? A controlled evaluation of protective efficacy. Am J Med 88:131–136, 1990.
17. Van der Meer JT, Thompson J, Valkenburg HA, Michel MF: Epidemiology of bacterial endocarditis in The Netherlands II. Antecedent procedures and use of prophylaxis. Arch Intern Med 152:1869–1873, 1992.

18. Gould IM, Buckingham JK: Cost effectiveness of prophylaxis in dental practice to prevent infective endocarditis. Br Heart J 70:79–83, 1993.
19. Bronzwaer SL, Cars O, Buchholz U, et al: A European study on the relationship between antimicrobial use and antimicrobial resistance. Emerg Infect Dis 8:278–282, 2002.
20. Priest P, Yudkin P, McNulty C, Mant D: Antibacterial prescribing and antibacterial resistance in English general practice: Cross sectional study. BMJ 323:1037–1041, 2001.
21. DeNeeling AJ, Overbeek BP, Horrevorts AM, et al: Antibiotic use and resistance of Streptococcus pneumoniae in The Netherlands during the period 1994–1999. J Antimicrob Chemother 48:441–444, 2001.
22. Devereux RB, Frary CJ, Kramer-Fox R, et al: Cost-effectiveness of infective endocarditis prophylaxis for mitral valve prolapse with or without a mitral regurgitant murmur. Am J Cardiol 74:1024–1029, 1994.

HOT TOPICS

Screening for and Treatment of Latent Tuberculosis Infection

chapter 9

Paul A. Kinniry, M.D.

With the introduction of antituberculosis antibiotics in the late 1940s, the United States saw a steady decline in tuberculosis, and many thought the disease would be eradicated in the United States. From 1985 to 1992, the incidences of tuberculosis cases increased by 20%.[1] Today, tuberculosis is again on the decline, but cases continue to occur in every state, and the incidence of multidrug-resistant tuberculosis continues to be a concern.[2] The recent decline in tuberculosis is largely due to increased control efforts, particularly with the use of the tuberculin skin test. Identifying patients with latent tuberculosis infection with this test is an important part of the control of the disease. Primary care practitioners are on the front lines of this screening effort. This makes screening for latent tuberculosis infection a "hot topic" in the field of infectious diseases.

Definition of Latent Tuberculosis

Patients with a positive tuberculin skin test without active tuberculosis are identified as having latent tuberculosis infection. After an initial, often clinically silent infection with tuberculosis, infection with tuberculosis can remain dormant, with the potential to progress to active infection at a later time. Approximately 5% of patients with latent tuberculosis will develop active infection in the first 2 years after primary infection, and an additional 5% will develop active infection later in life.[1] In addition, patients who are immunocompromised will develop active infection at a much higher rate. Progression from latent to active tuberculosis in those who have coexisting human immunodeficiency virus (HIV) infection is approximately 10% per year.[1] The only clinical indicator of latent tuberculosis infection in a patient may be a positive tuberculin skin test. Administration of the tuberculin skin test allows the identification of individuals with latent tuberculosis, and these people will benefit from treatment of their infection.[2]

The terms *prophylaxis* or *preventative therapy* have previously been

85

used to describe what is now more accurately called *treatment of latent tuberculosis infection.* This change in nomenclature was made to help foster a better understanding of the need for tuberculin skin testing and treatment of latent tuberculosis infection.[2]

Tuberculin Skin Testing

The Mantoux tuberculin skin test is the only preferred method of testing patients for latent tuberculosis infections. An intradermal injection of 0.1 ml of purified protein derivative (PPD), which contains 5 tuberculin units, is applied to the forearm. Trained health care workers should read the reaction 48 to 72 hours after the injection.[3] If the patient fails to return before 72 hours, a positive result can be interpreted up to 1 week after the injection; however, if the result is negative after 72 hours, the test should be repeated.[3]

It is the diameter of induration, and not the diameter of erythema, that determines the result of the tuberculin skin test. The diameter of induration perpendicular to the long axis of the forearm should be recorded. Interpretation of the result is dependent upon the size of the induration and the characteristics of the patient.[3] Table 1 provides an overview of the interpretation of the tuberculin skin test.

Tuberculin testing in patients with a prior history of bacillus Calmette-Guérin vaccination is not contraindicated. In these patients, the tuberculin skin test should be interpreted in the same fashion as patients without prior vaccination, and the prior history of bacillus Calmette-Guérin

---

TABLE 1. Interpretation of the Result of the Tuberculin Skin Test Based on the Diameter of Induration

A reaction equal to or greater than 5 mm is consider positive in:
  HIV-positive patients
  Recent contacts of tuberculosis cases
  Persons with fibrotic changes on chest radiograph consistent with old tuberculosis
  Patients with organ transplants and other immunosuppressed patients

A reaction equal to or greater than 10 mm is consider positive in:
  Recent arrivals from high-prevalence countries
  Injection drug abusers
  Residents and employees in high-risk settings
  Patients with medical conditions that place them at high risk
  Children younger than 4 years or children and adolescents exposed to high-risk adults

A reaction equal to or greater than 15 mm is consider positive in:
  All healthy adults; however, this patient population should not be screened

Adapted from American Thoracic Society, Centers for Disease Control and Prevention 1999: Targeted tuberculin testing and treatment of latent tuberculosis infection. Am J Respir Crit Care Med 161(Suppl): S221–247, 2000.

vaccination should be ignored for purposes of interpreting the skin test.[1,2,4]

Two-stage skin testing should be considered in instances in which patients are tested regularly. The reactivity to the skin testing may decrease over time but may be boosted by regular skin testing. If this effect is unrecognized, a patient may be incorrectly classified as a recent converter. If the first tuberculin skin test result is negative or is reactive but less than 10 mm in diameter, a repeat skin test in 1 week is recommended. If the skin test is greater than or equal to 10 mm at that time, the patient is not considered a recent converter.[2,3]

Anergy panels are no longer used in the interpretation of the results, even in those infected with HIV.[2] Patients with HIV who have a negative tuberculin skin test and a negative anergy panel result do not benefit from treatment with isoniazid.[5] The results of a negative anergy panel, therefore, do not aid in the decision of treatment. In patients with no known risk factors, a reaction greater than or equal to 15 mm is considered positive. However, targeted testing programs should exclude these patients from being tested.

Targeted Testing

As the cases of tuberculosis in the United States have declined, the disease has become concentrated in specific populations. It is these populations that targeted testing is directed toward. Targeted testing is the use of tuberculin skin testing to identify patients at high risk of tuberculosis who would benefit from treatment of latent tuberculosis infection. Targeted testing concentrates resources where they are most needed. It should be performed in two main high-risk groups[2]:

- Patients at higher risk for tuberculosis infection (Table 2)
- Patients at higher risk for developing disease once infected (Table 3)

Approach to the Positive Tuberculin Skin Test Result

If a patient's tuberculin skin testing is positive, that patient should be considered a candidate for treatment of latent tuberculosis infection. However, the possibility of active tuberculosis should first be ruled out prior to the initiation of treatment.[1–3] A chest radiograph should be obtained to evaluate for active disease. Patients with chest radiograph findings suggestive of prior, healed tuberculosis should have three consecutive sputum samples obtained to evaluate for active disease. Sputum is not routinely obtained in the absences of chest radiograph changes.

The clinician should also consider the possibility of coexisting HIV infection, and testing should be recommended, if appropriate. In the

TABLE 2. Patients at Higher Risk for Tuberculosis Infection

Close contacts of persons known or suspected to have tuberculosis
Foreign born persons, including children, from areas that have high tuberculosis incidence or prevalence
Residents and employees of high-risk congregate settings (e.g., correctional institutions, nursing homes, homeless shelters, mental institutions)
Health care workers who serve high-risk clients
Medically underserved, low-income populations
High-risk racial or ethnic minority populations, defined locally as having increased prevalence of tuberculosis (Asian and Pacific Islanders, Hispanics, African Americans, Native Americans, migrant farm workers, or homeless persons)
Infants, children, and adolescents exposed to adults in high-risk categories
Person who inject illicit drugs, and any other high-risk substance users (e.g., crack cocaine users)

Adapted from American Thoracic Society, Centers for Disease Control and Prevention 1999: Targeted tuberculin testing and treatment of latent tuberculosis infection. Am J Respir Crit Care Med 161(Suppl): S221–247, 2000.

presence of active pulmonary tuberculosis, patients with HIV may have either an abnormal appearance on chest radiograph or a normal chest radiograph. Thus, HIV patients with respiratory symptoms should have a sputum sample taken for testing, even with a normal chest radiograph.[1,2]

Evaluating a patient with a positive tuberculin skin test should also include determining whether there were preexisting medical conditions

TABLE 3. Persons at Higher Risk for Tuberculosis Disease Once Infected

• Patients with HIV infection
• Patients who were recently infected with tuberculosis (within the last 2 years)
• Patients who have medical conditions known to increase the risk for disease if infection occurs:
   Diabetes mellitus
   Silicosis
   Prolonged corticosteroid therapy
   Other immunosuppressive therapy
   Cancers of the head and neck
   Hematologic diseases
   End-stage renal disease
   Intestinal bypass or gastrectomy
   Chronic malabsorption syndromes
   Low body weight (less than 10% of ideal)
• Patients who inject illicit drugs, and other high-risk substance abusers
• Patients with history of inadequately treated tuberculosis

Adapted from American Thoracic Society, Centers for Disease Control and Prevention 1999: Targeted tuberculin testing and treatment of latent tuberculosis infection. Am J Respir Crit Care Med 161(Suppl): S221–247, 2000.

or medical regimens that would be a contraindication to treatment. In addition, information about prior medical therapy for tuberculosis infection should also be obtained.

Treatment of Latent Tuberculosis

Isoniazid

Daily treatment with isoniazid for 12 months was shown to reduce the risk for active tuberculosis by more than 90%.[2] A shorter 6-month regimen can also provide a reduced risk (approximately 70%) against the development of active infection. A 9-month regimen provides even greater protection than the 6-month regimen[6] and is considered the optimal length of therapy. A 6-month regimen is an acceptable, but less effective, regimen for adults. However, a 6 month regimen should not be used in HIV patients,[2,7] those younger than 18 years of age, and those with fibrotic lesions suggestive of old tuberculosis on chest radiograph.[2]

The dose of isoniazid is 300 mg daily in adults and 10 to 15 mg/kg per day (not to exceed 300 mg daily) in children. Twice-weekly dosing is also an acceptable alternative and may be useful when directly observed therapy is undertaken. The twice-weekly dose is 900 mg (20 to 40 mg/kg in children). The length of treatment is for 9 or 6 months as outlined above for the once- daily therapy.[2]

Pregnant women who are at high risk of developing active disease (for example, those who are HIV positive) should be offered isoniazid even in the first trimester. Isoniazid is not teratogenic, even if taken in the first trimester.[8] For women whose risk of active disease is lower, waiting until after delivery to start isoniazid treatment is also acceptable.

Baseline measurement of liver-associated enzymes and bilirubin is not uniformly recommended but should be obtained in patients with known or suspected liver disease (due to hepatitis B or C, chronic alcohol abuse, or other chronic liver disease), HIV infection, and in pregnant or postpartum women. Active hepatitis and end-stage liver disease are considered contraindications to therapy with isoniazid for latent tuberculosis infection.

Rifampin and Pyrazinamide

The combination of rifampin and pyrazinamide for 2 to 3 months is considered a less preferable alternative. Trials of this regimen have included only HIV-positive patients, and the efficacy of this regimen in HIV-negative patients has not been confirmed.[2] There are recent case reports of severe and fatal hepatitis in patients on rifampin and pyrazinamide, and, therefore, this regimen should be particularly avoided in those with underlying liver disease or alcohol abuse.[9] If these agents are used, liver enzymes should be measured at baseline and then monitored closely every 2 weeks.[2,9] For patients with HIV, the use of rifampin may be contraindicated with certain protease inhibitors and non-nucleoside reverse transcriptase inhibitors used in antiretroviral therapy.[1,2] A substitution of rifabutin for rifampin is recommended in these instances. Rifabutin should not be used with the protease inhibitor ritonavir, the non-nucleoside reverse transcriptase inhibitor delavirdine, or the hard gel of saquinavir, and cautions should be used with patients taking the soft gel form of saquinavir.[2]

Rifampin

Rifampin alone can be used in both HIV-positive and HIV-negative patients who cannot tolerate isoniazid or pyrazinamide. A 4-month course of rifampin is administered at a dose of 600 mg daily.[2] The efficacy of this regimen has been less extensively evaluated.

Monitoring Response to Therapy

Patients who are being treated for latent tuberculosis should be monitored periodically for the following:
- Signs and symptoms of active tuberculosis
- Adherence to the prescribed regimens
- Complications from the medical regimens, especially hepatitis

Patients should be educated on the signs and symptoms of hepatitis and should be instructed to stop medications and seek medical attention immediately for such an event. Patients on isoniazid should be monitored at least monthly. Routine monitoring of liver enzymes for patients on isoniazid is indicated when baseline liver readings are elevated or when risk factors for liver disease are present. Patients on pyrazinamide and rifampin should be seen every 2 weeks, and testing of liver enzymes and bilirubin should be obtained. If signs or symptoms of hepatoxicity develop, the liver enzymes should be tested and the medical regimen should be discontinued.[2] Approximately 10% to 20% of patients taking isoniazid will develop some mild asymptomatic elevation of liver-associated enzymes. These are usually self-limited and do not necessitate discontinuation of therapy. If elevations in liver-associated enzymes exceed five times the upper limit of normal or the patient notes abdominal symptoms, then the drug should be discontinued, and the patient followed closely for signs of hepatotoxicity.

Key Points: Screening for and Treatment of Latent Tuberculosis Infection in the United States

☞ Screening for latent tuberculosis with the tuberculin skin test should be limited to targeted patient populations.

☞ Patients who are tuberculin skin test positive should be evaluated for possible active disease, prior history of tuberculosis, and prior therapies, as well as for any coexisting medical conditions that may complicate treatment.

☞ Coexisting HIV infection should be considered in all tuberculin skin test positive patients.

☞ Daily isoniazid therapy for 9 months is the preferred treatment regimen for patients with latent tuberculosis infection.

☞ Hepatotoxicity is a known complication of isoniazid therapy and is a serious complication of therapy with rifampin and pyrazinamide.

References

1. Small PM, Fujiwara PI: Management of tuberculosis in the United States. N Engl J Med 345:189–200, 2001.
2. American Thoracic Society, Centers for Disease Control and Prevention 1999: Targeted tuberculin testing and treatment of latent tuberculosis infection. Am J Respir Crit Care Med 161(Supple):S221–247, 2000.
3. Centers for Disease Control and Prevention: Core Curriculum on Tuberculosis, 4th ed. Xxx, CDC, 2000.
4. Centers for Disease Control and Prevention: The role of BCG vaccine in the prevention and control of tuberculosis in the United States: A joint statement by the Advisory Council for the Elimination of Tuberculosis and the Advisory Committee on Immunization Practices. MMWR Morbid Mortal Wkly Rep 45:1–18, 1996.
5. Gordin FM, Matts JP, Miller C, et al: A controlled trial of isoniazid in persons with anergy and human immunodeficiency virus infection who are at high risk for tuberculosis. N Engl J Med 337:315–320, 1997.
6. International Union against Tuberculosis Committee on Prophylaxis: Efficacy of various durations of isoniazid preventive therapy for tuberculosis: Five years of follow up. Bull World Health Organization 60:555–564, 1982.
7. Centers for Disease Control and Prevention: Prevention and treatment of tuberculosis among patients infected with human immunodeficiency virus: Principles of therapy and revised recommendations. MMWR Morbid Mortal Wkly Rep 47(RR-20): 1–58, 1984.
8. Scheinhorn DJ, Angelillo VA: Antituberculosis therapy in pregnancy: Risk to the fetus. West J Med 127:195–198, 1977.
9. American Thoracic Society: Update: Fatal and severe liver injuries associated with rifampin and pyrazinamide for latent tuberculosis infection, and revisions in American Thoracic Society/CDC recommendations. MMWR Morbid Mortal Wkly Rep 50:733–735, 2001.

Management of Pulmonary Tuberculosis

Paul A. Kinniry, M.D.

chapter

10

From 1985 to 1992, the incidences of tuberculosis cases in the United States increased by 20%.[1,2] Today, tuberculosis is again on the decline, and the declining case rate has resulted in decreased attention and expertise in the diagnosis and treatment of active tuberculosis. Tuberculosis continues to be diagnosed in every state in the nation and remains a threat to public health. However, as the incidence of tuberculosis has decreased, many clinicians have lost their expertise in diagnosing and managing this once ubiquitous disease. This makes tuberculosis a "hot topic" in infectious diseases once more.

Pathogenesis

Tuberculosis is spread from infected individuals through the air by tiny droplets (1–5 μm in diameter) that contain *Mycobacterium tuberculosis*. These droplets are aerosolized when an infected patient coughs, sneezes, or speaks.[1–3] Particles larger than this size are deposited in the upper airway and tend not to cause infection.[2] After inhalation, droplets are deposited in the respiratory bronchioles or the alveoli, where the organisms can multiply. They can then spread via the lymphatics to the hilar lymph nodes and through the bloodstream to more distant sites.[1,3] Multiplication continues until the replicating mycobacteria are of a sufficient size to elicit a host immune response. In normal individuals, the growth of *M. tuberculosis* is halted once cell-mediated immunity develops.[2] This usually requires 2 to 12 weeks and corresponds temporally with the development of reaction to the tuberculin skin test.[1] Once cell-mediated immunity develops, granulomas consisting of macrophages and activated T lymphocytes can form and arrest the growth of the organisms. A small number of viable mycobacteria may persist inside the granulomas, typically in the necrotic center.[1] Often, this primary infection is clinically silent, but it may manifest as a mild pneumonic illness.[1,2] Primary infection can occasionally overcome the host defenses, resulting in primary progressive disease.[3] In most patients, however, the mycobacteria remain arrested inside the granulomas, with the potential for reactivation in the future. Reactivation occurs to create active disease.

About 10% of infected persons will develop active tuberculosis, with the highest risk of developing active disease in the first 2 years after infection.[2] Certain host factors are associated with an increased risk of developing active disease (see Table 2, Chapter 9). Patients with the human immunodeficiency virus (HIV) have a greatly increased risk of developing active tuberculosis and may progress from latent disease to active disease at a rate of 10% per year.[2]

Clinical Features of Pulmonary Tuberculosis

Cough is the most common presenting symptom associated with pulmonary tuberculosis. It may be nonproductive initially, but, as the disease progresses, the cough is usually productive of sputum.[1–3] Pleuritic chest pain may be identified if inflammation of the pulmonary parenchyma extends to adjacent pleural surfaces.[1] Systemic symptoms are also common, including fever, weight loss, night sweats, and weakness. Hemoptysis is rare and is not necessarily an indicator of active disease.[1]

Physical findings of pulmonary tuberculosis are nonspecific. Evidence of consolidation, including increased tactile fremitus, dullness to percussion, and inspiratory crackles, may be identified over the involved lung areas. There may be physical findings suggestive of pleural effusion, such as decreased tactile fremitus, dullness to percussion, and diminished breath sounds.[1]

Diagnosis

The chest radiograph is an invaluable tool in the diagnosis of pulmonary tuberculosis. Pulmonary tuberculosis typically demonstrates a number of abnormalities on chest radiographs. Primary pulmonary tuberculosis most commonly reveals hilar lymphadenopathy, which may cause right middle lobe compression and atelectasis. [1] Pulmonary infiltrates may be seen in primary tuberculosis, typically in the middle or lower lobes, but cavitary lesions are uncommon.[1] Pleural effusions may also be present in cases of primary infection.

In contrast, the radiographic appearance of reactivation tuberculosis is commonly that of disease of the upper lobes. Upper lobe infiltrates are routinely identified, and cavitation is common.[1] Atypical presentations of reactivation tuberculosis include lower lobe infiltrates, pulmonary nodules, isolated pleural effusions, or isolated hilar lymphadenopathy.

Rarely, chest radiographs may be normal in the patient with culture-proven tuberculosis, especially in immunosuppressed patients.[4] In those with HIV, the incidence of active tuberculosis with a normal chest radiograph is more common and may be close to 20% for patients with CD4 counts less than 200.[5]

Definitive diagnosis of tuberculosis relies on isolation of the organism from a clinical specimen. A patient with appropriate clinical findings and a chest radiograph suggestive of pulmonary tuberculosis should have sputum sent for mycobacterial stains and cultures. Sputum is best obtained by collecting the first sample expectorated by the patient in the morning. If the patient has evidence of pulmonary involvement by radiographs but continues to have nondiagnostic sputum samples, then bronchoscopy should be considered to confirm the diagnosis. The diagnostic yield of bronchoscopy may be greater than 90%.[6]

Distinguishing Mycobacterium tuberculosis from Mycobacterium avium complex is important, particularly in the patient who is mycobacteria smear positive with cultures that are pending or negative. The development of nucleic acid amplification tests in the United States may achieve this goal. Some practitioners recommend the use of nucleic acid amplification test to rapidly diagnosis tuberculosis in patients who are mycobacterial smear positive.[7] Nucleic acid amplification may also be used for patients with high clinical suspicion of pulmonary tuberculosis who remain smear-negative. Up to 50% of smear-negative cases that ultimately are culture positive can be rapidly diagnosed with these tests.[7] The general use of nucleic acid amplification tests should be limited to these conditions. More advanced techniques for diagnosis of tuberculosis are likely to become available in the near future.

Extrapulmonary Tuberculosis

In the HIV-negative patient, extrapulmonary disease is uncommon, occurring in about 15% of cases.[1] With HIV infection, the incidence of extrapulmonary disease has dramatically increased, and as the level of immunosuppresion progresses, the incidence of extrapulmonary tuberculosis rises. The locations of extrapulmonary disease in HIV-negative and HIV-positive patients are similar, with different severities and presentations.[1]

Central nervous system involvement with tuberculosis manifests typically as an indolent basilar meningitis, with neck stiffness, cranial nerve involvement, and delirium. Computed tomography (CT) of the brain may reveal hydrocephalus. The lumbar puncture typically reveals high protein levels, low glucose levels, and a mononuclear cell pleocytosis, although early in the course of disease, spinal fluid may show a predominance of neutrophils. Rarely, central nervous system involvement may be in the form of tuberculomas. These are one or more ring-enhancing lesions seen on CT scan or magnetic resonance imaging (MRI) scan of the brain. Biopsy is necessary for definitive diagnosis.[1]

Miliary tuberculosis results from the failure of the immune response to locally contain either a latent or a newly acquired infection. The chest radiograph reveals a "miliary" pattern consisting of multiple small nodules, approximately the appearance of millet seeds. Disseminated disease is common in miliary tuberculosis, occurring hematogenously, and multiorgan involvement is typical. The clinical presentation is nonspecific, with fevers, weight loss, night sweats, and weakness. More specific symptoms are dependent on the severity of specific organs involved. The central nervous system may be involved in miliary tuberculosis, and this involvement manifests as described above. Bone marrow involvement may also occur, resulting in pancytopenia.[1] Gastrointestinal involvement may also be seen, most often manifesting as right upper quadrant or diffuse abdominal pain. Liver-associated enzymes may reveal an elevated alkaline phosphatase level or elevated tranaminase level. Pancreatitis and cholestasis may also result.

Pleural tuberculosis most often results from a hypersensitivity response to tuberculosis infection. In approximately 30% of cases, there is no radiographic evidence of parenchymal tuberculosis. Tuberculous effusions are typically unilateral and moderate in size. Pleural fluid analysis reveals an exudative effusion with a lymphocyte-predominant pleocytosis. The pleural fluid protein level is typically elevated, and the glucose level is often greater than 60 mg/dL. Because of the low organism load in the pleural space, mycobacterial smears are typically negative, and diagnosis often relies on demonstrated granulomas on pleural biopsy specimens. Less commonly, a large number of organisms gain entrance into the pleural space, causing a tuberculous empyema.

The patient with skeletal tuberculosis typically presents with pain localizing to the site of the infection. Systemic symptoms are not common. Joint involvement may manifest as a monoarthritis. Spinal tuberculosis, also known as Pott's disease, can cause spinal cord compression and permanent neurologic injury. An MRI scan of the spine should be obtained when there is suspicion of spinal infection. Bone biopsy is often required to make the diagnosis.[1]

Genitourinary tract infection with tuberculosis often manifests without systemic involvement. Symptoms localizing to the genitourinary tract are often subtle and include dysuria, hematuria, and frequent urination. Urinalysis results are abnormal in more than 90% of patients, with hematuria or sterile pyuria. The diagnosis is confirmed with mycobacterial cultures of the urine. The yield for mycobacteria on smears of urine is low.[1]

A patient with tuberculous peritonitis often presents with abdominal swelling suggestive of ascites and prominent systemic symptoms of fever, anorexia, and weight loss. Physical examination may suggest an intra-abdominal infection, although signs and symptoms of peritonitis may be subtle. Paracentesis may suggest a cause for the ascites other than portal hypertension, although coexisting cirrhosis may obscure the diagnosis. Laparoscopy with peritoneal biopsy is often required to secure the diagnosis.[1]

Patients with pericardial tuberculosis present with prominent systemic symptoms. Chest pain may be present, and symptoms of dyspnea, orthopnea, cough, and ankle swelling suggestive of pericardial tamponade or constriction typically occur late. Diagnosis requires pericardiocentesis and often pericardial biopsy.[1]

Disease Reporting

Tuberculosis community control programs are the responsibility of both state and local governments, but clinicians have a role in the control effort. The reporting of tuberculosis is required by law in every state. All new cases and highly suspected cases of tuberculosis should be reported to the local health department without delay. Once reported, the health department will undertake an investigation to identify patient contacts to determine who might have active or latent infection and require therapy. These efforts help both the individual patient and the community.[3]

Treatment of Pulmonary Tuberculosis

The preferred antitubercular regimen in susceptible cases consists of an initial 2-month treatment with four drugs (isoniazid, rifampin, pyrazinamide, and either ethambutol or streptomycin) followed by a 4-month phase of isoniazid and rifampin. Total treatment time is typically 6 months.[1-3] If the local prevalence of isoniazid resistance is less than 4%, and the patient is not from an area with a high prevalence of drug resistance, then ethambutol (or streptomycin) may be withheld from the first phase. If cultures show that the organism is fully drug susceptible, then the ethambutol (or streptomycin) may be discontinued.[1-3]

Prior to the initiation of therapy, patients should have sufficient material obtained for culture to particularly ensure that susceptibility testing can be undertaken. In addition, baseline laboratory studies should be performed, including measurement of liver-associated enzymes, total bilirubin, and a complete blood cell count. All patients diagnosed with tuberculosis should be offered HIV testing.[8] If treatment with pyranzinamide is considered, a baseline uric acid level should be obtained, and if ethambutol is to be used, both visual acuity and color perception should be evaluated.

A number of different options are available for the treatment of tuberculosis, and these are listed in Table 1.

Directly Observed Therapy

Studies have shown that clinicians are unable to predict patient compliance.[9] Patient compliance is one of the key factors in treatment success and in the prevention of drug resistance. Directly observed therapy implies that a health care provider is present when the patient takes the medications. Although labor intensive, directly observed therapy is effective, especially when intermittent dosing regimens are chosen (see Table 1). It may take place in an office or clinic setting, or may consist of outreach workers who travel to the patient's residence. If the patient remains noncompliant with therapy, the local health department should be contacted to mobilize additional resources.

HIV Infection

Treatment of tuberculosis in the HIV-infected patient is complicated by drug interactions, particularly for patients on antiretroviral therapy. The administration of rifampin with certain protease inhibitors and non-nucleoside reverse transcriptase inhibitors can cause elevations in levels of rifampin, and subtherapeutic levels of the antiretroviral agents. One should not discontinue antiretroviral therapy so that rifampin can be used to treat tuberculosis.[1,3] Instead, rifabutin can be substituted for rifampin and used in combination with the protease inhibitors indinavir or nelfi-

TABLE 1. Dosing of Drugs Commonly Used for Tuberculosis		
Drug	Daily Dose (maximum)	Twice Weekly Dose (maximum)
Isoniazid	Children: 10 mg/kg (300 mg) Adults: 300 mg (300 mg)	Children: 20–70 mg/kg (900 mg) Adults: 15 mg/kg (900 mg)
Rifampin	Children: 10–20 mg/kg (600 mg) Adults: 600 mg (600 mg)	Children: 10–20 mg/kg (600 mg) Adults: 600 mg (600 mg)
Pyrazinamide	Children: 20–30 mg/kg Adults: <50 kg, 1.5 g 51–74 kg, 2.0 g >75 kg, 2.5 g	Children: 40–50 mg/kg Adults: <50 kg, 1.5 g 51–74 kg, 2.0 g >75 kg, 2.5 g
Ethambutol	Children and adults: 15–25 mg/kg (2.6 g)	Children: 30–50 mg/kg Adults: 50 mg/kg
Streptomycin	Children: 20–30 mg/kg Adults: 15 mg/kg	Not Recommended

Adapted from Small PM, Fujiwara PI: Management of tuberculosis in the United States. N Engl J Med 345:189–200, 2001.

navir as well as most available non-nucleoside reverse transcriptase inhibitors.[10] Rifabutin should not be used with the protease inhibitor ritonavir or the non-nucleoside reverse transcriptase inhibitor delavirdine.[2] If a regimen that does not contain rifabutin or rifampin is desired, a regimen consisting of isoniazid, pyrazinamide, and streptomycin for 9 months, with ethambutol added for the first 2 months, is recommended.[3] Given the complexities of antiretroviral therapy and the potential for drug interactions, patients with HIV infection and tuberculosis should be referred to clinicians who are experienced in the treatment of both infections.

Pregnancy

Pregnant women diagnosed with tuberculosis should be treated promptly. The preferred initial regimen is isoniazid, rifampin, and ethambutol.[3] Streptomycin should not be used because of known teratogenic effects. The safety of pyrazinamide in pregnancy is unknown, and this drug should be avoided.[3] Once the organism is known to be susceptible, ethambutol can be discontinued. The duration of treatment with regimens without pyranzinamide is typically 9 months.[3]

Treatment of Extrapulmonary Tuberculosis

The treatment of extrapulmonary tuberculosis is similar to that of pulmonary tuberculosis with certain exceptions. For meningitis, miliary tuberculosis, and bone or joint involvement, the duration of treatment should be lengthened to 12 months, with the additional months occurring during the two-drug phase.[11]

Drug-Resistant Tuberculosis

Drug-resistant tuberculosis represents a special concern. Treatment of multidrug-resistant tuberculosis is particularly challenging, and therapy needs to be altered depending on the drug resistance profile. Tuberculosis resistant to isoniazid can be treated with rifampin, pyrazinamide, and ethambutol for 6 months.[2,3] Isolated rifampin resistance can be treated with isoniazid and ethambutol for 18 months or isoniazid, pyrazinamide, and streptomycin for 9 months.[2,3]

Many second-line medications are available for the treatment of multidrug-resistant tuberculosis. These treatment regimens are complex, and therapy must be based on the resistance profile and factors related to the patient. Care of the patient with multidrug-resistant tuberculosis should be undertaken only with the assistance of a clinician who is experienced in treating such patients.[12]

Monitoring and Follow-Up Care

Patients with tuberculosis should be followed monthly to monitor possible complications of therapy, compliance, and success of treatment. Sputum should be sent at monthly intervals until mycobacterial smears become negative. Patients with multidrug-resistant tuberculosis should have sputum sent monthly for the duration of their treatment regimen.[3] Patients should be counseled regarding the signs and symptoms of adverse drug reactions and should be specifically alerted to the signs and symptoms of hepatitis, such as nausea, vomiting, jaundice, malaise, or persistent fevers.[3] Patients should be instructed to stop medications and seek medical attention if these symptoms do occur.[3] If the patient has abnormal baseline values, has signs or symptoms of hepatitis, or is at increased risked of adverse drug reaction, then monitoring of liver-associated enzymes is warranted.

Besides hepatotoxicity, there are other common adverse reactions associated with specific antitubercular agents. Peripheral neuropathy is a known complication of therapy with isoniazid, but it rarely occurs in doses used to treat tuberculosis. Patients should be given pyridoxine to prevent the development of peripheral neuropathy.[3] Rifampin and, to a lesser extent, rifabutin can induce activity of the cytochrome P-450 enzyme and are associated with a number of drug–drug interactions. The interaction with protease inhibitors and non-nucleoside reverse transcriptase inhibitors has been previously discussed. In addition, rifampin and rifabutin may increase the metabolism of many drugs, including coumadin, digoxin, oral hypoglycemic agents, corticosteriods, anticonvulsants, antifungal agents, and oral contraceptives.[3] Care must be taken with these medications to ensure proper dosing. Pyrazinamide may cause hyperuricemia. Acute gout is uncommon, and an asymptomatic elevation of uric acid level does not necessitate discontinuation of therapy. Streptomycin can cause ototoxity or nephrotoxicity. Patients should be monitored for these events and should be counseled to discontinue the medication if vertigo or hearing loss is noted. Ethambutol has been associated with optic neuritis, which may be unilateral. Baseline and monthly testing of visual acuity and color vision is recommended.

Treatment Failure

Patient noncompliance and the development of drug resistance are the two most common reasons for failure of an appropriate tuberculosis regimen. If a patient continues to have positive results of mycobacterial smears or cultures at 3 months, an investigation into the cause of the treatment failure should be undertaken. It is often very difficult to evaluate patient compliance, and if a patient is self-administering medications, a switch to directly observed therapy should be made. To evaluate for drug resistance, repeat cultures with drug susceptibilities should be undertaken. If the possibility of drug resistance is suspected, adding two or more agents (to which the organism is likely to be susceptible) is recommended. A single drug should never be added to a failing regimen. If second-line agents are required, three or more drugs should be added to the treatment regimen.

Inappropriate initial regimens, inadequate dosing, and adding a single drug to a failing regimen have all been associated with treatment failure, the development of drug resistance, and poor patient outcomes.[14] This has been shown to occur more frequently when the patient is treated by a private physician, who typically have less experience in treating tuberculosis, then by public clinics that are more experienced in the management of tuberculosis.

Key Points: Management of Pulmonary Tuberculosis

- Tuberculosis is a complex disease that typically manifests as a pulmonary disease, but can occur with many other clinical syndromes in the presence or absence of pulmonary disease.
- HIV can complicate the clinical presentation, disease course, and management of tuberculosis.
- Excellent medical regimens exist for the treatment of tuberculosis.
- If treatment regimens are used properly, patients typically have a good response, but if used improperly, the potential for harm is enormous.

References

1. American Thoracic Society: Diagnostic standards and classification of tuberculosis in adults and children. Am J Respir Crit Care Med 161:1376–1395, 2000.
2. Small PM, Fujiwara PI: Management of tuberculosis in the United States. N Engl J Med 345:189–200, 2001.
3. United States Department of Health and Human Service, Centers for Disease Control and Prevention: Core Curriculum on Tuberculosis, 4th ed. CDC, 2000.
4. Marciniuk DD, McNab BD, Martin WT, Hoeppner VH: Detection of pulmonary tuberculosis in patients with a normal chest radiograph. Chest 115:445–452, 1999.
5. Greenberg SD, Frager D, Suster B, et al: Active pulmonary tuberculosis in patients with AIDS: Spectrum of radiographic findings (including a normal appearance). Radiology 193:115–119, 1994.
6. Neiderman MS, Sarosi GA: Respiratory tract infections. Chest Medicine 4th ed. Philadelphia, Lippincott Williams & Wilkins, 409–414, 2000.
7. Schluger NW: Changing approaches to the diagnosis of tuberculosis. Am J Respir Crit Care Med 164:2020–2024, 2001.

8. Horsburgh CR Jr, Feldman S, Ridzon R: Practice guidelines for the treatment of tuberculosis. Clin Infect Dis 31:633–639, 2000.
9. Mushlin AI, Appel FA: Diagnosing potential noncompliance. Arch Intern Med 137:318–321, 1977.
10. Havlir DV, Barnes PF: Tuberculosis in patients with human deficiency virus infection. N Engl J Med 340:367–373, 1999.
11. Bass JB, Farer LS, Hopewell PC, et al: Treatment of tuberculosis and tuberculosis infection in adults and children. Am J Respir Crit Care Med 149:1359–1374, 1994.
12. Iseman MD: Treatment of multidrug-resistant tuberculosis. N Engl J Med 329:784–791, 1993.
13. American Thoracic Society: Update: Fatal and severe liver injuries associated with rifampin and pyrazinamide for latent tuberculosis infection, and revisions in American Thoracic Society/CDC recommendations. MMWR Morbid Mortal Wkly Rep 50:733–735, 2001.
14. Rao SN, Mookerjee AL, Obasanjo OO, Chaisson RE: Errors in the treatment of tuberculosis in Baltimore. Chest 117:734–737, 2000.

Acute Infectious Diarrheal Diseases

Leanne Beers, M.D.

chapter

11

Worldwide, acute infectious diarrhea is the second leading cause of morbidity and mortality and is one of the most common diagnoses in outpatient practice in the United States. An overwhelming majority of the 3 to 5 billion episodes of diarrhea and more than 3 millions deaths per year occur in developing countries.[1] In the developed world, more than 350,000 episodes of diarrhea require hospital admission, incurring nearly $800,000 in medical costs and lost productivity each year.[2] Many more patients visit outpatient practices or do not seek medical attention at all. The prevalence of acute diarrheal illness is estimated at 1 to 1.5 episodes per person per year, and although most cases are self-limited, the severity of illness can vary markedly depending on characteristics of both the pathogen and the host.[3] Management of each episode, therefore, varies based on cause, severity of illness, the host, and the host's comorbid illnesses.

Prompt recognition, diagnosis, and treatment of infectious diarrhea may have public health implications. The primary care physician is instrumental in early control of local outbreaks as well as in preventing secondary transmission, most importantly in health care workers, day care workers, and food handlers. Stool testing for diagnosis of specific pathogens can abbreviate illness, reduce morbidity, decrease development of antimicrobial resistance through pathogen-directed treatment, and help identify and trace public health outbreaks. However, because the vast majority of patients with acute diarrhea have a self-limited illness that requires only supportive therapy, laboratory testing and antimicrobial treatment in such cases can be fruitless and costly. Additionally, inappropriate treatment can be detrimental through promotion of antimicrobial resistance and, in some cases, prolonged infectivity. Only 1.5% to 5.8% of all submitted stool cultures are positive, making the cost per positive test around $1000.[2,4] Pursuit of a microbiologic diagnosis, therefore, must be initiated on a case-by-case basis. This chapter discusses the major etiologic agents of acute infectious diarrhea, presents an overall diagnostic approach, and reviews the current treatment strategies for the primary care physician.

Definitions

Historically, diarrhea has been defined as more than 200 grams of stool per day, but practically, this definition is limiting. The Infectious Disease Society of America defines diarrhea as "an alteration in a normal bowel movement characterized by an increase in the water content, volume, or frequency of stools."[4] The American College of Gastroenterology's definition of acute diarrhea is "the passage of a greater number of stools of decreased form from the normal lasting less than 14 days."[3] It is generally accepted that an increase in frequency to three or more loose stools per day for less than 14 days constitutes an acute diarrheal episode. Episodes lasting longer than 30 days qualify as "chronic diarrhea" and are more rarely associated with infectious causes.[3,4]

Pathophysiology

Enteropathogens gain access to the intestinal tract via oral contamination and cause diarrhea by disrupting intestinal and colonic mucosa through a variety of mechanisms. Bacteria such as *Staphylococcus aureus, Bacillus cereus,* and *Clostridium botulinum* release enterotoxins, which invoke intestinal secretion. Other pathogens, such as *Shigella* and enteroinvasive *Escherichia coli,* express invasins, which allow tissue invasion and disruption of mucosa. Many other bacteria elicit cytotoxic mediators that directly damage enteric and colonic mucosa.[2] Enteropathogenic mechanisms of disease, therefore, are the basis for the two common clinical syndromes: inflammatory and noninflammatory diarrhea (Table 1).

Inflammatory diarrheal syndromes often manifest clinically as dysentery, characterized by fever, tenesmus, abdominal pain, and frequent, small-volume stools that are often bloody. Organisms such as *Shigella, Campylobacter jejuni,* and enteroinvasive *E. coli* produce an inflammatory reaction that yields fecal leukocytes and blood on laboratory examination of stool. Patients with an inflammatory acute diarrheal illness can be quite toxic appearing and often require antibiotic treatment.

Conversely, noninflammatory diarrheal syndromes are usually self-limited and more often do not require antimicrobial therapy.[5] Enteropathogens such as *Vibrio parahaemolyticus, Cryptosporidium parvum,* and *Giardia lamblia* as well as viral agents and toxin-producing bacteria, such as *Staphylococcus aureus, Clostridium difficile,* and enterotoxigenic *E. coli,* typically induce watery, non-bloody diarrhea without fever or significant abdominal pain. Stool examination is notable for the

TABLE 1.	Inflammatory Versus Noninflammatory Diarrhea	
	Inflammatory	Noninflammatory
Key characteristics	Small, frequent stools	Voluminous stools: >1 L/day
	Bloody/mucoid stools	Watery stool
	Fever	Absence of fever
	Abdominal pain	Absence of severe abdominal pain
	Stool leukocytes or lactoferrin	Minimal/no stool leukocytes
Likely pathogens	**Bacteria**	**Bacteria**
	Salmonella species	Vibrio species
	Shigella species	Staphyloccoccus aureus
	Campylobacter jejuni	
	Escherichia coli	**Viruses**
	(enterohemorrhagic,	Rotavirus
	interoinvasive)	Norwalk
	Clostridium difficile	
	Yersinia enterocolitica	**Parasites**
		Giardia lamblia
	Parasites	Cryptosporidium parvum
	Entamoeba histolytica	
Antimicrobial therapy	More likely	Less likely

absence of leukocytes and blood.[6] Typically, more than 1 L of watery stool is passed each day, and volume depletion may be profound.

Common Pathogens

A summary of several medically important causes of acute infectious diarrhea is presented here. Table 2 presents a summary of the characteristics of the common stool pathogens and various clinical syndromes.

Salmonella. *Salmonella typhi* and *Salmonella paratyphi* most commonly cause typhoid, or enteric fever, in which an acute febrile illness is preceded by ingestion of the organism and a short course of diarrhea, which resolves before the onset of fever. Nontyphoidal *Salmonella,* however, is the most common cause of foodborne diarrhea in the United States, transmitted via contaminated meats, poultry, eggs, and dairy products.[7] Food handlers can be reservoirs. Rarely, outbreaks are water-borne or from pet reptiles, which are frequently carriers.[8] Patients with nontyphoidal illness often present with nausea, vomiting, and diarrhea 6 to 48 hours after ingestion of contaminated food. Abdominal pain and fever are common, but bloody stools occur less frequently. Stool examination reveals leukocytes, and routine cultures will be positive in 58% of cases.[8]

Most cases of gastroenteritis resolve without treatment in 3 to 7 days.

TABLE 2. Selected Etiologic Agents of Acute Infectious Diarrhea

Pathogen or Syndrome	History	Symptoms	Laboratory Diagnosis*	Treatment	Other
Dysentary	Varies	Fever, bloody stools, abdominal pain	+Fecal leukocytes +Blood Routine stool culture	Quinolone × 3–5 days	Empiric treatment while awaiting lab studies
Traveler's diarrhea	Symptoms at destination or days after return	Fever, bloody stools, abdominal pain	+/– Fecal leukocytes +/– Blood Routine stool culture +Ova/parasite studies	Quinolone × 2–5 days	No treatment or lab studies needed if patient is improving
Persistent diarrhea	Diarrhea persisting >2 weeks.	Malabsorption if post infectious or *Giardia*	+/– Fecal leukocytes +/–Blood Routine stool culture +Ova/parasite studies	Quinolone trial	If diarrhea persists, consider noninfectious etiology
Shigella	Travel, institutional, day care, sick contact homosexuals	Mild diarrhea to severe dysentery	+Fecal leukocytes +/– Blood Routine stool culture	Quinolone × 3–5 days TMP/SMX Ampicillin	
Salmonella	Ingestion or handling of poultry, eggs, milk products.	Mild diarrhea to dysentery	+Fecal leukocytes +/– Blood Routine stool culture	TMP/SMX × 5–7 days Quinolone	Therapy usually not required and may prolong fecal shed.
Campylobacter	Ingestion or handling of contaminated poultry	Fever, abdominal pain, watery or bloody diarrhea	+Fecal leukocytes +Blood Routine stool culture	Erythromycin × 5 days Quinolone × 5 days	Therapy usually not required Quinolone resistance reported
Enterotoxigenic *Escherichia coli*	Consumption of water, fruit, vegetables in travel	Cramps, explosive watery or bloody diarrhea	–Fecal leukocytes +/–Blood	Quinolone × 2–5 days	Enterotoxin mediated Therapy not required if resolving or mild

Organism	Source	Clinical	Diagnosis	Therapy	Comments
Enterohemorrhagic Escherichia coli (O157:H7)	Contaminated meat, petting zoo	Bloody stools, abdominal pain, rarely fever	+Fecal leukocytes +/- Blood Requires O157:H7 culture		Therapy associated with increased risk of complications
Enteropathogenic Escherichia coli	Pediatrics, day care centers, nurseries	Watery diarrhea	-Fecal leukocytes -Blood	TMP/SMX × 5 day	Indistinguishable from viral syndrome
Enteroinvasive Escherichia coli	Rare in the United States	Dysentery or watery diarrhea	+Fecal leukocytes	TMP/SMX if in USA Quinolone if traveler	Resistance is common Therapy not required if mild
Yersinia enterocolitica	Pediatrics, raw milk, contaminated fresh water. Fall, winter	Mild diarrhea/dysentery; right lower quadrant pain	+Fecal leukocytes Requires Yersinia culture	Quinolone × 7–10 days TMP/SMX Doxycycline	Therapy not shown to alter course but may decrease spread
Vibrio species	Raw shellfish, cirrhotics at risk	Severe, profuse watery diarrhea	+Fecal leukocytes if V. parahemolyticus -Fecal leukocytes if V. cholera Requires Vibrio culture	No therapy for V. parahaemolyticus Consider quinolone or doxycycline for V. cholera-	Toxin-mediated
Aeromonas	Late summer, fall. Private well water, shellfish. Young children.	Usually self-limited Rarely prolonged	+/- Fecal leukocytes +/- Blood Routine stool culture	TMP/SMX × 5 days Quinolone	Treat if immune suppressed or symptoms last >7 days
Plesiomonas	Water, seafood (oysters), chickens, tropical travel	Abdominal pain Usually self-limited Rarely prolonged.	+/- Fecal leukocytes +/- Blood	TMP/SMX × 5 days Quinolone	Treat severe cases only Risk of sepsis in asplenic patients

(continued)

TABLE 2. Selected Etiologic Agents of Acute Infectious Diarrhea (*Continued*)

Pathogen or Syndrome	History	Symptoms	Laboratory Diagnosis*	Treatment	Other
Clostridium difficile	Exposure to antibiotics	Crampy abdominal pain, fever, diarrhea	+Fecal leukocytes +/− Blood Requires cytotoxin assay for toxin A/B	Metronidazole × 10 days or Vancomycin (oral)	Stop antibiotic therapy Requires contact isolation
Staphylococcus aureus	Eggs, mayonnaise 1–6 hour incubation	Vomiting, cramps, watery diarrhea	−Fecal leukocytes −Blood	No treatment	Toxin-mediated
Bacillus cereus	Fried rice, 8–16 hr incubation	Vomiting, cramps, diarrhea	−Fecal leukocytes −Blood	No treatment	Toxin-mediated
Viruses	Person-to-person contact	Nausea, vomiting, watery diarrhea	−Fecal leukocytes −Blood	No treatment	Requires viral identification for diagnosis
Giardia lamblia	Camping, travel to mountains	Short or prolonged diarrhea, flatus, malabsorption,	−Fecal leukocytes +Ova/parasite studies +Enzyme immunoassay	Metronidazole 250 mg orally 4 times daily × 7 days	May be difficult to eradicate
Cryptosporidium parvum	HIV, day care, water-borne outbreaks	Watery diarrhea, weight loss, wasting, abdominal pain	−Fecal leukocytes −Blood +Ova/parasite studies +Enzyme immunoassay	Paromomycin	Antiretroviral therapy is beneficial for patients with HIV/AIDS

* Laboratory Diagnosis: +, usually present; +/−, may or may not be present; −, usually absent
TMP/SMX, trimethoprim-sulfamethoxazole 160/800 mg (DS tab) PO bid.
Quinolone, Norfloxacin 400 mg orally twice daily ofloxacin 400 mg orally twice daily, ciprofloxacin 500 mg orally twice daily, levofloxacin 500 mg orally once daily.

Symptoms of colitis may persist for several weeks. Treatment can prolong the fecal excretion of organisms and should be avoided in mild cases.[1,8] Antibiotics should be given to patients with severe symptoms, at extremes of age, with immunosuppression, with cardiovascular disease, or with a prosthesis, as the organism has a propensity to infect vascular aneurysms and prosthetic joints. Carriage of nontyphoidal salmonella can persist for 4 to 5 weeks after resolution of diarrhea. Fluoroquinolones, ampicillin, and trimethoprim-sulfamethoxazole are acceptable agents to treat *Salmonella* infection. Length of treatment is usually 1 week, but if the patient is bacteremic or focally infected, longer courses are necessary.[8]

Shigella. *Shigella* species require an inoculum of only 10 to 100 organisms and thus is highly communicable. Outbreaks have been traced to food and water, but most infections are transmitted person-to-person. *Shigella* is, therefore, a major pathogen in day care centers and nursing homes. Variable in its morbidity, *Shigella* produces Shiga toxin, which causes fever, malaise, cramping, tenesmus, and voluminous diarrhea that is initially watery and often becomes bloody. Because most cases are self-limited and resistance is increasing, antimicrobial therapy may not be indicated, especially if the patient is improving at presentation. But, in cases of moderate to severe illness, patients at the extremes of age, and patients with comorbid illness, antibiotic therapy should not be withheld because it may decrease symptoms and shorten fecal excretion.[8] Trimethoprim-sulfamethoxazole, ampicilline, tetracyclines, and fluoroquinolones are acceptable agents, but resistance is becoming more common.

Escherichia coli. There are five types of *E. coli*. Enterotoxogenic *E. coli* (ETEC) is the most frequent cause of diarrhea in travelers returning to the United States. By means of an enterotoxin that stimulates massive fluid secretion, patients present with cramping and explosive watery as well as bloody diarrhea that yields low-level or negative fecal leukocytes on stool testing. Because an overwhelming majority of cases of traveler's diarrhea are due to ETEC, empiric treatment with a fluoroquinolone without bacteriologic identification of a causative organism is appropriate. Enteropathogenic *E. coli* is a frequent cause of childhood diarrhea and causes watery diarrhea that is usually indistinguishable from viral infection. Enteroinvasive *E. coli,* which is rare in the United States, occasionally causes a dysentery-like syndrome with destruction and severe inflammation of the bowel mucosa and bloody diarrhea. More typically, the diarrhea is watery and self-limited, not requiring treatment. Enterohemorrhagic *E. coli* usually causes a hemorrhagic colitis without fever or significant inflammation and is associated with hemolytic uremic syndrome (HUS) and thrombocytopenic thrombotic purpura, particularly in pediatric patients. Serotype 0157:H7 is the most well known subtype. The organism is found in undercooked ground beef, and outbreaks have been linked to fast food chains, farms, and petting zoos. It is not identified with routine stool culture media; special cultures can identify the 0157:H7 subtype only. Treatment is not recommended because antibiotics do not appear helpful and may increase the incidence of complications such as HUS.[1,3,4,8]

Campylobacter. Most cases of inflammatory diarrhea in the United States are caused by *Campylobacter jejuni* and are acquired through ingestion of contaminated poultry. Stool samples are positive for leukocytes and blood in 75% and 50% of samples, respectively.[8] If started promptly, antibiotics may shorten the course of illness, which can persist for 1 to several weeks without treatment. Erythromycin, clindamycin, and ciprofloxacin have been used, but fluoroquinolone resistance is becoming prevalent.

Clostridium difficile. *C. difficile* colitis (pseudomembranous colitis) accounts for 10% to 20% of cases of antibiotic-associated diarrhea and the majority of cases of antibiotic-associated colitis.[9] Complications include toxic megacolon, hypoalbuminemia, prolonged hospital stays, and increased costs. Antibiotic usage disrupts bowel flora, permitting the proliferation of *C. difficile,* which elicits a toxin and causes colitis and inflammatory diarrhea. The most common antibiotics implicated are clindamycin (highest incidence), cephalosporins (highest in number of cases), and extended-spectrum penicillins.[9] However, any antibiotic has the potential to induce disease regardless of course length. Hospitalized patients not on antibiotics may acquire disease through person-to-person contact; thus, isolation of infected patients is essential. Diagnosis is made by a cytotoxin assay that identifies either toxin A or toxin B secreted by the bacteria. Assays are very specific but have a 5% to 10% false-negative rate, and two stool samples should be sent to maximize sensitivity. Available assays detect toxin A or both toxin A and B. One to 2% of *C. difficile* organisms produce only toxin B, and thus, the latter test may be needed to identify infection in some patients. Metronidazole or oral vancomycin for 10 days is ideal treatment, although relapses occur and can be problematic.[9]

Sexually Transmitted Diseases. *Chlamydia trachomatis, Neiserria gonorrhoeae, Treponema pallidum,* and herpes simplex virus can produce proctitis and proctocolitis in men and women either via anal intercourse or via autoinoculation from infected vaginal secretions.[8] Constipation may alternate with diarrheal episodes, and rectal pain, irritation, fullness, and bleeding are often predominant complaints. Special cultures or endoscopy may be required for diagnosis.

Viruses. Viral infection by rotaviruses, Norwalk agent, adenovirus, and astroviruses are easily spread and frequent causes of diarrhea in children. Most cases are waterborne or foodborne, and after an incubation period of more than 12 hours, symptoms of nausea, vomiting, and watery diarrhea predominate. Bouts are self-limited, and treatment should include antidiarrheals and rehydration. **Parasites.** *Giardia lamblia, Entamoeba histolytica, Cryptosporidium,* and *Cyclospora* are the most common parasites causing diarrhea in travelers, patients with acquired immunodeficiency syndrome (AIDS), and people in day care centers. Persistent diarrhea lasting longer than 2 weeks and travel to underdeveloped or mountainous regions should prompt evaluation for parasites in the appropriate patient.[3] *Giardia* infection may be self-limited or chronic and is diagnosed by microscopic visualization, direct immmunofluorescence, or, more commonly, enzyme-linked immunosorbent assay (ELISA). Empiric treatment may be justified in patients with persistent diarrhea without further testing.[3] Preferred treatment is metronidazole or albendazole. *Cryptosporidium parvum* is transmitted fecal-orally, through contact with farm animals, food, or water, and is resistant to chlorination. Diagnosis is made by identification of oocysts in fresh stool or by ELISA. Patients with human immunodeficiency virus (HIV) infection whose CD_4 count is less than 200 are at increased risk for chronic infection, severe dehydration, wasting, and death.[10] In immunocompetent individuals, the disease is self-limited. Trials are currently underway to find an appropriate treatment. *E. histolytica* can cause a variety of illnesses, including bloody diarrhea, ulcerative colitis, and metastasis with liver abscesses and involvement of lungs, heart, and brain. Identification of cysts or trophozoites or positive ELISA findings should prompt treatment with metronidazole followed by diloxanide or paromomycin—the latter two agents for prevention of systemic invasion by remaining cysts.[10]

Diagnostic Approach

History

A complete and thorough history is essential in the initial evaluation of a patient with acute diarrhea. The physician should elicit a detailed description of the diarrheal syndrome, including length of symptoms, quantity and quality of stool, presence of fever, and abdominal symptoms. The history should address recent travel to underdeveloped countries, potential exposures to raw or undercooked food, sick contacts, contact with children, and employment in health care facilities. A sexual history may elicit risk factors for herpes simplex, *Chlamydia, Neisseria gonorrhoeae,* or *Treponema pallidum* proctitis.

Establishing the immune status of the host is essential. Patients with immune deficiencies due to organ transplant, HIV, and certain drugs (particularly steroids, chemotherapeutic agents, and immunosuppressants) can be more susceptible to less typical gastrointestinal pathogens. Such patients may also exhibit more severe symptoms and experience a more fulminant course, lowering the threshold for antimicrobial therapy and hospitalization.

Recent hospitalization or antimicrobial therapy increases the likelihood of *C. difficile* infection or antibiotic-associated diarrhea. Other medications may cause diarrhea or other adverse gastrointestinal effects.

Patients presenting with diarrhea after international travel often are infected with bacteria or parasites, most frequently enterotoxigenic *E. coli*. Recent camping, travel to mountainous areas, or a prolonged diarrheal illness lasting more than 14 days suggests *Giardia* infection.[3]

Physical Examination

Physical examination should concentrate on assessment of volume status with particular attention to heart rate, blood pressure, and mental status, especially in the very young and elderly. A directed examination of the abdomen may qualify the illness, but sensitivity and specificity for agents of infectious diarrhea is extremely low. A rectal examination may reveal hemoccult or grossly positive blood or mucus and may elicit tenderness, indicating proctitis.

Laboratory Studies

Because most diarrheal illnesses are self-limited and mild, physicians must use their clinical judgment to determine whether diagnostic testing will be helpful in managing each patient. Laboratory testing may include fecal leukocytes, lactoferrin, routine stool culture, toxin assays, ova and parasites, and specific bacterial cultures or studies, depending on the suspected cause of diarrhea. Laboratory testing should be considered in the following situations[3]:

- Inflammatory diarrhea (bloody stools, fever)
- Persistent symptoms for more than 3 days
- Recent travel
- Immunosuppressed host
- Nosocomial diarrhea
- Potential community outbreak
- Potential foodborne outbreak

Fecal Leukocytes and Lactoferrin. Microscopic identification of fecal leukocytes or a positive immunoassay for the neutrophil marker lactoferrin can confirm a suspected inflammatory origin.[3] One study found that fecal leukocytes were absent in all cases of viral diarrhea and present in 89% of cases of bacterial diarrhea.[2] Negative results would justify watchful waiting in place of further diagnostic testing that is likely to be unhelpful. Because stool cultures may take several days to grow, stool positive for leukocytes or lactoferrin justifies the use of empiric antibiotics in patients with infectious diarrhea.[3,4] Physicians should keep in mind that stool tested in cases of diarrhea due to toxin-mediated disease will usually be negative, and suspected cases need a specialized approach. Certain situations mandate that empiric antibiotics be used despite negative fecal leukocytes and lactoferrin, as in traveler's diarrhea caused by enterotoxogenic *E. coli*.[3,4] Lactoferrin may be a more sensitive test, but fresh stool (less than 24 hours old) will increase the sensitivity of fecal leukocytes.[4]

Routine Cultures. Routine stool cultures in most laboratories screen for *Salmonella, Shigella, Campylobacter,* and, usually, *Aeromonas* and *Plesiomonas.* Most other bacteria can either be cultured by special requests (*Yersinia, Vibrio*) or are identified only in research laboratories. The Centers for Disease Control and Prevention recommend special testing for *E. coli* 0157:H7 in all patients with acute bloody diarrhea or HUS because of public health implications. Other types of enterohemorrhagic *E. coli* cannot be readily cultured; however, toxin can be detected in stool samples. Routine bacterial stool cultures should not be requested for patients who develop diarrhea after 3 days of hospitalization because studies have shown an extremely low yield.[6] These patients should have stool evaluated for *Clostridium difficile* toxin with up to three stool specimens for maximal sensitivity.

Ova and Parasites. Microscopy by trained microbiologists can identify a parasitic origin, and specific immunoflorescent testing is available for *Giardia* and *Cryptosporidium.* Testing should be reserved for patients with a longer duration of diarrhea, recent travel to mountainous regions, exposure to infants, and AIDS, and in patients with dysentery who have few fecal leukocytes on fecal examination.[2]

Selected Hosts

Immunosuppressed Patients. Infection with HIV and other immunocompromised states such as receiving chemotherapy, steroids, or other immunsuppressive agents usually necessitate empiric antimicrobials for all bacterial causes of diarrhea, as these patients are at increased risk for certain infections and may exhibit more severe illness. Alcoholics and patients with cirrhosis should avoid raw shellfish because of increased risk for severe infections due to *Vibrio* species. *Listeria monocytogenes* may be found in soft cheeses, cold deli meats, and raw dairy products. Infection is fecal-oral, and bacteremia or meningitis is often preceded by enteritis. All immunocompromised patients and pregnant women should avoid such foods.

Travelers. Travelers to underdeveloped countries are exposed to a variety of novel bacteria and parasites and are often subject to poor food and water handling. The likelihood of acquiring diarrhea in certain geographic areas is as high as 50%.[5] The most common pathogen is ETEC, but other bacteria and parasites cause disease as well. Strategies for prevention include avoidance of water, fresh fruits, and vegetables. The use of antimicrobial prophylaxis is usually not recommended, except in patients with at-risk comorbidities, but may be considered in travelers to high-risk areas who have underlying illnesses or those in whom diarrhea would prove problematic (short trips for important business, politicians, honeymooners). If preventive medicine is requested by the traveler, bismuth subsalicylate (2 tablets with meals and before bed) is 62% effective in eliminating diarrhea.[3]

The Hospitalized Patient. Routine stool samples for culture as well as ova and parasite studies in hospitalized patients who develop diarrhea after their third day of admission are rarely positive and are not cost effective. Stool should be sent for *C. difficile* toxin assay, and if found negative, noninfectious causes such as medication and enteric feeding should be considered.

Treatment

Treatment options for patients with acute infectious diarrhea include supportive care (hydration, antimotility agents) and antimicrobial agents (empiric and agent specific). In all cases, the physician should encourage aggressive oral hydration to prevent dehydration and recognize the need for intravenous fluid replacement. Oral rehydration solutions are available over the counter, or home remedies may be used. Patients should consume glucose-containing electrolyte solutions and avoid hyperosmolar fluids, which can exacerbate symptoms and fluid loss. Milk and lactose-containing products and caffeine can exacerbate diarrhea and should be avoided.[5]

Antidiarrheal agents such as opiates (loperamide), which slow intestinal transit time, and adsorbant agents (Kaopectate) may provide symptomatic relief. Use of agents that decrease intestinal transit time in infectious diarrhea is controversial, but concerns about the slow clearance of pathogens have not been supported.[11] Bismuth subsalicylate has direct antidiarrheal and antibacterial effects and is generally safe.

The use of empiric antibiotics is appropriate while awaiting bacteriologic identification in patients in whom inflammatory diarrhea is likely and are slow to improve, in returning travelers, when diarrhea persists for more than 2 weeks, and when *Giardia* is suspected.[3,4] Because many bacterial causes of diarrhea vary in clinical course and degree of morbidity, a decision to treat should be influenced greatly by the patients' comorbidities, immune state, and clinical appearance, calling for clinical judgment on the part of the physician after a complete history and physical evaluation. Specific recommendations for antibiotic treatment have been addressed here as well as in Table 2. In general, the vast majority of cases of infectious diarrhea do not require antimicrobial therapy because there is no effective agent for the organism or because the illness is mild and self-limited (or both). Patients who are improving and have mild illness need no chemotherapeutic intervention. Severe illness, dysentery, persistent symptoms, or immunosuppression mandate an attempt to identify an enteropathogen to provide specific and appropriate treatment. Particular attention should be given to resistance patterns within the community, and antibiotics should be chosen accordingly. Finally, knowledge of the potential for antibiotics to increase complication rates (HUS in EHEC) and prolong shedding and infectivity (*Salmonella*) is essential when debating the pros and cons of antimicrobial therapy.

Key Points: Acute Infectious Diarrheal Diseases

- ⟳ Acute infectious diarrhea is a common complaint in the outpatient practice.
- ⟳ Most cases of diarrhea are mild and self-limited, but severe and life-threatening illness can occur with certain pathogens and in certain demographic groups, most notably the immunosuppressed, the very old, and the very young.
- ⟳ A detailed history may elicit clues to identify potential causative agents, and the decision to pursue laboratory testing, prescribe empiric antibiotics, or manage conservatively depends on both the suspected enteropathogen and the host.
- ⟳ Because most death from diarrhea is secondary to dehydration, physicians must counsel patients to be diligent with oral replacement therapy and recognize individuals who are not maintaining adequate hydration so that intravenous therapy can be initiated.
- ⟳ Physicians should encourage frequent hand washing to prevent the spread of disease, especially among day care workers, employees of nursing homes, and food handlers, who may need to abstain from their activities.
- ⟳ When diarrhea persists and diagnostic testing fails to identify a pathogen, noninfectious or extraintestinal causes of diarrhea should be considered, which may prompt further laboratory work, imaging, endoscopy, and referral to a gastroenterologist.

Key Points (*Continued*)

☞ Further research is needed to develop more concrete algorithms for the diagnosis and treatment of acute diarrhea. Primary care physicians must employ a sound knowledge of epidemiologic risk factors, potential etiologic agents, pathophysiology, and at-risk patients to provide cost-effective care to the many patients seen each year with acute infectious diarrhea.

References

1. Oldfield EC, Wallace MR: The role of antibiotics in the treatment of infectious diarrhea. Gastroenterol Clin North Am 30:817–836, 2001.
2. Ilnychkyj A: Clinical evaluation and management of acute infectious diarrhea in adults. Gastroenterol Clin 30:599–609, 2001.
3. DuPont HL: Guidelines on acute infectious diarrhea in adults. Am J Gastroenterol 92:1962–1975, 1997.
4. Guerrant RL, Van Gilder T, Steiner TS, et al: Practice guidelines for the management of infectious diarrhea. Clin Infect Dis X: 331–350, 2001.
5. Aranda-Michel J, Giannella RA: Acute diarrhea: A practical review. Am J Med 106: 670–676, 1999.
6. Hines J, Nachamkin I: Effective use of the clinical microbiology laboratory for diagnosing diarrheal diseases. Clin Infect Dis 23:1292–1301, 1996.
7. Wanke CA: Epidemiology and causes of acute diarrhea. In: UptoDate version 10.3. www.uptodateonline.com. Accessed November 5, 2002.
8. Goldsweig CD, Pacheco PA: Infectious colitis excluding *E. coli* 0157:H7 and *C. difficile*. Gastroenterol Clin 30:709–733, 2001.
9. Bartlett JG: Antibiotic-associated diarrhea. N Engl J Med 346:334–339, 2002.
10. Okhuysen PC: Traveler's diarrhea due to intestinal protozoa. Clin Infect Dis 33: 110–114, 2001.
11. Schiller LR: Advances in gastroenterology: Diarrhea. Med Clin North Am 84:1259–1274, 2000.
12. Powell DW: Approach to the patient with diarrhea. In Yamada T, ed: Textbook of Gastroenterology, 3rd ed. Philadelphia: Lippincott Williams & Wilkins, 1999:858–909.
13. Turgeon DK, Fritsche TR: Laboratory approaches to infectious diarrhea. Gastroenterol Clin 30:693–707, 2001.

Management of Chronic Hepatitis C

Vincent Lo Re III, M.D., and
Jay R. Kostman, M.D.

chapter

12

Infection with the hepatitis C virus (HCV) is one of the leading causes of liver disease in the United States.[1] This disorder was initially recognized in the mid-1970s and was categorized as "non-A, non-B hepatitis."[2] HCV was subsequently identified as an RNA virus in 1989 and was found to account for the majority of cases of non-A, non-B hepatitis.[3] The virus can cause persistent infection in susceptible hosts after parenteral or percutaneous transmission.[4] Progression to chronic disease occurs in the majority of HCV-infected people, and infection is a major cause of cirrhosis, end-stage liver disease, and hepatocellular carcinoma.[1,5] Infection with HCV also accounts for the main indication for liver transplantation.[6]

Chronic HCV is a growing health care concern in the United States. The primary care physician plays a key role in the management of these patients by (1) identifying those chronically infected with HCV, (2) educating such individuals about the nature of the disease (particularly transmission, progression, and interaction with alcohol), and (3) assisting in treatment decisions.[7] To better assist clinicians in this endeavor, this chapter reviews the epidemiology, natural history, and clinical characteristics of HCV infection. The diagnostic evaluation and current treatment modalities are also discussed.

Scope of the Problem

Hepatitis C virus infection is a major public health problem in the United States. An estimated 3.9 million Americans are infected with HCV (1.8% prevalence in the general population), making this the most common bloodborne infection nationally, but most of these people are asymptomatic and do not know that they are infected.[8] Approximately 35,000 new HCV infections occur each year, and 8000 to 10,000 annual deaths result from HCV-associated chronic liver disease. The burden of this infection on the health care system is expected to rise in the near future. Many cases are likely to come to medical attention in the next decade, and a fourfold increase in the number of adults diagnosed with chronic HCV infection is projected from 1990 to 2015.[9]

Risk Factors for HCV Infection

Hepatitis C virus is transmitted primarily through large or repeated percutaneous exposures to blood.[1] During a medical evaluation, it is important to obtain a history of high-risk practices associated with transmission of the virus. Risk factors for HCV infection include the following:

- **Injection and other illegal drug use**—Currently, most new HCV infections are associated with injection drug use, and this accounts for 60% of HCV transmission in the United States.[1,7] Approximately 50% to 60% of these individuals are infected within 3 months of initiation of injection behavior.[7] Even individuals who infrequently used injection drugs in the remote past may be at risk for infection with HCV. Intranasal cocaine use has also been associated with the acquisition of HCV.[10]

- **Transfusion and organ transplantation**—Improved screening of blood and organ donors has made transmission of HCV by transfusion or transplantation rare. The introduction of HCV antibody detection testing in 1992 significantly reduced the risk of disease by these routes. With the implementation of this testing in blood banks, the risk for HCV infection from blood transfusion is now less than 1 in 103,000 transfused units.[11] The residual risk results from blood donations that occur in the period between infection and the development of detectable antibodies.[6]

- **Hemodialysis**—The prevalence of HCV antibody among hemodialysis patients is approximately 10%, and the infection is presumed to have been transmitted by inadequate infection control practices.[1]

- **Health care workers**—The prevalence of HCV infection among health care workers is similar to that in the general population (approximately 2%).[1] Needle-stick injury is the primary risk factor for HCV transmission, and the incidence of seroconversion after such an injury is 3% to 4%.[6,12] Transmission of HCV from blood splash to the conjunctiva has also been reported.[13,14]

- **Sexual activity**—Transmission of HCV does occur through sexual activity, but at low frequency. In the United States, the estimated seroprevalence of HCV is 2% to 3% among partners of HCV-infected individuals who are in long-term monogamous relationships.[9] Thus, monogamous couples do not need to use barrier protection but should be advised that condoms may reduce the risk of HCV transmission. HCV-infected individuals who have multiple sexual partners or who are in short-term relationships should be advised to use condoms to prevent the transmission of HCV (as well as other sexually transmitted disease).

- **Household contact**—HCV transmission by normal household contact is extremely uncommon. There is no evidence that casual contact, such as kissing, hugging, or sharing eating utensils, is associated with HCV transmission. However, sharing household items that may be contaminated with blood, such as razors, toothbrushes, or nail care tools, should be avoided.[1]
- **Tattooing/body piercing**—These activities have been associated with HCV transmission, and contaminated equipment or supplies have been implicated.[15,16]
- **Vertical transmission**—Among infants born to HCV-positive, human immunodeficiency virus (HIV)–negative women, the incidence of HCV infection is 5% to 6%, but the incidence is higher among children born to HCV and HIV coinfected mothers (14–20%).[1,9] Infants born to HCV-positive women should have their blood tested for either HCV RNA at approximately 6 months of age or HCV antibody at 15 months of age (after maternal antibodies have waned).[9] Breastfeeding does not appear to transmit HCV. Current therapeutic modalities for HCV are contraindicated during pregnancy, and no studies have evaluated the use of elective cesarean section for the prevention of mother-to-infant HCV infection.

Natural History and Clinical Features

Acute Infection

The incubation period for HCV infection ranges from 2 weeks to 6 months, with an average incubation period of 6 to 7 weeks.[5,17] Most cases (60–70%) of acute HCV infection produce no discernible symptoms.[17] In approximately 20% to 30% of cases, patients may develop jaundice accompanied by fatigue, anorexia, and abdominal pain.[5,17] Acute HCV infection, however, is rarely fulminant.[18] Elevations in serum alanine aminotransferase (ALT) may be identified and reflect hepatocyte injury. Symptomatic disease usually subsides after several weeks as ALT levels decline.[9] In approximately 15% of cases, acute HCV infection completely resolves, and this appears to be associated with a younger age at infection, female gender, and certain major histocompatibility complex genes.[1,9,17] However, most patients (85%) develop chronic infection, which has been primarily attributed to the propensity of HCV to mutate and evade host defenses.[1,5,6,9,17]

Chronic Infection

Hepatitis C virus infection becomes chronic in the majority of cases, manifested by the persistence of detectable virus in the serum. Chronic infection is usually characterized by a prolonged period in which there are no symptoms or only fatigue. No clinical features of acute disease or risk factors for infection have been found to be predictive of chronicity. Patients are often incidentally found to have elevated ALT levels on "routine" biochemical tests or a positive anti-HCV antibody result at the time of blood donation.[5] Serum ALT levels typically fluctuate over time and may even be normal on occasion.[5] The major complication of chronic HCV infection is progressive hepatic fibrosis leading to cirrhosis, which develops in approximately 15% to 20% of those infected with HCV.[9]

Progression of chronic liver disease is insidious in most patients. The average time from viral acquisition to the development of clinically significant hepatitis, cirrhosis, or hepatocellular carcinoma is 10 to 18 years, 21 years, and 29 years, respectively.[5] Patients with persistently normal levels of serum ALT have a lower risk for fibrotic progression.[7] However, a number of factors can accelerate progression to advanced liver disease, most notably alcohol consumption,[19] coinfection with HIV[20] or hepatitis B virus,[21] and older age at the time of infection.[9] In particular, excessive alcohol use has an additive effect on liver injury and can significantly promote the development of progressive liver disease.[19] Even lower amounts may increase the risk of liver damage associated with HCV. Death from HCV typically occurs because of decompensated cirrhosis but may also be due to hepatocellular carcinoma.

Hepatocellular Carcinoma

Like infection with hepatitis B virus, chronic HCV infection is associated with an increased risk of hepatocellular carcinoma. Hepatocellular carcinoma occurs primarily in the setting of HCV-induced cirrhosis and rarely in patients with chronic HCV infection who do not have cirrhosis.[5] Once cirrhosis is established, the risk of hepatocellular carcinoma is 2% to 5% per year.[22] The risk for development of hepatocellular carcinoma is increased in patients who have chronic hepatitis B or consume alcohol.[5]

Extrahepatic Manifestations

In addition to hepatic disease, there are important extrahepatic manifestations of HCV infection.[23–25] These are primarily associated with autoimmune or lymphoproliferative states. HCV is the main cause of essential mixed cryoglobulinemia (type II cryoglobulinemia), with up to 90% of affected individuals having HCV viremia.[6] Cryoglobulins can be found in up to half of patients with HCV infection, although only 10%

to 15% have symptomatic disease (primarily weakness, arthralgias, and purpura).[6] Membranoproliferative glomerulonephritis and porphyria cutanea tarda are also common extrahepatic manifestations. A higher incidence of non-Hodgkin's lymphoma has been observed in association with HCV infection.[6] Other extrahepatic conditions, including Sjögren's syndrome, autoimmune thyroiditis, lichen planus, and Mooren's corneal ulcers, have been reported in patients with HCV infection, but no definitive associations have been established.[5,6,9]

Diagnostic Evaluation

A number of tests can be used to diagnose and monitor HCV infection.

Serologic Assays. The detection of HCV antibodies is useful for screening at-risk populations and is recommended as the initial test for the identification of HCV in patients with clinical liver disease.[9,26] Once individuals seroconvert, they usually remain positive for HCV antibody.[6] Thus, the presence of HCV antibody may reflect remote or current infection.[26]

The primary serologic test used for the detection of HCV antibody is an enzyme immunoassay, which is relatively inexpensive, is reproducible, and carries a high sensitivity (99%) and specificity (99%).[9] It can detect antibodies 4 to 10 weeks after infection.[6] A negative enzyme immunoassay finding is sufficient to exclude the diagnosis of HCV infection in immunocompetent patients.[9] However, the test can be falsely negative in those with immunodeficiencies or end-stage renal disease.[6,9] A recombinant immunoblot assay is another serologic test for HCV, and this detects the antibody response to individual HCV proteins.

RNA Assays. Assays based on the molecular detection of HCV using polymerase chain reaction techniques can be qualitative or quantitative. A qualitative HCV RNA test should be used to confirm viremia in a patient with a positive enzyme immunoassay finding. This test can also confirm infection in patients with negative results on enzyme immunoassay in whom infection is still suspected.[6] A single negative result does not necessarily exclude viremia, since viral levels may transiently drop below the limit of detection of the assay. Repeat testing should be performed to confirm the absence of active HCV replication in these instances.

Quantitative assessment of the HCV viral load can help predict the likelihood of response to treatment (patients with HCV RNA levels exceeding 2 million copies/mL respond less well) and is useful in monitoring HCV therapy.[6,7,9,27] However, these tests provide no information about disease severity or progression. Therefore, serial monitoring of viral loads in untreated patients is unnecessary.

Alanine Aminotransferase Levels. ALT levels may be useful in monitoring HCV infection but are insensitive in predicting disease progression to cirrhosis.[9] ALT levels may be normal or fluctuate in those with HCV infection, and a single normal value does not eliminate active infection, progressive liver disease, or cirrhosis.[6,17] HCV-positive patients with normal transaminase values should undergo serial ALT measurements over 6 to 12 months to confirm the persistence of normal levels.[9,17] Serial measurements of ALT levels may also be helpful in monitoring the effectiveness of HCV therapy in the intervals between molecular testing, and the resolution of elevated ALT values appears to be an important indicator of disease response.[9]

Liver Biopsy. Since ALT abnormalities do not accurately predict the degree of hepatic inflammation and fibrosis, histologic evaluation of a liver biopsy specimen remains the gold standard for reliably estimating the prognosis and likelihood of disease progression in patients with HCV.[27] Biopsy specimens are graded on a scale of 0 to 4, representing the degree of hepatic inflammation and necrosis, and staged on a similar scale, signifying the degree of fibrosis.[27] Histologic grade and stage correlate with the risk of subsequent progression to cirrhosis.[17,27] Concurrent disease processes (steatohepatitis, iron overload) that can contribute to hepatic injury may also be identified. In addition, liver biopsy aids in the selection of HCV-positive patients for treatment and helps to correctly time various therapeutic interventions.[27] However, it is not always considered mandatory prior to the initiation of therapy, and patients infected with genotypes 2 or 3, in particular, may not need liver biopsy to make a decision to treat.

Genotype. Worldwide, six genetically distinct groups of HCV isolates, called *genotypes,* and multiple subtypes have been identified.[6,9,17,27] The known genotypes have been numbered from 1 through 6, and the subtypes have been labeled a, b, and c, in order of discovery. In the United States and western Europe, genotypes 1a and 1b are the most common, followed by genotypes 2 and 3.[1] The other genotypes are rarely found in these countries but may be identified in other areas, such as Egypt in the case of genotype 4, South Africa in the case of genotype 5, and Southeast Asia in the case of genotype 6.[1] The genotype is the strongest predictor of response to current therapy and is useful in determining the duration of HCV treatment.[9]

Hepatocellular Carcinoma Screening. Many clinicians screen patients with HCV-induced cirrhosis for hepatocellular carcinoma with serum alfa-fetoprotein and abdominal ultrasonography every 6 months, but data on the clinical utility of this practice are lacking.

HIV Screening. Many risk factors for HCV infection are shared by HIV infection. Patients with HCV who are at risk for HIV infection should be offered testing with appropriate pretest and post-test counseling.

Hepatitis B Screening. Since coinfection with hepatitis B virus accelerates the progression to cirrhosis[21] and increases the risk of hepatocellular carcinoma,[5] patients with HCV should also be tested for antibodies to hepatitis B virus.

Treatment of Chronic HCV Infection

Indications for HCV Therapy

Treatment is typically recommended for patients with chronic hepatitis C who are at the greatest risk for progression to cirrhosis.[9] The risks and benefits of treatment must be assessed for each patient, particularly given the slow course of natural infection. In general, treatment may be recommended for patients with the following conditions:

- **Moderate liver disease** –Persistently elevated ALT levels, HCV viremia, and liver biopsy demonstrating at least moderate inflammation (at least grade 2) and fibrosis (at least stage 1).
- **Mild liver disease**—Elevated ALT levels, HCV viremia, and only mild inflammatory changes (grades 1 to 2, stage 0) on liver biopsy. Observation may also be reasonable in these instances.
- **Compensated cirrhosis**—These patients may have a higher rate of side effects from therapy.
- **HIV coinfection**

Patients with persistently normal ALT levels and minimal or no histologic evidence of inflammation have an excellent prognosis without therapy.[9] Patients with decompensated cirrhosis should not be treated, since they are unlikely to have a response and their condition may worsen with therapy. Pregnancy is an absolute contraindication to HCV treatment. Little is known about the treatment of HCV in children and adolescents, and further research is needed.

Interferon and Ribavirin

Interferons are natural glycoproteins that are produced by cells in response to viral infections, and they possess intrinsic antiviral activity. Initially, interferon-alfa was the only therapy available for the treatment of chronic HCV, and the drug needed to be given by intradermal injection three times per week. Administration of interferon-alfa resulted in a sustained virologic response (defined as complete HCV suppression 24 weeks after cessation of therapy) in only 15% to 20% of patients after 48 weeks of treatment.[28] Subsequently, two large randomized trials demonstrated that the combination of interferon-alfa and the nucleoside analogue ribavirin was more effective than interferon alone, resulting in a sustained virologic response in 38% to 43% of patients after 48 weeks of therapy.[29,30] Histologic improvement was noted in patients treated with combination therapy. Both studies also showed that patients with genotypes 2 or 3 had a higher sustained virologic response (64–69%) and required only 24 weeks to achieve this outcome, whereas those with genotype 1 had a much lower rate of sustained virologic response (28–31%) and required a full 48 weeks of therapy.[29,30]

The attachment of polyethylene glycol (PEG) to interferon results in a compound that has a much longer half-life than unmodified interferon, requiring only one intradermal injection per week. Two types of pegylated interferons (peginterferon alfa-2a and 2b), which differ in their pharmacokinetic and chemical properties, have been developed. Subsequently, randomized trials showed that once-weekly treatment with peginterferon alfa-2a had a higher rate of sustained virologic response (44–69%) than conventional interferon alfa-2a given three times per week (14–28%) after 48 weeks of therapy.[31,32] In addition, peginterferon alfa-2b plus ribavirin was shown to produce a higher rate of sustained virologic response (54%) compared with interferon alfa-2b plus ribavirin (47%) after 48 weeks of therapy.[33] Recently, peginterferon alfa-2a plus ribavirin was found to produce significant improvements in the rates of sustained virologic response (56%) compared with interferon alfa-2b plus ribavirin (44%) or peginterferon alfa-2a alone (29%) after 48 weeks of therapy.[34]

Contraindications to HCV therapy are reviewed in Table 1, and the side effects of interferon and ribavirin are listed in Table 2. These must be reviewed and discussed with patients prior to the initiation of treatment. Therapy is usually discontinued if no response to combination

TABLE 1. Contraindications to Therapy with Interferon-Alfa and Ribavirin	
Interferon-alfa	Severe depression
	History of psychotic disorder
	Decompensated cirrhosis
	Active substance abuse (particularly alcohol)
	Autoimmune disorders
	Neutropenia
	Thrombocytopenia
	Hyperthyroidism
Ribavirin	Anemia
	Hemoglobinopathies
	Coronary artery disease
	End-stage renal disease
	Pregnancy
Adapted from Lauer GM, Walker BD: Hepatitis C virus infection. N Engl J Med 345:41–52, 2001.	

TABLE 2. Possible Side Effects of Interferon-Alfa and Ribavirin Therapy	
Interferon-alfa	**Ribavirin**
Influenza-like symptoms (headaches, fatigue, fever, myalgias, anorexia)	Hemolytic anemia
Leukopenia	Nausea
Thrombocytopenia	Pruritus
Injection site pain/erythema	Gout
Depression	
Diarrhea	
Loss of libido	
Hypothyroidism	
Retinopathy	
Alopecia	
Autoantibodies	
Adapted from Lauer GM, Walker BD: Hepatitis C virus infection. N Engl J Med 345:41–52, 2001.	

therapy has been observed after 24 weeks.[9] Referral to an infectious disease physician or hepatologist should be performed to ensure appropriate treatment and monitoring.

Immunization Against Hepatitis A and B

Acute infection with hepatitis A or B in patients with underlying chronic HCV infection can result in high morbidity and mortality.[5,21] Hepatitis A and B vaccinations have been shown to be safe and effective in patients with chronic hepatitis C and may prevent poor outcomes.[7]

References

1. Centers for Disease Control and Prevention: Recommendations for prevention and control of hepatitis C virus (HCV) infection and HCV-related chronic diseases. MMWR Morbid Mortal Wkly Rep 47(RR-19):1–39, 1998.
2. Feinstone SM, Kapikian AZ, Purcell RH, et al: Transfusion-associated hepatitis not due to viral hepatitis type A or B. N Engl J Med 292:767–770, 1975.
3. Alter HJ, Purcell RH, Shih JW, et al: Detection of antibody to hepatitis C virus in prospectively followed transfusion recipients with acute and chronic non-A, non-B hepatitis. N Engl J Med 321:1494–1500, 1989.
4. Liang TJ, Rehermann B, Seeff LB, Hoofnagle JH: Pathogenesis, natural history, treatment, and prevention of hepatitis C. Ann Intern Med 132:296–305, 2000.
5. Sharara AI, Hunt CM, Hamilton JD: Hepatitis C. Ann Intern Med 125:658–668, 1996.
6. Lauer GM, Walker BD: Hepatitis C virus infection. N Engl J Med 345:41–52, 2001.
7. Herrine SV: Approach to the patient with chronic hepatitis C infection. Ann Intern Med 136:747–757, 2002.
8. Alter MJ, Kruszon-Moran D, Nainan OV, et al: The prevalence of hepatitis C virus infection in the United States, 1988 through 1994. N Engl J Med 341:556–562, 1999.
9. National Institutes of Health: Consensus Development Conference Statement—

Management of hepatitis C: 2002. http://www.consensus.nih.gov. Accessed October 1, 2002.

10. Conry-Cantilena C, VanRaden M, Gibble J, et al: Routes of infection, viremia, and liver disease in blood donors found to have hepatitis C virus infection. N Engl J Med 334:1691–1696, 1996.

11. Schreiber GB, Busch MP, Kleinman SH, Korelitz JJ: The risk of transfusion-transmitted viral infections. N Engl J Med 334:1685–1690, 1996.

12. Sulkowski MS, Ray SC, Thomas DL: Needlestick transmission of hepatitis C. JAMA 287:2406–2413, 2002.

13. Sartori M, LaTerra G, Aglietta M, et al: Transmission of hepatitis C via blood splash into conjunctiva [letter]. Scand J Infect Dis 25:270–271, 1993.

14. Rosen HR: Acquisition of hepatitis C by a conjunctival splash. AJIC Am J Infect Control 25:242–247, 1997.

15. Ko YC, Ho MS, Chiang TA, et al: Tattooing as a risk of hepatitis C virus infection. J Med Virol 38:288–291, 1992.

16. Tsang TH, Horowitz E, Vugia DJ: Transmission of hepatitis C through tattooing in a United States prison [letter]. Am J Gastroenterol 96:1304–1305, 2001.

17. Moyer LA, Mast EE, Alter MJ: Hepatitis C: Part I. Routine serologic testing and diagnosis. Am Fam Phys 59:79–88, 1999.

18. Farci P, Alter HJ, Shimoda A, et al: Hepatitis C virus-associated fulminant hepatic failure. N Engl J Med 335:631–634, 1996.

19. Wiley TE, McCarthy M, Breidi L, Layden TJ: Impact of alcohol on the histological and clinical progresion of hepatitis C infection. Hepatology 28:805–809, 1998.

20. Soto B, Sánchez-Quijano A, Rodrigo L, et al: Human immunodeficiency virus infection modifies the natural history of chronic parenterally-acquired hepatitis C with an unusually rapid progression to cirrhosis. J Hepatol 26:1–5, 1997.

21. Zarski JP, Bohn B, Bastie A, et al: Characteristics of patients with dual infection by hepatitis B and C viruses. J Hepatol 28:27–33, 1998.

22. Colombo M, de Franchis R, Del Ninno E, et al: Hepatocellular carcinoma in Italian patients with cirrhosis. N Engl J Med 325:675–680, 1991.

23. Pawlotsky JM, Roudot-Thoraval F, Simmonds P, et al: Extrahepatic immunologic manifestations in chronic hepatitis C and hepatitis C virus serotypes. Ann Intern Med 122:169–173, 1995.

24. Koff RS, Dienstag JL: Extrahepatic manifestations of hepatitis C and the association with alcoholic liver disease. Semin Liver Dis 15:101–109, 1995.

25. Zignego AL, Bréchat C: Extrahepatic manifesations of HCV infection: Facts and controversies. J Hepatol 31:369–376, 1999.

26. Moyer LA, Mast EE, Alter MJ: Hepatitis C: Part II. Prevention counseling and medical evaluation. Am Fam Phys 59:349–354, 1999.

27. Rosenberg PM: Hepatitis C: A hepatologist's approach to an infectious disease. Clin Infect Dis 33:1728–1732, 2001.

28. Carithers RL Jr, Emerson SS: Therapy of hepatitis C: Meta-analysis of interferon alfa-2b trials. Hepatology 26(Suppl 1):S83–88, 1997.

29. Poynard T, Marcellin P, Lee SS, et al: Randomised trial of interferon α2b plus ribavirin for 48 weeks or for 24 weeks versus interferon α2b plus placebo for 48 weeks for treatment of chronic infection with hepatitis C virus. Lancet 352:1426–1432, 1998.

30. McHutchison JG, Gordon SC, Schiff ER, et al: Interferon alfa-2b alone or in combination with ribavirin as initial treatment for chronic hepatitis C. N Engl J Med 339:1485–1492, 1998.

31. Zeuzem S, Feinman SV, Rasenack J, et al: Peginterferon alfa-2a in patients with chronic hepatitis C. N Engl J Med 343:1666–1672, 2000.

32. Heathcote EJ, Shiffman ML, Cooksley WGE, et al: Peginterferon alfa-2a in patients with chronic hepatitis C and cirrhosis. N Engl J Med 343:1673–1680, 2000.
33. Manns MP, McHutchison JG, Gordon SC, et al: Peginterferon alfa-2b plus ribavirin compared with interferon alfa-2b plus ribavirin for initial treatment of chronic hepatitis C: A randomised trial. Lancet 358:958–965, 2001.
34. Fried MW, Shiffman ML, Reddy KR, et al: Peginterferon alfa-2a plus ribavirin for chronic hepatitis C virus infection. N Engl J Med 347:975–982, 2002.

Intra-Abdominal Infections

Carolyn V. Gould, M.D.

chapter
13

Intra-abdominal infections may involve the peritoneum or intra-abdominal organs, and patients may present with syndromes ranging from diffuse peritonitis to a localized abscess. Abdominal pain is, in most cases, a common feature of intra-abdominal infection, and primary care doctors play a leading role in the initial assessment of patients with abdominal pain. Early diagnosis and management, which often involves surgical consultation or immediate referral in the case of acute abdominal infections, is essential in reducing morbidity and mortality.[1] This chapter focuses on the key features and management of various intra-abdominal infections, including primary, secondary, and tertiary peritonitis as well as peritonitis in the setting of peritoneal dialysis, intra-peritoneal and visceral abscesses, appendicitis, and diverticulitis.

Primary Peritonitis

Primary peritonitis is defined as an ascitic fluid infection that occurs in the absence of a surgically treatable intra-abdominal source of infection. It occurs almost exclusively in patients with ascites, usually in the setting of hepatic dysfunction or nephrotic syndrome. Because most cases are due to bacterial infection, it is often referred to as *spontaneous bacterial peritonitis* (SBP).

Causes of Primary Peritonitis

In adults, SBP is most commonly associated with cirrhosis and ascites and develops in up to 25% of this population.[2] However, it has also been reported to occur in patients with a number of other conditions, such as congestive heart failure, metastatic malignant disease, chronic active hepatitis, acute viral hepatitis, systemic lupus erythematosus (with no obvious ascites), and rarely in adults with no predisposing disease.[3] Primary peritonitis may also occur in children without ascites, usually in girls younger than 10 years of age, but is usually associated with nephrotic syndrome.

In cirrhotic patients, hematogenous seeding of the ascitic collection is thought to be the most likely route of infection.[2] This occurs because of intrahepatic shunting, which prevents clearance of bloodborne bacteria by the hepatic reticuloendothelial system. Enteric bacteria may also enter the peritoneal cavity by migration across the intact intestinal wall due to intestinal bacterial overgrowth and edema of the bowel wall in patients with cirrhosis. Patients with severe liver disease also have deficient bactericidal activity of the peritoneal fluid.[4]

Primary peritonitis may occur as a result of transfallopian spread of organisms into the peritoneum. This mechanism may explain cases of peritonitis in women with intrauterine devices and cases of perihepatitis due to *Chlamydia trachomatis* or *Neisseria gonorrhoeae* (Fitz-Hugh-Curtis syndrome), although hematogenous spread in the latter condition is possible.

Tuberculous peritonitis may result from hematogenous seeding from another focus of tuberculosis or direct seeding of the peritoneal cavity from lymph nodes, intestine, or genital tract, when these organs are actively infected.

Flora

Primary peritonitis is almost always monomicrobial, so growth of more than one organism should raise the suspicion for secondary peritonitis. Gram-negative enteric organisms make up about 60% of SBP infections, with *Escherichia coli* and *Klebsiella pneumoniae* being most frequently isolated.[4] Gram-positive organisms, most often *Streptococcus pneumoniae* and other streptococcal species, account for about 25% of episodes. Patients receiving selective intestinal decontamination (SID), usually with fluoroquinolone antibiotics, may have a higher frequency of gram-positive SBP episodes. Despite the predominantly anaerobic flora of the colon, anaerobic organisms are rarely isolated from peritoneal fluid and, when present, correlate strongly with polymicrobial infection.[5] Bacteremia occurs in up to 75% of SBP cases when the infection is due to a single aerobic species, but it is rare in patients with peritonitis due to anaerobes.[2]

The most common infecting organisms in children with primary peritonitis are *S. pneumoniae* and group A streptococci. Uncommon organisms isolated in cases of primary peritonitis include *N. gonorrhoeae, C. trachomatis, Mycobacterium tuberculosis,* and *Coccidioides immitis.*[2]

Clinical Presentation

Primary peritonitis in children may mimic acute appendicitis, with fever, abdominal pain, nausea, vomiting, diarrhea, diffuse abdominal tenderness, rebound tenderness, and hypoactive or absent bowel sounds. In cirrhotic patients, the presentation is often atypical and may present insidiously with no signs of peritoneal irritation.[2] The most frequent symptoms are fever (69%) and abdominal pain (59%).[4] Other signs and symptoms include hepatic encephalopathy (54%), abdominal tenderness (49%), diarrhea (32%), ileus (30%), shock (21%), and hypothermia (17%). Approximately 10% of patients with SBP have no signs or symptoms.[4] Because of the variable clinical picture, patients with cirrhosis who have unexplained deterioration, especially hepatic encephalopathy, should undergo a diagnostic paracentesis.

Tuberculous peritonitis usually appears gradually, with fever, malaise, weight loss, night sweats, and abdominal distension. The abdomen is often described as being "doughy" on palpation. Surgery or laparoscopy typically reveals multiple nodules over the peritoneal and omental surfaces with adhesions.[2] C. immitis causes a granulomatous peritonitis and manifests variably.

Diagnosis

The diagnosis of peritonitis is based on analysis of ascitic fluid obtained by abdominal paracentesis. Paracentesis has been found to be safe, even in cirrhotic patients with coagulopathy. There is an approximately 1% chance of abdominal wall hematoma, 0.01% chance of hemoperitoneum, and 0.01% chance of iatrogenic infection.[4]

The ascitic fluid should be sent for cell count, differential, Gram stain, and bacterial culture. Ten to 20 mL of fluid should be inoculated into blood-culture bottles at the bedside, which yields bacterial growth in about 80% of cases of neutrocytic (neutrophil-predominant) ascites, compared to less than 50% with conventional culture techniques.[6] If there is a suspicion for tuberculous peritonitis, fluid should be sent for mycobacterial smear and culture, although the sensitivity of these tests is very low. In contrast, a peritoneal biopsy for tuberculosis approaches a sensitivity of 100%.[7] Measurement of adenosine deaminase activity in peritoneal fluid has been found to be an insensitive test for tuberculous peritonitis in the United States, especially in cirrhotic patients, but is helpful if the result is positive.[7]

The diagnosis of SBP is confirmed by an ascitic fluid polymorphonuclear (PMN) count of 250 cells/mm³ or greater and a positive bacterial culture. Two other variants of primary peritonitis exist that do not meet these criteria:
- **Culture-negative neutrocytic ascites** (CNNA) is present when there is a PMN count of 250 cells/mm³ or greater but a negative bacterial culture. This may also occur in the setting of peritoneal carcinomatosis, pancreatitis, and tuberculous peritonitis, and these conditions must be ruled out. CNNA has similar clinical and prognostic features as SBP and is treated in the same way.[4]

- **Bacterascites** is defined as the isolation of bacteria in ascitic fluid cultures with a PMN count of less than 250 cells/mm³. The clinical course of bacterascites depends on whether or not the patient is symptomatic. If signs and symptoms of infection are present, the clinical course, mortality, and treatment are similar to SBP and CNNA. In the absence of symptoms, the colonization usually resolves without antibiotics.[4]

Treatment

Initial treatment of primary peritonitis is often empiric, since the Gram stain is frequently (60% to 80% of the time) negative. Broad antimicrobial coverage should be started until the results of culture and susceptibilities are available (Table 1). The combination of ampicillin plus an aminoglycoside has generally gone out of favor for patients with cirrhosis, given the potential for nephrotoxicity in this group. Third-generation cephalosporins are often recommended, but many other agents, including carbapenems (particularly, imipenem) and beta-lactam/beta-lactamase-inhibitor combinations (e.g., ampicillin-sulbactam) are alternative options. Anaerobic coverage (metronidazole or clindamycin) should be added, unless a beta-lactam/beta-lactamase inhibitor combination is used. If cultures remain sterile but there is a strong clinical suspicion of primary peritonitis (CNNA), antibiotics should be continued. Treatment is usually continued for 10 to 14 days, although a shorter course of therapy for 5 days has been found to be effective in patients

TABLE 1.	Empiric Therapy of Spontaneous Bacterial Peritonitis in Adults
Antibiotic Choice	**Adult Doses***
First Option	Ceftriaxone 1–2 g IV daily
	Cefotaxime 1 g IV every 8 hours
Second Option	Ampicillin-sulbactam 3 g IV every 6 hours
	Ticarcillin-clavulanate 3.1 g IV every 4–6 hours
	Pipercillin-tazobactam 3.375 g IV every 4–6 hours
	Imipenem-cilastin 500 mg IV every 6 hours
	Clindamycin 600 mg IV every 8 hours plus fluoroquinolone[†]
Penicillin-allergic	Clindamycin plus fluoroquinolone[†]
Prophylaxis	Norfloxacin 400 mg PO daily
	Ciprofloxacin 750 mg PO every week
	Trimethoprim-sulfamethoxazole 1 double-strength tablet PO daily for 5 days each week

*Adjust doses for renal insufficiency
[†]Fluoroquinolone options include ciprofloxacin 400 mg IV every 12 hours, levofloxacin 500 mg IV every 24 hours, or gatifloxacin, 400 mg IV every 24 hours
Adapted from Loutit J: Intra-abdominal infections. In: Wilson WR, Sande MA, eds: Current Diagnosis and Treatment in Infectious Diseases. New York: McGraw-Hill, 2001:164–176.

who are clinically well with a declining ascitic fluid leukocyte count and negative cultures after this period of therapy.[8] Clinical improvement as well as a decline in the ascitic fluid white blood cell count should occur by 48 hours of treatment if the diagnosis is correct; otherwise, further evaluation to rule out other pathologic conditions should be done. While treatment is successful in more than 50% of cirrhotic patients, the overall mortality rate of SBP is high, between 57% and 70%, primarily because of the underlying disease.[8] Patients with the poorest prognosis include patients with renal insufficiency, hypothermia, hyperbilirubinemia, and hypoalbuminemia.[9]

Prevention

Antimicrobial prophylaxis (SID) is recommended after treatment of SBP in cirrhotic patients because of a high recurrence rate (43% at 6 months, 69% at 1 year).[4] Both oral norfloxacin (400 mg daily) and ciprofloxacin (750 mg once weekly) have been shown to decrease significantly the incidence of SBP.[10] However, the potential disadvantage of these agents is the selection of gram-positive organisms, such as *Staphylococcus aureus*, and resistant gram-negative bacteria. Trimethoprim-sulfamethoxazole (one double-strength dose given once daily for 5 days each week) also reduces the incidence of SBP and is well tolerated.[11] Neither of these agents has been shown to improve survival.

Secondary Peritonitis

The diagnosis of secondary peritonitis is made when there is an ascitic fluid infection in the presence of a surgically treatable intra-abdominal source of infection. This process involves a breach of the gastrointestinal or genitourinary mucosal barrier, allowing spillage of microorganisms into the peritoneal space. It may occur as a complication of appendicitis, diverticulitis, cholecystitis, penetrating wound of the bowel, perforation of a gastric or duodenal ulcer, or a post-surgical anastomotic leak.[2] Secondary infection can involve generalized peritonitis or a localized abscess.

Flora

Gastrointestinal perforation typically leads to a polymicrobial infection. The types of organism involved depend on the level of perforation. Intestinal flora may also be altered by previous antimicrobial therapy or severe underlying disease. The normal flora of the stomach, duodenum, and proximal small bowel are sparse and similar to oropharyngeal flora.[12] Low numbers of α-hemolytic streptococci, lactobacilli, *Candida* species, and anaerobes predominate. The distal small bowel contains larger numbers of organisms, including Enterobacteriaceae, *Enterococcus* species, and anaerobes.

Colonic perforation leads to hundreds of different species being introduced into the peritoneal cavity. However, once infection is established, the number is narrowed down to an average of five pathogens.[2] The colon contains enormous numbers of bacteria ($\sim 10^{12}$/g), with more than 99.9% being obligate anaerobes, mostly of the *Bacteroides fragilis* group.[12] *B. fragilis* and *E. coli* are the most frequently isolated organisms.[12] Facultative organisms include *E. coli, Proteus, Klebsiella,* and *Enterococcus* species. *E. coli* has been shown to be responsible for sepsis and mortality in early peritonitis, while *B. fragilis,* in conjunction with *E. coli* and other flora, causes late abscess formation.[13]

Clinical Presentation

Abdominal pain, nausea, vomiting, altered bowel habits, fever, and tachycardia are often present in patients with secondary peritonitis. Patients typically avoid movement and may keep their hips and knees flexed. Abdominal examination often reveals tenderness, involuntary guarding, and rebound tenderness. Hypotension due to sepsis and hypovolemic shock may occur with diffuse peritonitis, whereas patients with a localized abscess usually have minimal vital sign abnormalities.

Diagnosis

Patients with suspected intra-abdominal infection should have a peripheral leukocyte count, urinalysis, and blood cultures performed. The leukocyte count is elevated in most cases.

Radiologic evaluation in cases of suspected secondary peritonitis is invaluable. An upright chest radiograph or left lateral decubitus radiograph often reveals free air in patients with perforated gastric or duodenal ulcers. Although ultrasonography is very useful in evaluating the gallbladder, biliary tract, and pelvic structures, computed tomography (CT) with intravenous, oral, and rectal contrast is the most definitive diagnostic test overall in detecting abdominal sources of infection.[12]

Patients with ascites and suspected intra-abdominal infection should have a paracentesis performed. When a source of intra-abdominal infection is not clear, analysis of ascitic fluid may help differentiate secondary peritonitis from SBP. Fluid cultures in secondary peritonitis are usually polymicrobial, and the PMN count is 250 cells/mm³ or greater, although it may be markedly elevated (>10,000 cells/mm³). Other parameters may also be helpful. Unlike in SBP, the ascitic fluid analysis in secondary peritonitis usually meets at least two of the following criteria: (1) a total protein level of more than 1 gm/dL, (2) a glucose concentration of less than 50 mg/dL, or (3) a lactate dehydrogenase (LDH) level of more than 225 U/mL.[4]

Treatment

Patients with evidence of secondary peritonitis should be referred immediately for surgical evaluation. Prompt surgery is the mainstay of treatment for patients with secondary peritonitis to control the source of contamination and to remove necrotic tissue, blood, or intestinal contents from the peritoneal cavity.[12] Medical management consists of antimicrobial therapy and physiologic support of the patient. The mortality rate of secondary peritonitis approaches 100% if treatment does not include surgical intervention.[14]

The choice of antimicrobial agents is generally made empirically, based on the likely pathogens. Although no clinical trials have demonstrated the superiority of one antimicrobial regimen over the other, it is known that both anaerobes and gram-negative aerobes should be covered.[12] Combination antimicrobial therapy has traditionally been used, although single broad-spectrum agents, including beta-lactam/beta-lactamase inhibitor combinations and the carbapenems, are alternatives. Recommendations for empiric therapy depend on the severity of illness and whether the infection was acquired in a community or hospital setting (Table 2). The duration of antimicrobial therapy after surgery is usually 5 to 7 days, depending on the severity of the infection, clinical response, and normalization of the white blood cell count.

The role of enterococci in secondary peritonitis is not clearly defined, as most cases of secondary peritonitis are cured with regimens that do not have activity against enterococcus. However, regimens that include specific enterococcal coverage are recommended if these organisms grow in a pure culture from an intra-abdominal source of infection or from the blood.[2]

Tertiary Peritonitis

Tertiary peritonitis is considered a later stage of secondary peritonitis, when clinical signs of peritonitis and systemic signs of sepsis persist after treatment. Culture of the peritoneal fluid usually reveals either no organisms or low-virulence organisms (typically enterococci, *Candida* species, and coagulase-negative staphylococci). These may be present due to selection from the initial polymicrobial infection by antibiotic therapy, contamination from surgical procedures, or translocation from the gut in patients with impaired host defenses and multiorgan dysfunction.[2]

Peritonitis Complicating Peritoneal Dialysis

Continuous ambulatory peritoneal dialysis (CAPD) creates another mechanism for the development of peritonitis. The incidence of peritonitis is 1.3

TABLE 2. Empiric Therapy of Secondary Bacterial Peritonitis in Adults	
Indication	**Adult Doses***
Community-acquired infection: Mild to moderate severity	Ampicillin-sulbactam 3 g IV every 6 hours Ticarcillin-clavulanate 3.1 g IV every 4–6 hours Cefoxitin 2 g IV every 4–6 hours Cefotetan 2 g IV every 12 hours Clindamycin 600 mg IV every 8 hours plus fluoroquinolone[†]
Community-acquired infection: Penicillin allergy	Anti-anaerobe[‡] plus fluoroquinolone[†]
Hospital-acquired infection	Piperacillin-tazobactam 3.375 g every 4–6 hours Meropenem 1 g IV every 6 hours Clindamycin 600 mg IV every 8 hours plus aztreonam 1–2 g IV every 8 hours Anti-anaerobe[‡] plus aminoglycoside[§] Anti-anaerobe[‡] plus third-generation cephalosporin[¶]
Hospital-acquired infection: Penicillin allergy	Anti-anaerobe[‡] plus fluoroquinolone[†] Anti-anaerobe[‡] plus aminoglyoside[§] Clindamycin 600 mg IV every 8 hours plus aztreonam 1–2 g IV every 8 hours

*Adjust doses for renal insufficiency.
[†]Fluoroquinolone options include ciprofloxacin 400 mg IV every 12 hours, levofloxacin 500 mg IV every 24 hours, or gatifloxacin 400 mg IV every 24 hours.
[‡]Anti-anaerobic options include clindamycin 600 mg IV every 8 hours or metronidazole 500 mg IV every 12 hours.
[§]Aminoglycoside options include gentamicin or tobramycin 5 mg/kg IV every 24 hours.
[¶]Third-generation cephalosporin options include cefotaxime or ceftazidime 1 g IV every 8 hours; cefepime 1–2 g IV every 12 hours; ceftriaxone 1–2 g IV every 24 hours.
Adapted from Loutit J: Intra-abdominal infection. In: Wilson WR, Sande MA, eds: Current Diagnosis and Treatment in Infectious Diseases. New York: McGraw-Hill, 2001:164–176.

to 1.4 episodes per CAPD patient per year.[8] The most common route of access by organisms into the peritoneal cavity is via the dialysis catheter, followed by hematogenous seeding and transmural penetration through the intestinal wall.[15]

Flora

A single pathogen is isolated in CAPD peritonitis in most cases. Gram-positive cocci account for 60% to 70% of cases, with coagulase-negative staphylococci being the most common, followed by S. aureus and Streptococcus species. Gram-negative bacilli account for 20% to 30% of cases, with Enterobacteriaceae implicated in the majority of cases. Fungal infections have become increasingly important, with Candida species accounting for 80% to 90% of fungal cases, although molds such as Aspergillus, Mucor, and Rhizopus species have been reported.

Mycobacterial infections make up less than 3% of cases of CAPD peritonitis.[8]

Diagnosis

Any two of the following criteria are required to establish the diagnosis of CAPD peritonitis: (1) symptoms of peritoneal inflammation, (2) cloudy dialysate fluid (leukocyte count of >100 cells/mm^3 with >50% neutrophils), and (3) a positive fluid Gram stain or bacterial culture.[15]

Treatment

Empiric therapy should cover both gram-positive and gram-negative organisms until culture results are available. Third-generation cephalosporins and vancomycin are generally recommended. The use of intraperitoneal antibiotics has allowed most patients to be treated on an ambulatory basis. The duration of therapy is usually 10 to 14 days.

Intraperitoneal Abscess

Intraperitoneal abscesses may develop as a consequence of diffuse peritonitis with localization of pus in dependent regions such as the pelvis, paracolic gutters, and subphrenic areas, or by direct extension of infection from a diseased organ (especially periappendiceal or diverticular abscesses). Almost half of all intraperitoneal abscesses occur in the right lower quadrant due to rupture of the appendix.[8] Postoperative anastomotic leaks also account for a large percentage of intra-abdominal abscesses. The microbiology is generally the same as that involved in secondary and tertiary peritonitis, and the antibiotics used in management are similar. Both aerobic and anaerobic organisms are required for abscess formation.

Computed tomography and ultrasonography have simplified the diagnosis of intra-abdominal abscess. CT is generally superior to ultrasonography, with an overall sensitivity for detecting abscesses of 78% to 100%, compared with 75% to 82% for ultrasonography.[12] CT is more accurate and sensitive than ultrasonography; with the exception of detecting lesions in the pelvis and right upper quadrant.

The main therapy for any intraperitoneal abscess is drainage. Although conventional therapy has involved surgical drainage, recent years have seen the successful use of percutaneous drainage as an alternative to surgery, made possible by refined imaging techniques.[16]

Subphrenic Abscess

Subphrenic abscesses most commonly develop after surgery involving the duodenum, stomach, biliary tract, or appendix, or after rupture of a hollow viscus, such as a perforated peptic ulcer or acute appendicitis. Patients may present with fever and abdominal pain in the right or left upper quadrants. Other symptoms may include hiccups, jaundice, shoulder pain, chest pain, cough, dyspnea, or a pleural effusion.[8] The syndrome may be an acute, febrile illness, or a more chronic, insidious process with intermittent fevers, weight loss, and other constitutional symptoms. The chronic form develops most often in patients who have previously received antibiotics. The diagnosis of subphrenic abscess should always be considered in patients presenting with fever of unknown origin, especially if they have a history of abdominal surgery within the preceding few months.[8]

Computed tomographic scan and ultrasonography are the best methods for diagnosing a subphrenic abscess. An initial plain radiograph may give clues to the diagnosis, often showing a pleural effusion, an elevated hemidiaphragm, and concomitant lower lobe atelectasis or pneumonia.[8,16]

The primary treatment is drainage, via either a percutaneous procedure or an open laparotomy. Empiric antibiotic therapy is aimed at the organisms likely to be involved, depending on the mechanism of infection, and is the same as that recommended for secondary peritonitis (see Table 2).

Liver Abscess

Pyogenic liver abscesses are relatively uncommon, with an incidence of 0.005% for all hospital admissions.[8] The most common cause of pyogenic liver abscess is biliary tract disease leading to ascending cholangitis. Other routes of infection include the portal vein (draining an intra-abdominal infection), the hepatic artery (with systemic bacteremia), direct extension from a contiguous focus of infection (e.g., cholecystitis, subphrenic abscess), or penetrating trauma to the liver.[17] One quarter of all hepatic abscesses are cryptogenic, with no direct cause found.[16]

The etiologic organisms are primarily enteric bacteria, with *E. coli* and *K. pneumoniae* being most common. Enterococci and viridans streptococci are also likely, particularly in cases of polymicrobial abscesses.[17] Two thirds of liver abscesses are polymicrobial, and one third involve anaerobes. *S. aureus* is more common in children and in patients with bacteremia. *Entamoeba histolytica* is responsible for 10% of liver abscesses.[8]

A minority of patients present with the classic triad of fever, jaundice, and right upper quadrant pain (Charcot's triad).[17] More often, fever and constitutional symptoms, including malaise, fatigue, anorexia, and weight loss, are present. Patients often have an enlarged liver and may have point tenderness. Suspicion of an amoebic liver abscess may be elicited by a history of travel or diarrhea, although impaired immunity also appears to be a risk factor in the absence of a travel history.[18]

Peripheral leukocytosis is common, as are elevated serum alkaline phosphatase levels, usually without an elevation in bilirubin. Stool examination to look for *E. histolytica* trophozoites or cysts is usually not helpful, since most patients do not have detectable parasites in the stool.[18] Serologic testing with enzyme immunoassays specific for *E. histolytica* is often useful.

Computed tomography is the most accurate imaging technique in the diagnosis of liver abscess, with a sensitivity of 95% or greater.[17] Ultrasonography is the study of choice in patients with suspected biliary tract disease or in patients who must avoid intravenous contrast agents. An amoebic liver abscess is more likely to be solitary than pyogenic abscesses and is usually limited to the right lobe of the liver.[16,18]

Treatment of a pyogenic liver abscess requires drainage as well as antibiotics. The initial procedure of choice is percutaneous drainage, which has a success rate of almost 90%.[8] Surgical drainage is usually reserved for cases that do not resolve with the percutaneous approach. Empiric therapy for pyogenic liver abscess is the same as that recommended for secondary peritonitis (see Table 2). Amoebic liver abscess can usually be treated with medical management alone. Metronidazole is the drug of choice and is given as 750 mg three times a day for 10 days. This should be followed by a luminal agent (typically paromomycin or diloxanide furoate) to treat asymptomatic colonization.[18]

Pancreatic Abscess

Pancreatic abscess most often occurs after an episode of acute pancreatitis but may also develop as a result of secondary infection of an established pancreatic pseudocyst. One to 9% of cases of acute pancreatitis are complicated by pancreatic abscess.[16] Secondary infection of necrotic pancreas, possibly by reflux of contaminated bile, is the most likely pathogenesis. Up to one half of infections are polymicrobial, typically involving *E. coli* and other gram-negative facultative organisms, enterococci, viridans streptococci, anaerobes, and occasionally *S. aureus*.

Pancreatic abscesses may result in two different clinical syndromes. In the first, the patient recovers from the initial acute pancreatitis but then develops fever, nausea, vomiting, and abdominal pain 1 to 5 weeks following the episode. These patients are usually found to have a well-defined abscess on CT scan. In the second group, patients never recover from the initial episode of pancreatitis and develop fever and hemodynamic instability.

Computed tomography is the best study to detect pancreatic abscesses. Treatment requires early surgical débridement and drainage; percutaneous drainage appears to be inadequate in most cases.[16] Initial empiric antibiotic therapy is the same as that recommended for secondary peritonitis (see Table 2).

Complications of pancreatic abscesses include intra-abdominal hemorrhage, spread of infection to the lesser sac, and fistula formation. There is a 100% mortality rate in patients with undrained pancreatic abscesses and a 53% to 86% survival rate in those who undergo surgery.[16]

Splenic Abscess

Splenic abscesses are uncommon lesions that are usually the result of hematogenous dissemination, as a result of bacteremia or septic embolization. Infected splenic infarcts and contiguous spread of infection are also potential mechanisms.

Patients often present with fever, chills, and left upper quadrant abdominal pain. Irritation of the diaphragm may lead to pleuropulmonary symptoms and referral of pain to the left shoulder.[8,16] A quarter of cases involve a polymicrobial infection. Causative organisms include *S. aureus* and *Streptococcus* species (usually in cases of bacterial endocarditis), as well as *Salmonella* species and other enteric bacteria, including anaerobes. Fungi, especially *Candida* species, are important causes of splenic abscesses in immunocompromised hosts.[8,16]

Broad-spectrum empiric antimicrobial therapy, as recommended for secondary peritonitis (see Table 2), is required. Although the treatment of choice is generally splenectomy, percutaneous drainage may be considered in some cases.

Acute Appendicitis

Acute appendicitis is the most common surgical condition of the abdomen, with a lifetime risk of 7%, and a peak incidence occurring between the ages of 10 and 30 years.[19] The primary care physician plays a leading role in the prompt diagnosis of acute appendicitis, which can prevent the complications of appendiceal rupture. Cases of obvious appendicitis require urgent referral, whereas equivocal cases frequently warrant surgical consultation and further evaluation.

Obstruction of the appendiceal lumen initiates the process of acute appendicitis. Obstruction can arise from a variety of mechanisms, including primary lymphoid hyperplasia or secondary lymphoid hyperplasia, which may be caused by upper respiratory infections, gastroenteritis, mononucleosis, Crohn's disease, or parasitic infections, along with fecaliths, foreign bodies, or tumors.[20]

The most common symptoms in acute appendicitis are abdominal pain, anorexia, nausea, and vomiting. Patients presenting early may experience a vague, constant pain referred to the perumbilical or epigastric region, which subsequently localizes to the right lower quadrant at or near McBurney's point. Low-grade fever, rebound tenderness, voluntary guarding, and subsequent abdominal rigidity are common features. However, it is important to note that this classic presentation occurs in only 50% of patients.[19]

Variations in the anatomic location of the appendix lead to differences in the location of pain and physical findings. For example, patients with a retrocecal appendix may have flank or back pain and tenderness and pain on extension of the right thigh (psoas sign). A pelvic appendix will cause suprapubic pain with pain on internal rotation of the right thigh (obturator sign) or during rectal examination. Because many gynecologic conditions can mimic appendicitis, all women with abdominal pain should have a pelvic examination.

If allowed to progress, the appendiceal inflammation ultimately compromises arterial blood flow, resulting in infarction, gangrene, and perforation, which usually occurs between 24 and 36 hours.[20] The adjacent viscera and omentum may wall off the spillage to the periappendiceal area, resulting in a localized abscess that may be felt as a mass in the right lower quadrant. If the process is not completely walled off, spreading diffuse peritonitis will occur.

Patients at the extremes of age are at highest risk for perforation due to delayed diagnosis. Older patients may have more subtle manifestations and often treat themselves with analgesics before seeking medical attention, resulting in misdiagnosis rates of 50% and perforation rates ranging from 40% to 70%.[20] Young children may be misdiagnosed in more than one half of cases, with perforation rates as high as 90% in some series.[20] Children are more likely to present with diffuse rather than localized or referred pain, and those misdiagnosed have a higher incidence of vomiting, diarrhea, constipation, dysuria, and respiratory symptoms.[21] Patients during pregnancy may be misdiagnosed, often presenting atypically during the second or third trimester with right upper quadrant or flank pain mimicking biliary colic or pyelonephritis. Early diagnosis and surgery during pregnancy is essential, since fetal mortality rates may be as high as 35% in patients with perforation and peritonitis.[20]

The white blood cell count is almost always elevated in patients with acute appenditis, typically with neutrophilia, although not necessarily in immunocompromised patients. Urinalysis findings are often abnormal; however, the presence of more than 30 red blood cells or 20 white blood cells suggests the presence of urinary tract disease. Serum electrolytes, blood urea nitrogen, and creatinine are helpful in evaluating patients for dehydration or associated electrolyte abnormalities.

The use of appendiceal CT scans has improved the diagnosis of appendicitis. Appendiceal CT scans have an accuracy of 98% and have been shown to prevent unnecessary appendectomies and reduce the use of hospital resources.[22] However, surgical consultation is still mandatory, as the use of CT scans prior to surgical evaluation may result in less accuracy.[23]

In the presence of perforation or abscess formation, antibiotics should be initiated, primarily directed against gram-negative anaerobes and Enterobacteraceae. Empiric antibiotic therapy is the same as that recommended for secondary peritonitis (see Table 2).

Diverticulitis

Diverticulitis occurs as a result of impaction of diverticula with fecaliths, which create an inflammatory process, sometimes leading to erosion and perforation of the colonic wall. Simple diverticulitis, which occurs in the majority of patients, is not associated with complications; these patients usually respond to medical therapy. Complicated diverticulitis involves perforation, obstruction, abscess, or fistula. This occurs in a quarter of patients with the first episode and requires surgery.[24]

Most patients with acute sigmoid diverticulitis have left lower quadrant pain, fever, and leukocytosis. A mass may be palpated on pelvic and rectal examination. CT scanning is the diagnostic technique of choice and typically reveals thickening of the bowel wall, streaky mesenteric fat, and associated abscess.[25]

Patients with mild symptoms in the absence of systemic signs and symptoms may be treated on an outpatient basis with a low-residue diet and broad-spectrum oral antibiotics for 7 to 10 days.[25] Hospitalization is required for significant fever, more severe signs and symptoms, or inability to tolerate an oral diet. Treatment consists of bowel rest, intravenous antibiotics, and intravenous fluids. Persistent fever and leukocytosis after 48 hours suggest an unresolving abscess. Up to one third of patients will go on to have a second episode of diverticulitis, and elective surgery should be considered in these patients.

Surgery is mandatory for patients with complications of diverticulitis. Percutaneous drainage of an abscess may be used preoperatively to simplify a subsequent surgery, or in some cases eliminate the need for surgery.[25] The antibiotic regimens recommended for secondary peritonitis (see Table 2) are also appropriate for antimicrobial management of diverticular complications.

References

1. Pitcher WD, Musher DM: Critical importance of early diagnosis and treatment of intra-abdominal infections. Arch Surg 117:328–333, 1982.
2. Johnson CC, Baldesarre J, Levison ME: Peritonitis: Update on pathophysiology, clinical manifestations, and management. Clin Infect Dis 24:1035–1047, 1997.
3. Conn HO, Fessel JM: Spontaneous bacterial peritonitis in cirrhosis: Variations on a theme. Medicine (Baltimore) 50:161–190, 1971.

4. Such J, Runyon BA: Spontaneous bacterial peritonitis. Clin Infect Dis 27:669–676, 1998.

5. Sheckman P, Onderdonk AB, Bartlett JG: Anaerobes in spontaneous peritonitis [letter]. Lancet 2:1223, 1977.

6. Runyon BA, Canawati HN, Akriviadis EA: Optimization of ascitic fluid culture technique. Gastroenterology 95:1351–1355, 1988.

7. Hillebrand DJ, Runyon BA, Yasmineh W, et al: Ascitic fluid adenosine deaminase insensitivity in detecting tuberculous peritonitis in the United States. Hepatology 24:1408, 1996.

8. Loutit J: Intra-abdominal infections. In: Wilson WR, Sande MA, eds: Current Diagnosis and Treatment in Infectious Diseases. New York: McGraw-Hill, 2001:164–176.

9. Weinstein MP, Iannini PB, Stratton CW, Eickhoff TC: Spontaneous bacterial peritonitis: A review of 28 cases with emphasis on improved survival and factors influencing prognosis. Am J Med 64:592–598, 1978.

10. Rolachon A, Cordier L, Bacq Y, et al: Ciprofloxacin and long-term prevention of spontaneous bacterial peritonitis: Results of a prospective controlled trial. Hepatology 22:1171–1174, 1995.

11. Singh N, Gayowksi T, Yu VL, Wagener MM: Trimethoprim-sultamethoxazole for the prevention of spontaneous bacterial peritonitis in cirrhosis: A randomized trial. Ann Intern Med 122:595–598, 1995.

12. McClean KL, Sheehan GJ, Harding GK: Intra-abdominal infection: A review. Clin Infect Dis 19:100–116, 1994.

13. Weinstein WN, Onderdonk AB, Bartlett JG, Gorbach SL: Experimental intra-abdominal abscesses in rats: development of an experimental model. Infect Immun 10:1250–1255, 1974.

14. Akriviadis EA, Runyon BA: The value of an algorithm in differentiating spontaneous from secondary bacterial peritonitis. Gastroenterology 98:127, 1990.

15. Vas S, Oreopoulos DG: Infections in patients undergoing peritoneal dialysis. Infect Dis Clin North Am 15:743–774, 2001.

16. Levison ME, Bush LM: Peritonitis and other intra-abdominal infections. In: Mandell GL, Bennett JE, Dolin R, eds: Mandell, Douglas, and Bennett's Principles and Practice of Infectious Diseases, 5th ed. Philadelphia: Churchill Livingstone, 2000: 2474–2489.

17. Johannsen EC, Sifri CD, Madoff LC: Pyogenic liver abscesses. Infect Dis Clin North Am 14:547–563, 2000.

18. Hughes MA, Petri WA Jr: Amebic liver abscess. Infect Dis Clin North Am 14:565–582, 2000.

19. Hardin DM: Acute appendicitis: Review and update. Am Fam Phys 60:2027–2034, 1999.

20. Graffeo CS, Counselman FL: Appendicitis. Emerg Med Clin North Am 14:653–671, 1996.

21. Rothrock SG, Skeoch G, Rush JJ, et al: Clinical features of misdiagnosed appendicitis in children. Ann Emerg Med 20:45, 1991.

22. Rao PM, Rhea JT, Novelline RA, Mostafavi AA, McCabe CJ: Effect of computed tomography of the appendix on treatment of patients and use of hospital resources. N Engl J Med 338:141–146, 1998.

23. Morris KT, Kavanagh M, Hansen P, et al: The rational use of computed tomography scans in the diagnosis of appendicitis. Am J Surg 183:547–550, 2002.

24. Young-Fadok TM, Pemberton JH: Treatment of acute diverticulitis. UpToDate 2002. www.uptodateonline.com. Accessed November 15, 2002.

25. Young-Fadok TM, Roberts PL, Spencer MP, Wolff BG: Colonic diverticular disease. Curr Probl Surg 37:457, 2000.

Biliary Infections

Vincent Lo Re III, M.D.

chapter
14

A significant proportion of adult patients who have abdominal pain are found to have a biliary infection. Infections of the biliary system commonly arise as a result of obstruction, and the clinical presentation varies with the level of obstruction.

Acute Calculous Cholecystitis

Approximately 15% of persons with gallstones develop acute cholecystitis.[1] Acute calculous cholecystitis accounts for more than 90% of cases of cholecystitis.[2]

Pathogenesis

Acute inflammation of the gallbladder wall usually follows obstruction of the infundibulum or cystic duct by a stone.[1] This obstruction of bile leads to an increase in pressure in the gallbladder that damages the mucosa and causes release of inflammatory mediators. Continued distention of the gallbladder wall can lead to a compromise of its blood supply, resulting in gangrene or perforation. Bacteria can proliferate in the inflamed gallbladder, and infection develops in up to one half of cases.[2,3]

Clinical Manifestations

Initial obstruction of the infundibulum or cystic duct may be accompanied only by mild epigastric pain, nausea, and anorexia.[3] Vomiting may occur and contribute to intravascular volume depletion. As the episode continues, the pain of acute cholecystitis becomes more localized to the right upper quadrant (RUQ) of the abdomen and may radiate to the right scapula or shoulder.[4]

On physical examination, low-grade fevers, rigors, hypoactive bowel sounds, and RUQ abdominal tenderness may be present. Murphy's sign, characterized by the sudden cessation of inspiration due to the pain induced by RUQ palpation, may also be identified. Approximately 20% of patients have a palpable mass in the RUQ due to irritation of the omentum overlying the inflamed gallbladder.[2,3] Localized rebound tenderness and guarding may also be found if gallbladder perforation and early peritonitis have occurred. Jaundice, it should be noted, is unusual early in the course of acute cholecystitis but may occur when inflammation involves the adjacent bile ducts.

Diagnosis

The differential diagnosis of acute calculous cholecystitis is quite broad (Table 1), but the condition should be suspected on the basis of clinical history and examination findings. Laboratory data may further suggest the diagnosis but are nonspecific. Leukocytosis with bandemia is typically present. The serum bilirubin level is elevated in 45% of patients, and 25% to 40% have a mild transaminitis.[3,4] A plain radiograph of the abdomen may show radiopaque stones in up to 15% of cases, but this is not helpful in obtaining a diagnosis.[1]

Abdominal ultrasonography is the test of choice. Acute calculous cholecystitis is suggested by a thickened (>5 mm) and edematous gallbladder wall, a positive Murphy sign induced by the ultrasound probe, and pericholecystic fluid in the presence of stones.[2] Biliary scintigraphy with a HIDA (hepatobiliary iminodiacetic acid) scan may also be useful in detecting acute calculous cholecystitis.[1] The radionuclide material is injected intravenously into the patient, concentrated in the liver, and then excreted into the bile, resulting in visualization of the hepatobiliary system. Since the cystic duct is occluded in cases of acute calculous cholecystitis, the gallbladder is not visualized, but the common bile duct and duodenum can be identified. The main drawbacks of this test include the necessity for injection of a radiopharmaceutical and the time required for the test. An abdominal computed tomography (CT) scan may demonstrate findings consistent with acute calculous cholecystitis, but this should not

TABLE 1. Differential Diagnosis of Right Upper Quadrant Abdominal Pain
Acute hepatitis
Appendicitis
Diseases of the right kidney (pyelonephritis, nephrolithiasis)
Fitz-Hugh-Curtis syndrome (perihepatitis due to gonococcal infection)
Intestinal obstruction
Myocardial infarction
Pancreatitis
Perforating peptic ulcer
Pyogenic liver abscess
Right lower lobe pneumonia
Right-sided intra-abdominal abscess

be the initial test used for diagnosis. Magnetic resonance cholangiopan-creatography (MRCP) is a relatively new noninvasive technique for eval-uating the intrahepatic and extrahepatic biliary ducts, but its role in the diagnosis of acute calculous cholecystitis is currently under investigation.

Treatment

In approximately 75% of cases, acute calculous cholecystitis will sub-side with conservative therapy, which consists of maintenance of a fast-ing state, intravenous fluid hydration, and analgesia.[4] Although acute calculous cholecystitis is primarily an inflammatory process, secondary bacterial infection of the gallbladder can occur, particularly when com-plications ensue (see later). The organisms found in the biliary tract in these instances are typically the same as normal intestinal flora.[2] The most frequently isolated bacteria that are involved in biliary infections are listed in Table 2. Empiric antimicrobial therapy should be directed at these organisms (Table 3). When the results of antimicrobial susceptibil-ity testing become available, more specific antibiotic therapy should be substituted. Antibiotics are typically not required for the treatment of un-complicated cholecystitis, since they do not appear to affect the outcome of the attack or decrease the incidence of local infectious complications.[5]

The selection and timing of surgical intervention depend on the severity of symptoms and the patient's overall risk of surgery. Surgical intervention should be considered in patients with a known or suspected complication (gangrene, pericholecystic abscess, perforation with peritonitis) or in those with intractable pain and progressive fever despite supportive therapy. Con-sultation with a general surgeon should be obtained to assist in the selec-tion of definitive therapy. Although open cholecystectomy had been con-sidered the gold standard for the treatment of acute calculous cholecystitis, laparoscopic cholecystectomy has become the operative procedure of choice.[1] In unstable patients in whom surgical intervention is contraindi-cated, drainage of the gallbladder may be performed with an ultrasound-

TABLE 2. Common Bacteria Involved in Biliary Infections in Adults	
Aerobes	**Anaerobes**
Gram-positive	Gram-positive
Enterococcus species	*Peptostreptococcus* species
Viridans streptococci	*Clostridium perfringens*
Gram-negative	Gram-negative
Escherichia coli	*Bacteroides fragilis*
Klebsiella pneumoniae	*Fusobacterium* species
Proteus mirabilis	
Pseudomonas aeruginosa	

TABLE 3. Options for Empiric Antimicrobial Therapy of Acute Cholangitis in Adults*	
Standard	**For Penicillin-Allergic Patients**
Ampicillin[†] 2 g IV every 6 hours *and* Gentamicin[‡] 2 mg/kg IV load, then 1.7 mg/kg IV every 8 hours *and* Metronidazole 500 mg IV every 12 hours	Levofloxacin 500 mg IV daily *or* Ciprofloxacin 400 mg IV every 12 hours *and* Metronidazole 500 mg IV every 12 hours *or* Clindamycin 600 mg IV every 8 hours
Ampicillin/sulbactam 1.5–3.0 g IV every 6 hours	
Piperacillin/tazobactam 3.375 g IV every 6 hours	Aztreonam 1–2 g IV every 8 hours *and* Metronidazole 500 mg IV every 12 hours
Piperacillin 4 g IV every 6 hours *and* Metronidazole 500 mg IV every 12 hours	
Imipenem 500 mg IV every 6 hours	

*Drug dosages are based on normal renal function.
[†]Ampicillin should be used with caution given the emergence of ampicillin-resistant *Escherichia coli* in community-acquired infections.[3]
[‡]Aminoglycosides must be used with caution, especially after the fifth day of use, due to their potential for nephrotoxicity. Peak and trough serum levels of these drugs should be monitored to ensure proper dosing.

guided percutaneous cholecystostomy.[6] This involves placing a catheter into the gallbladder with the patient under local anesthesia. Complications include bacteremia, bleeding, and peritonitis due to bile leak.

Acute Acalculous Cholecystitis

Infection of the gallbladder may occur in the absence of gallstones in approximately 10% of patients with acute cholecystitis, and this is termed *acalculous cholecystitis*.[7] Although it is less common than acute calculous cholecystitis, it is much more serious, accounting for an overall mortality rate of approximately 40%.[8] Failure to diagnose and treat acute acalculous cholecystitis early enough can lead to gangrene or perforation of the gallbladder wall. Cases of this disease are typically found in elderly patients with multiple comorbid conditions or in the critically ill who have undergone major surgery, suffered serious trauma or burns, or are receiving parenteral nutrition.[3] The clinical conditions that predispose to acute acalculous cholecystitis are listed in Table 4.

Pathogenesis

The pathogenesis of acute acalculous cholecystitis is poorly understood but is likely associated with bile stasis and gallbladder dysfunction.[8]

TABLE 4.	Conditions that Predispose to Acute Acalculous Cholecystitis
	Burns
	Coronary artery disease
	Childbirth (especially if labor is prolonged)
	Diabetes mellitus
	Elderly
	Immunosuppression
	Infection (salmonellosis, *Campylobacter jejuni*, leptospirosis, cholera)
	Mechanical ventilation
	Sepsis
	Surgery
	Trauma

Impaired gallbladder contractile function may occur in the elderly or critically ill, leading to biliary stasis, gallbladder wall inflammation, and ischemia. Necrosis and bacterial invasion of the gallbladder mucosa can subsequently occur.

Clinical Manifestations

The clinical findings of acute acalculous cholecystitis are usually indistinguishable from those of acute calculous cholecystitis.[2,3] Fever, RUQ abdominal pain, nausea, and anorexia are common. In some situations, however, fever, leukocytosis, and vague abdominal pain may be the only clues. A RUQ mass may be palpable, and jaundice is seen in up to 20% of patients due to partial biliary obstruction induced by inflammation extending into the common bile duct.[7,8]

Diagnosis

The clinical diagnosis of acalculous cholecystitis can be extremely difficult and requires a high index of suspicion. Leukocytosis, conjugated hyperbilirubinemia, and mild elevations in transaminases are common.[8]

As with acute calculous cholecystitis, abdominal ultrasonography is considered the first-line study and usually demonstrates a large, tense gallbladder without stones. Other findings include a thickened (>5 mm) and edematous gallbladder wall, pericholecystic fluid, biliary sludge, and a sonographic Murphy sign.[7,8] Abdominal CT scan can also be used to confirm the diagnosis.

Treatment

Prompt institution of therapy is essential. After blood cultures have been drawn, intravenous antibiotics that cover the biliary flora should be started (see Table 3). The definitive treatment is either open or laparoscopic cholecystectomy. With unstable patients in whom surgery is contraindicated, ultrasound-guided cholecystostomy should be considered.

Chronic Cholecystitis

The constant presence of gallstones can lead to chronic inflammation of the gallbladder wall due to persistent mechanical irritation.[4] Chronic cholecystitis may be asymptomatic for years or may progress to acute cholecystitis with or without complications.

Complications of Cholecystitis

A number of complications have been associated with acute and chronic cholecystitis:

- *Empyema*—occurs when superinfection of stagnant bile leads to pus filling the gallbladder. This complication carries a high risk of gram-negative sepsis.[4]
- *Gangrene*—results from chronic ischemia of the gallbladder wall leading to complete tissue necrosis.[2] There is a high risk of perforation associated with this complication.
- *Perforation (with or without peritonitis)*—may be either localized (contained by the omentum and serosa of contiguous organs) or free (frank rupture of the gallbladder into the peritoneal cavity).[3] Fever and a palpable RUQ mass may be present when a localized perforation has occurred. A free perforation produces the clinical findings of diffuse peritonitis.
- *Emphysematous cholecystitis*—occurs when gas-producing bacteria invade a gangrenous gallbladder wall. The clinical manifestations are usually more severe but may be indistinguishable from nongaseous cholecystitis.[4] An abdominal plain radiograph may reveal gas within the gallbladder lumen, gas in a ring along the contours of the gallbladder wall, or a gas-fluid level in the gallbladder.
- *Cholecystenteric fistulas*—can form with chronic inflammation and can connect areas of bowel adjacent to the gallbladder wall. Fistulas from the gallbladder to the duodenum are the most common.[4]
- *Gallstone ileus*—refers to the mechanical intestinal obstruction resulting from passage of a large gallstone through the bowel lumen. If a significantly sized gallstone (>2.5 cm in diameter) passes through a fistula into the intestines, it can cause obstruction, typically at the ileocecal valve. An abdominal plain radiograph reveals intestinal obstruction, gas in the biliary tree, and a calcified gallstone in the bowel lumen.
- *Porcelain gallbladder*—can occur in the setting of chronic cholecystitis when calcium salts deposit within the chronically inflamed gallbladder wall. Cholecystectomy is recommended in these cases because of the association of carcinoma of the gallbladder.

- *Pericholecystic abscess*—consists of a localized pus collection adjacent to the gallbladder.
- *Intra-abdominal abscess*—can occur following a perforation of the galbladder (usually a free perforation).
- *Bacteremia*—results from translocation of bacteria from the gallbladder into the bloodstream.

Acute Cholangitis

First described by Jean Marie Charcot in 1877, acute (ascending) cholangitis occurs in an infected and usually obstructed biliary system, typically at the level of the common bile duct.[2,9] This illness is characterized by fever, abdominal pain, and jaundice and is an important cause of the "acute abdomen." If the biliary obstruction is not relieved, persistently elevated intraductal pressures can cause reflux of biliary contents and bacteremia, ultimately leading to sepsis.

Pathogenesis

Bile is normally sterile because of the constant flow into the duodenum, flushing the biliary system, and the antibacterial properties of Immunoglobulin A and bile salts in the bile itself.[9,10] The sphincter of Oddi also helps to prevent intestinal contents from refluxing onto the common bile duct.[9] Obstruction of the common bile duct causes a rise in pressure that leads to edema and necrosis of the walls of the biliary tree. Obstructions is primarily due to gallstones in the majority of cases, and these may arise from the gallbladder or spontaneously form in the common bile duct after cholecystectomy.[2] Other reasons for biliary obstruction include malignancy, benign strictures, congenital abnormalities, cysts, parasites (*Ascaris, Clonorchis,* or *Echinococcus* species), pancreatitis, or extrinsic compression.[9] In the presence of any of these causes of obstruction, bacteria may reach the biliary tree by either reflux from the duodenum or translocation from the portal circulation.[10] The bacteriologic findings in cholangitis are similar to those in acute cholecystitis (see Table 2).[11]

Clinical Manifestations

Patients with acute cholangitis usually have a prior history of biliary tract disease, particularly cholelithiasis or choledochelithiasis. The onset of cholangitis is usually acute, with high fevers, rigors, and abdominal pain. The classic Charcot triad of fever, RUQ abdominal pain, and jaundice can be found in up to 70% of cases.[2] Patients with acute obstructive suppurative cholangitis, in which there is pus in the biliary tree, may additionally present with altered mental status and hypotension

(Reynold's pentad).[2] These extra findings are typically due to the presence of gram-negative sepsis, particularly by *Escherichia coli* or *Klebsiella pneumoniae*. A pyogenic liver abscess is a rare complication of acute cholangitis.[10]

Diagnosis

Most patients with acute cholangitis have marked leukocytosis, hyperbilirubinemia, and elevated alkaline phosphatase levels, but serum transaminases are usually only modestly elevated.[3] Up to one third of cases have hyperamylasemia caused by concomitant obstruction of the pancreatic duct.[2]

Ultrasonography is the preferred study to confirm the diagnosis because of its ability to identify dilated biliary ducts.[2,3,9,10] Significant biliary ductal dilatation in a patient with the appropriate clinical picture confirms the diagnosis. Ultrasonographic examination can also evaluate the gallbladder size, the presence of stones, masses associated with the bile ducts, and liver parenchymal changes.[10]

Endoscopic retrograde cholangiopancreatography (ERCP) provides the most accurate means of determining the cause and location of obstruction.[3] This is the procedure of choice if common bile duct stones are present, since stone extraction and biliary stent placement can be performed, decompressing the biliary system. MRCP may also allow visualization of the biliary tree but does not permit removal of the obstruction.[10]

An abdominal CT scan can demonstrate the presence and, potentially, the cause of biliary obstruction.[2] Plain radiography and HIDA scans are less useful in confirming the diagnosis.

Treatment

Antibiotics and biliary drainage are the mainstays of treatment of acute cholangitis. Other general measures include intravenous fluid hydration and correction of coagulation abnormalities with vitamin K and fresh frozen plasma.

Antibiotic treatment is considered complementary to the establishment of biliary drainage and is used to control sepsis and inflammation.[11] Conservative management with antibiotics may also help to suitably delay biliary drainage until the acute disease has subsided. Treatment with broad-spectrum antibiotics should be started promptly (see Table 3). The antibiotic regimen can be narrowed once blood culture results become known.

Decompression of the obstructed biliary tree is crucial to the management of acute cholangitis. Surgical exploration and placement of a T-tube can provide definitive therapy of acute cholangitis in patients with difficult ductal stones, but surgery is generally no longer the procedure of choice.[10] Drainage is preferably accomplished with ERCP or a percutaneous transhepatic biliary catheter, since these are both associated with less morbidity and mortality.[3] During percutaneous transhepatic biliary drainage, a catheter is placed into the biliary tree under ultrasonographic or CT guidance, decomprssing the biliary tree.[10] ERCP is advantageous because it allows for stone extraction and stent placement during the procedure. After drainage of the biliary ducts, antibiotic treatment is usually continued for 7 to 10 days.[11] A longer course may be recommended for recurrent or refractory disease.[3]

With appropriate therapy, the mortality rate from acute cholangitis is less than 10%.[3] However, it can exceed 50% in patients with acute obstructive suppurative cholangitis.[10]

References

1. Moscati RM: Cholelithiasis, cholecystitis, and pancreatitis. Emerg Med Clin North Am 14:719–737, 1996.
2. Eckburg PB, Montoya JG: Hepatobiliary infections. In: Wilson WR, Sande MA, eds: Current diagnosis and treatment in infectious diseases. New York: McGraw Hill, 2001:268–286.
3. Levison ME, Bush LM. Peritonitis and other intra-abdominal infections. In: Mandell GL, Bennett JE, Dolin R, eds: Mandell, Douglas, and Bennett's Principles and Practice of Infectious Diseases, 5th ed. Philadelphia: Churchill Livingstone, 2000:821–856.
4. Greenberger NJ, Isselbacher KJ: Diseases of the gallbladder and bile ducts. In: Fauci AS, Braunwald F, Isselbacher KJ, et al, eds: Harrison's Principles of Internal Medicine, 14th ed. New York: McGraw Hill, 1998: 1725–1736.
5. Kune GA, Burden JG: Are antibiotics necessary in acute cholecystitis? Med J Aust 2:627, 1975.
6. Teplick SK, Brandon JC, Haskin PH, et al: Percutaneous cholecystostomy in patients at high risk: Treatment of acute calculous cholecystitis. Postgrad Med 81:209–214, 1987.
7. Chung SC: Acute acalculous cholecystitis: A reminder that this condition may appear in a primary care practice. Postgrad Med 98:199–204, 1995.
8. Kalliafas S, Ziegler DW, Flancbaum L, Choban PS: Acute acalculous cholecystitis: Incidence, risk factors, diagnosis, and outcome. Am Surg 64:471–475, 1998.
9. Hanau LH, Steigbigel NH: Acute (ascending) cholangitis. Infect Dis Clin North Am 14:521–546, 2000.
10. Sinanan MN: Acute cholangitis. Infect Dis Clin North Am 6:571–599, 1992.
11. van den Hazel SJ, Speelman P, Tytgat GNJ, et al: Role of antibiotics in the treatment and prevention of acute and recurrent cholangitis. Clin Infect Dis 19:279–286, 1994.

Non-necrotizing Skin and Soft Tissue Infections

chapter

15

Barry E. Kenneally, M.D.

The skin, our largest organ, is crucial to preventing infection and maintaining homeostasis. As a barrier against infection, the skin is often exposed to bacterial, fungal, and viral pathogens in the environment. As such, skin infections are a very common presentation in the primary care setting. Cellulitis alone may account for 2.2% of primary care office visits.[1] This chapter reviews some of the common skin infections seen in primary care.

Cellulitis

Etiology

Cellulitis is a bacterial infection of the skin and subcutaneous tissues characterized by pain and erythema. The most common pathogens are *Staphylococcus aureus* and group A streptococci. *Escherichia coli, Proteus mirabilis, Acinetobacter, Enterobacter,* and *Pseudomonas aeruginosa* are more common in immunocompromised patients.[2] Children younger than 3 years of age may develop *Haemophilus influenzae* group B infections in the skin of the head and neck, commonly related to an underlying ear or sinus infection.

The most common site for cellulitis is the lower leg, which may be exposed to minor trauma. It also occurs in intact skin.

Signs and Symptoms

Patients with cellulitis generally complain of a very painful, red rash of acute onset. A prodrome of fever, chills, and malaise occasionally precedes the rash.

Cellulitic skin appears as a well demarcated, irregularly shaped, erythematous, and edematous plaque. Affected skin may be tender, warm, and indurated. Fluctuance suggests an abscess or furuncle (discussed later). Lymphatic streaks and lymphadenopathy may be noted proximally and reflect the spread of the infection.

Laboratory Tests

Wound cultures are low yield (approximately 45%) in cellulitis and are generally reserved for patients who are immunocompromised or have poor response to treatment.[2] Wound culture is performed by aspirating subcutaneous fluid with a 20-gauge needle (22-gauge for the face) on a tuberculin syringe. Some clinicians inject a small amount of sterile preservative-free saline before aspirating. It is best to aspirate at the point of maximum inflammation. Blood cultures yield a pathogen in only about 11% of cases of cellulitis.[3]

Treatment

Cellulitis should be treated with systemic antibiotics. Limited disease of the torso and extremities can be treated with oral antibiotics. Treatment choices include penicillinase-resistant penicillins, first-generation cephalosprins, amoxicillin-clavulonate, broad-spectrum macrolides, second-generation fluoroquinolones, or clindamycin (Table 1). Some clinicians administer an initial dose of intravenous antibiotics (i.e., cefazolin, ceftriaxone) to reduce the risk of progression before starting oral medication. A recent study demonstrated the effectiveness of home-administered once-daily intravenous cefazolin plus oral probenecid.[4]

Close follow-up is important once treatment is started. At the initial visit, the margin of the rash should be traced with a marker. Patients should be seen within 24 hours for reassessment. Most cases will improve after 1 day of treatment, but sometimes it may take several days to see regression. As long as the cellulitis does not progress, it is reasonable to continue the initial antibiotic and monitor patients closely. Once the infection has demonstrated significant regression, patients can be instructed to finish their antibiotics and return as needed.

TABLE 1.   Empiric Treatment of Bacterial Skin Infections
Minocycline or doxycycline 50–100 mg twice daily for 2 to 4 weeks
Dicloxacillin 500 mg four times daily for 7 to 10 days
Amoxicillin/clavulanate (Augmentin) 875/125 mg twice daily for 7 to 10 days
Cephalexin (Keflex) 500 mg four times daily for 7 to 10 days
Cefadroxil (Duricef) 500 mg–1 g twice daily for 7 to 10 days
Clarithromycin (Biaxin) 1 g daily or 500 mg twice daily for 7 to 10 days
Azithromycin (Zithromax) 500 mg once then 250 mg daily for 4 days
Levofloxacin (Levaquin) 500 mg daily for 7 to 10 days
Penicillin 500 mg four times daily for 10 days*

*For streptococcal infection (i.e. erysipelas, perinal cellulitis)
Adapted from Gilbert DN, Moellering RC Jr, Sande MA: The Sanford Guide to Antimicrobial Therapy 2002, 32nd ed; Martins CR: Folliculitis. In: Johns Hopkins Division of Infectious Diseases Antibiotic Guide. http://www.hopkins-abxguide.org/. Accessed Sept. 18, 2002; and Epocrates ID: Infectious Diseases. http://www.epocrates.com/. Accessed Sept. 22, 2002.

Erysipelas

Erysipelas is a more acute and inflamed variant of cellulitis. Although erysipelas is often described as distinct from cellulitis, the differences can be subjective. It is usually caused by group A streptococci and commonly occurs on the lower legs or the face. Erysipelas is redder, more sharply demarcated, and more superficial than typical cellulitis. Lymphatic streaking and systemic symptoms are common. Because erysipelas is more superficial, edema may be less prominent. Repeated episodes of erysipelas can lead to permanent lymphatic damage and chronic stasis.

Some clinicians use penicillin as the drug of choice for erysipelas.[5,6] Other organisms, especially *S. aureus,* may cause more than 20% of cases of erysipelas and these bacteria are often resistant to penicillin.[7,8] Unless streptococcal infection has been confirmed by culture, many clinicians use a broader spectrum antibiotic to cover *S. aureus* as well.[1]

Blistering Distal Dactylitis

Blistering distal dactylitis is a superficial infection of the anterior fat pad of the distal fingers. It is most commonly caused by group A beta-hemolytic streptococci. A painful vesicle or pustule forms in the skin adjacent to the nail bed. These pustules do not tend to protrude like those elsewhere on the body. They should be promptly incised and drained, followed by a 10-day course of antibiotics.

Perianal Cellulitis

Perianal cellulitis is another form of cellulitis caused by group A beta-hemolytic streptococci. It occurs most commonly in children. Patients may present with perirectal itching, rectal pain, or blood-streaked stools. Systemic symptoms are uncommon. On examination, marked circumferential erythema is noted extending as far as 3 cm from the anus. Because recurrences are common, culture should be performed before and after treatment with a 10-day course of oral antibiotics.[2]

Pseudomonas Cellulitis

Pseudomonas aeruginosa typically causes infections in the warm, moist areas that it colonizes: feet, nail beds (green nail), skin folds, foreskin (balanitis), ear canals, and burn sites. *P. aeruginosa* will not grow if normal, dry skin is inoculated.[9]

Pseudomonas infection is characterized by dusky red skin, blue-green purulence, and a fruity odor. *Pseudomonas* also fluoresces green-white under a Wood's lamp because it produces a compound called py-overdin. Neglected lesions can become eroded and even necrotic. Localized infection can be treated with 5% acetic acid compresses for 20 minutes, four times daily until resolution. For *Pseudomonas* balanitis, topical mercurochrome twice daily is effective.[2] These infections can also be treated with systemic first- or second-generation fluoroquinolones.

Impetigo

Epidemiology

Impetigo is a common superficial skin infection that is usually caused by *S. aureus*, but it can also be caused by group A beta-hemolytic strep-tococci or a combination of the two.[10,11] Bullous impetigo is usually caused by a toxigenic staphylococcus strain that causes epidermal cleavage. Impetigo is more commonly seen in children, especially those between 2 and 5 years of age. The rash usually occurs on intact skin, but streptococci require traumatized skin to cause infection. Two to 5% of impetigo cases are complicated by post-streptococcal glomeru-lonephritis, but clusters with rates as high as 15% have been reported.[2]

Signs and Symptoms

Impetigo typically occurs around the nose and mouth or on the limbs. It begins as a vesicle (<5 mm) or cloudy pustule that spontaneously rup-tures to expose a well-demarcated, red, weeping, shallow erosion. In bullous impetigo, vesicles progress to form bullae (>5 mm) before erod-ing. A characteristic honey-colored crust accumulates on the lesions. The infections spread both radially and by autoinoculation to form satellite lesions. Lesions are typically asymptomatic, but some patients may re-port mild pruritis. Regional adenopathy is common, but systemic symp-toms are unusual. Without treatment, lesions can persist for months.

Diagnosis

The diagnosis is based on clinical assessment. In recurrent or resistant cases, Gram stain and culture of the lesions should be performed. The differential diagnosis of impetigo includes varicella (chickenpox), her-pes simplex virus, candidiasis, atopic or contact dermatitis, scabies, and guttate psoriasis. Impetigo can also arise secondarily from these lesions.

Treatment

Treatment should provide coverage for both *S. aureus* and strepto-cocci. Topical treatment with mupirocin 2% ointment/cream (Bac-troban) works well for isolated lesions. It should be applied three times daily for 7 to 14 days or until the infection is clear. Oral antibiotics are favored by many experts, especially when impetigo is extensive.[5,12] Options for systemic treatment include cloxacillin, dicloxacillin, clindamycin, amoxicillin-clavulonate, azithromycin, clarithromycin, first- and second-generation cephalosporins, and second-generation fluoroquinolones. Patients should be warned to use contact precautions until lesions begin to heal.

Recurrent Impetigo

Recurrent impetigo has been linked to carriage of *S. aureus*, especially in the nares. Mupirocin ointment applied to the nares twice daily for 5 days can reduce nasal carriage and infection.[13,14] The 5-day treatment can be repeated monthly in difficult cases.

Ecthyma (Ulcerative Impetigo)

Ecthyma can be considered an ulcerative variation of impetigo. It is caused by streptococci and begins as vesicles or bullae, typically on the legs. These lesions progress to a deeper erosion and have a thick crust that is sometimes gray. Ecthyma arises in minor wounds that are neglected. It should be treated with systemic antibiotics to minimize scarring.

Folliculitis

Inflammation of hair follicles can be caused by a number of processes:
- Infection
  - Bacterial (especially staphylococcal)
  - Fungal
- Reaction to a chemical or allergen
  - Contact dermatitis
  - Follicular urticaria
- Trauma
  - Tight-fitting clothing, hats, or helmets
  - Pseudofolliculitis barbae (shaving)

Bacterial Folliculitis

Signs and Symptoms

Patients with folliculitis have scattered pustules and small red papules centered around hair follicles. Lesions may be mildly pruritic or painful. Systemic symptoms are very rare.

Pustules are confined to hair follicles, typically in one region of the body such as the chest, thighs, or back. However, follicles throughout the body can become infected over the course of a few days. In bacterial infections, most pustules still have a hair shaft protruding from the center. There may be some surrounding erythema and slight swelling.

Main Causes

Staphylococcal Folliculitis. Staphylococcal infection should be suspected if erythema, swelling, and tenderness are striking. If needed, culture should be performed by shaving a pustule with a scalpel and sending the whole pustule for culture. Oral antibiotics are preferred when staphylococcal infection is suspected.[2]

Gram-Negative Folliculitis. The gram-negative organisms *Klebsiella, Enterobacter,* and *Proteus* can also cause folliculitis. Infection typically occurs on the faces of acne patients treated with long-term antibiotics active against gram-positive organisms. Topical erythromycin is usually effective.[9] Severe cases are treated using amoxicillin-clavulonate (Augmentin) or even isotretinoin (Acutane).[1]

Hot Tub Folliculitis. Folliculitis acquired from wet objects such as hot tubs, whirlpools, loofah sponges, or wet suits is usually caused by *Pseudomonas aeruginosa.* Lesions appear on exposed areas of the trunk and extremities between 6 and 72 hours after contact. In immunocompetent patients, lesions typically resolve spontaneously within 10 days. Treatment is not required, but the source should be cleaned and new tub water properly sanitized. *Pseudomonas* in a loofah sponge is killed when the sponge is simply allowed to dry completely.[9] Soaks in 1% to 5% acetic acid,[9,15] topical silver sulfadiazine cream,[9] or garamycin cream[15] may be helpful. If needed, systemic fluoroquinolones can also be used.

Treatment

Topical antibiotics work well in most cases of superficial bacterial folliculitis (Table 2). Antibiotics should be targeted against the presumed etiologic organisms. Therapy should be continued until lesions resolve. If follicles are widely distributed, systemic antibiotics can be used (see Table 1).

Fungal Folliculitis

Fungal follicular infections tend to occur on the scalp (tinea capitis) and face (tinea barbae). Infection in areas other than the scalp or beard often follows the use of topical steroids on sites with superficial fungal infections. Tinea capitis occurs mainly in children and is the most contagious of the superficial fungal infections.[16] *Trichophyton tonsurans* causes more than 90% of cases in the United States. Other organisms include *Microporum canis* and *Microporum audouinii.*

Fungal folliculitis can be difficult to distinguish from bacterial. Tinea is not often suspected until a patient has failed treatment with anti-

TABLE 2. Topical Treatment of Superficial Folliculitis
Mupirocin cream 2% (Bactroban) cream, ointment three times daily
Clindamycin 1% (Cleocin T) gel, lotion, solution twice daily
Erythromycin 2% (T-Stat, ATS) gel, solution twice daily
Sodium sulfacetamide 10% (Klaron) lotion twice daily
Benzoyl peroxide 2.5–10% cream, gel, lotion, wash once or twice daily
Gentamycin 0.1% (Garamycin) cream, ointment
Adapted from Gilbert DN, Moellering RC Jr, Sande MA: The Sanford Guide to Antimicrobial Therapy 2002, 32nd ed; Martins CR: Folliculitis. In: Johns Hopkins Division of Infectious Diseases Antibiotic Guide. http://www.hopkins-abxguide.org/. Accessed September 18, 2002; Epocrates ID: Infectious Diseases. http://www.epocrates.com/. Accessed Sept. 22, 2002.

biotics. Hints toward tinea infection include a more insidious onset, alopecia, scaling, and fewer pustules than seen in bacterial folliculitis. Involved hairs in fungal infections can be removed with only gentle manipulation. Hairs that have broken close to the skin surface may appear as black dots. *M. audouinii* fluoresces under black light but *T. tonsurans* does not. Fungal culture of scales and several hairs can be performed for speciation.

Systemic antifungals are needed to penetrate the follicle. Although resistance is emerging, griseofulvin remains the drug of choice.[16,17] However, concerns regarding resistance and drug toxicity prompt many clinicians to use terbenifine, itraconazole or fluconazole instead.[5] Close contacts should be prophylactically treated with ketoconazole or selenium sulfide shampoo.[2]

Noninfectious Folliculitis

Follicular Urticaria

Follicular urticaria is a variant of urticaria, or hives. As with most cases of urticaria, the cause is usually not discovered. In follicular urticaria, lesions appear more vesicular than pustular and may have a surrounding wheal. Follicular urticaria is usually very pruritic but nontender. Treatment is the same as for typical urticaria (antihistamines, steroids, etc).

Pseudofolliculitis Barbae

Also called *razor bumps,* pseudofolliculitis is not an infection but a foreign body reaction to hair that has been shaved below the opening of the hair shaft. It is more common among African-Americans and typically appears as red follicular papules and pustules on the neck. Symptoms of pruritis continue until the hair grows above the surface or is dislodged. Treatment includes avoidance of shaving or changing shaving techniques. Because bacteria can aggravate the problem, antibiotics may speed recovery.[2]

Furuncle and Carbuncle

Furuncles, or boils, represent a progression of bacterial folliculitis. An abscess extends out from an infected follicle, forming a painful, red, firm nodule. Carbuncles are conglomerations of coalescing furuncles. Systemic symptoms may occur with carbuncles but not furuncles. *S. aureus* is the most common pathogen, but anatomically localized microflorae also play a role. For example, perianal abscesses can be caused by fecal flora and head-neck abscess may be due to anaerobes.

Furuncles and carbuncles are self-limited. With time, the lesions become fluctuant and will either point to the surface and open or be reabsorbed. Warm compresses are the mainstay of treatment. Topical antibiotics are of no use. Systemic antistaphylococcal antibiotics can be helpful in early cases before furuncles have pointed.[9] Many clinicians reserve antibiotics for carbuncles or for patients with fever or secondary cellulitis. Once lesions have pointed and become fluctuant, incision and drainage hastens recovery. It is harmful to incise deeper lesions.[15] Patients with recurrent furuncles or carbuncles can be treated to eradicate *S. aureus* carriage. This can be accomplished with nasal mupirocin ointment for 5 days or an oral penicillinase-resistant penicillin for 14 days.[9]

Superficial Fungal Infections

Tinea

Tinea infections are caused by dermatophytes from three genera, *Trichophyton, Microsporum,* and *Epidermophyton.* The lifetime risk of dermatophyte infection is between 10% and 20%.[18] These infections are typically named for the site that is infected.

Because other skin diseases mimic fungal infections, it is best to confirm the presence of fungus. Culture can be reserved for complicated cases, but it is very simple to perform a potassium hydroxide (KOH) preparation for microscopy. Scales should be scraped from the leading edge of lesions and placed on a microscope slide. One or two drops of KOH (10–20%) are added and a cover slip placed on top. The slide is then either heated or allowed to sit at room temperature for 10 to 15 minutes. A microscope is then used to search for the branching hyphae characteristic of dermatophyte infections. A drop of ink or fungal stain can make the hyphae easier to find.[2]

Tinea Pedis

Tinea pedis, or athlete's foot, is the most common dermatophytic infection.[18] Tinea pedis typically occurs in hot and humid weather when the patient is wearing occlusive footwear. It can present in three patterns (sometimes all in the same patient):

* Interdigital (especially third and fourth spaces) maceration and cracking
* Scaling, hyperkeratotic lesions in a ballet shoe or moccasin distribution
* Scattered, very pruritic, vesiculobullous lesions

Tinea Cruris

Tinea cruris, or jock itch, is a caused by *Epidermophyton floccosum* or *Trichophyton rubrum* infection of the intertriginous areas in male patients.

Tinea Corporis

Tinea corporis, or ringworm, is caused by *T. rubrum* or by *Trichophyton verrucosum*, or *Microsporum canis* (from animal contact). Tinea corporis can refer to tinea anywhere except the scalp, beard, hands, or groin. The classic ringworm appearance demonstrates annular plaques with erythema and scaling. The center clears to a dusky or brown color as the lesion extends radially. Unlike other tinea infections, tinea corporis occurs in exposed areas.

Treatment

First-line treatment for tinea is topical, with allylamines (naftifine, butenafine, terbinafine) being slightly more effective (Table 3).[19] Treatment should be continued for 1 week after cure. This will typically take 2 weeks for tinea corporis and tinea cruris. Tinea pedis may require 4 weeks of treatment. Chronic or resistant cases may require the use of oral agents such as itraconazole, terbinafine, griseofulvin, or once-weekly fluconazole.[18] Environmental factors are also important in treatment and prevention. Keeping clothing, shoes, and skin dry can be very helpful. Treating shoes with antifungal powder may also be helpful.[12] When tinea is especially inflamed and pruritic, some clinicians will use a topical steroid in conjunction with antifungal therapy, at least early in therapy. This approach helps to alleviate symptoms quickly and may even hasten resolution of the infection.[20]

Tinea Versicolor

Tinea versicolor is a misnomer because it is not actually a tinea or dermatophyte. The name *pityriasis* is more appropriate for this infection, which is caused by *Malassezia furfur*. Versicolor presents as hypopigmented macules (sometimes hyperpigmented) scattered on the shoulders, upper back, and chest. The macules may be pink, red, light-brown, or white and have a slight scale, which may only be seen after scratching.

TABLE 3. Topical Antifungal Medications		
Medication	Available Formulations	Dosing
Imidazoles		
Clotrimazole 1% (Lotrimin, Mycelex)*	C, S, L	Twice daily
Econazole 2% (Spectazole)	C	Daily
Ketoconazole 2% (Nizoral)	C, Sh	Daily Every 3 to 4 days for Sh
Miconazole 2% (Micatin, Monistat)*	C, P, Sp	Twice daily
Oxiconazole 1% (Oxistat)	C, L	Once to twice daily
Sulconazole 1% (Exelderm)	C, S	Once to twice daily
Allylamines		
Terbinafine 1% (Lamisil)*	C, S, Sp	Once to twice daily
Naftifine 1% (Naftin)	C, G	Once to twice daily
Butenafine 1% (Mentax)	C	Once daily
Miscellaneous		
Ciclopirox 1% (Loprox, Penlac)	C, L	Twice daily
Nystatin 1 million units/g (Mycolog)	C, O, P	Two to three times daily
Haloprogin 1% (Halotex)	C, S	Twice daily
Tolnaftate 1% (Tinactin)*	C, S, P	Twice daily
Amphotericin B 3% (Fungizone)	C, L, O	Two to four times daily
Undecylenic acid (Cruex, Desenex)*	C, S, P, G	Twice daily

*Nonprescription
C, cream; G, gel; L, lotion; P, powder; S, solution; Sh, shampoo; Sp, spray; O, ointment.
Adapted from Weinstein A, Berman B: Topical treatment of common superficial tinea infections. Am Fam Phys 65:2095–2102, 2002.

The hypopigmentation may only be noted after sun exposure. The macules are sometimes mistaken for vitiligo, but vitiligo is characterized by a complete loss of pigment. Versicolor will fluoresce a gold or orange-brown color under a Wood lamp. KOH preparation of scales reveals nonbranching hyphae and clusters of round spores, described as the "spaghetti-and-meatballs" pattern.

Pityriasis versicolor responds well to topical therapy with dandruff shampoos containing selenium sulfide (Selsun) or pyrithione zinc (Head & Shoulders). A lather should be applied to the affected skin and left to sit for 10 minutes daily for 1 week. Ketoconazole shampoo is another option that can be used twice weekly for 4 weeks. Topical antifungal agents are also recommended by some practitioners.[6,21]

Widespread or persistent cases can be treated with oral ketoconazole. Ketoconazole can be given as 200 mg daily for 7 to 10 days. Another option is 400 mg ketoconazole once, and some practitioners consider this the treatment of choice.[5] This should be followed by exercise to induce sweating, and the patient should wait 1 day before showering. This should be repeated in 1 week. Other oral regimens include fluconazole 300 to 400 mg once or itraconazole 400 g daily for 3 to 7 days.[5]

The discoloration of pityriasis versicolor does not resolve immediately following treatment. Normal pigmentation will not return until the skin is exposed to sunlight. Response to treatment is presumed when the scales disappear.

Onychomycosis

Onychomycosis is a fungal infection of the nail bed, matrix, or plate. It accounts for one third of fungal skin infections and one half of all nail dystrophies.[22] Infection is more common in toenails than fingernails and is usually associated with tinea pedis. Infection can be caused by dermatophytes and other molds as well as by yeasts.

Infection usually starts at the distal, free edge of the nail. The edge of the nail is discolored white-yellow-brown and an accumulation of subungual white hyperkeratosis lifts the nail from the bed. The nail surface itself can become rough, furrowed, and brittle, especially in *Candida* infections. If all nails are affected, the dystrophy is likely noninfectious (i.e., psoriasis, lichen planus, trauma). If diagnosis is in doubt, fungal infection can be confirmed by potassium hydroxide preparation or culture.

Treatment of onychomycosis can be very challenging. Topical treatment even with newer agents such as ciclopirox (Penlac), rarely achieves cure.[3,22] Systemic regimens can be effective, but relapses, drug interactions, and hepatic or hematpoietic toxicity are common. Terbinifine (Lamisil) 250 mg daily for 6 (fingernails) to 12 (toenails) weeks is very effective, but complete blood cell count and liver enzyme tests must be monitored. Itraconazole (Sporanox) is also effective in a 6- to 12-week regimen of 200 mg daily. Liver enzyme tests should be monitored with itraconazole as well, but not when using pulse therapy. Pulse therapy is itraconazole 200 mg daily for 1 week during each of 2 to 4 months. There is also an effective pulse therapy regimen using fluconazole (Diflucan), but this is not approved by the Food and Drug Administration. Fluconazole 150 to 450 mg once weekly is given for 3 to 12 months. Liver enzymes need not be monitored when prescribing fluconazole.

The true relapse rate of onychomycosis is difficult to measure. If culture was not initially performed, it should be done for relapses before another treatment is considered. Controlling moisture and tinea pedis may help prevent relapses.

Viral Skin Infections

Common Warts

Common warts, or verruca vulgaris, are caused by human papillomavirus infection, of which there are over 60 types. The virus infects keratinocytes by direct contact. Warts often resolve spontaneously.

Groups of hyperkeratotic, cylindrical projections form and often make up a distinct mosaic pattern when fused. The lesions are typically less than 1 cm in diameter and remain confined to the epidermis. Warts can be differentiated from other lesions (molluscum contagiosum, seborrheic keratosis) by the red to brown dots within them, which are actually thrombosed capillaries. Warts are diagnosed by visual inspection. A hand lens is often helpful, as is paring with a scalpel, which can reveal the black dots and mosaic pattern described above.

Treatment

Common warts can be treated a number of different ways, including salicylic acid, bichloroacetic acid cantharidin, podophyllin, liquid nitrogen, tretinoin cream, intralesional interferon, blunt dissection, and electrocautery. The site and size of the lesion should be considered when deciding upon therapy. For instance, treatment of plantar warts can be lengthy and painful. Warts often require several treatment sessions. Warts disrupt the normal "fingerprint lines" of the skin. Watching for the return of these lines is helpful in monitoring response to treatment.

Molluscum Contagiosum

Molluscum contagiosum is caused by a poxvirus. Like warts, this infection occurs by direct contact. Typically, the lesions will resolve spontaneously within 9 months.

The asymptomatic lesions are discrete papules measuring a few millimeters in diameter and are pink to pearly-white, dome-shaped, and umbilicated in the center. The periphery of the lesions is often erythematous. These lesions can be sexually transmitted, causing lesions on the genitals or the suprapubic area. The presence of extensive facial lesions should prompt suspicion of human immunodeficiency virus (HIV) infection. The diagnosis is usually made on inspection. If necessary, diagnosis can be confirmed by microscopic examination of the core of an individual lesion. The core is removed and placed on a slide with potassium hydroxide and heated. Infected epithelial cells lose their flat, rectangular shape and become dark, round, and nonadherent to their neighboring epithelial cells. Treatment options include liquid nitrogen, isotretinoin blunt dissection, electrocautery, and imiquimod (Aldara).[23]

Nongenital Herpes Simplex Infection

Although better known for causing genital herpes, the herpes simplex virus (HSV) can infect skin anywhere on the body. HSV type 1 is a more common cause of these nongenital infections. The major difference is that type 2 is more prone to recurrence.

The virus is spread by direct contact and respiratory droplets.[2] Primary infection occurs within 1 week of contact, frequently beginning with generalized symptoms such as fever, headache, and myalgias. Clusters of uniformly sized vesicles appear on an erythematous base. The vesicles erode and heal over a course of 2 to 6 weeks. During primary infection, virus ascends peripheral nerves to dorsal root ganglia, where it enters a latent stage. Secondary infection occurs through reactivation of these dormant clusters of virus. Secondary lesions are typically preceded by tingling, itching, or burning and are sometimes preceded by a prodrome of generalized symptoms.

There are a number of manifestations of HSV infection. Lesions that occur on the fingers are called herpetic whitlow. Herpes gladiatorum, classically described in wrestlers, occurs on abraded or traumatized skin. Vesicles can occur near the eye and should be taken very seriously, since ophthalmic infection can lead to permanent visual impairment. Prompt ophthalmology referral is crucial in such cases.

Nongenital herpes infections may be treated with acyclovir, valacyclovir, or famciclovir. Prophylaxis can be used for frequent recurrences (more than six per year). Prophylaxis should also be considered for patients in whom recurrence presents an occupational limitation (e.g., those in health care or athletics).

References

1. Stulberg DL, Penrod MA, Blatny RA: Common bacterial skin infections. Am Fam Phys 66:119–124, 2002.
2. Habif TP: Clinical Dermatology, 3rd ed. St. Louis: Mosby-Year Book, 1996.
3. Perl B, Gottehrer, Raveh D, et al: Cost-effectiveness of blood cultures for adult patients with cellulitis. Clin Infect Dis 29:1483–1488, 1999.
4. Grayson ML, McDonald M, Gibson K, et al: Once-daily intravenous cefazolin plus oral probenecid is equivalent to once-daily intravenous ceftriaxone plus oral placebo for the treatment of moderate-to-severe cellulitis in adults. Clin Infect Dis 34:1440–1448, 2002.
5. Gilbert DN, Moellering RC Jr, Sande MA: The Sanford Guide to Antimicrobial Therapy, 32nd ed. Hyde Park, VT, Antimicrobial Therapy, Inc., 2002.
6. Martins CR: Folliculitis. In: Johns Hopkins Division of Infectious Diseases Antibiotic Guide. Accessed Sept. 18, 2002 at http://www.hopkins-abxguide.org/.
7. Eriksson B, Jorup-Ronstrum C, Karkkonen K, et al: Erysipelas: Clinical and bacteriologic spectrum and serologic aspects. Clin Infect Dis 23:1091–1098, 1996.
8. Chartier C, Grosshans E: Erysipelas: An update. Int J Dermatol 35:779–781, 1996.
9. Rhody C: Bacterial infections of the skin. Primary Care Clin Office Pract 27:459–473, 2000.
10. Barton LL, Friedman AD: Impetigo: A reassessment of etiology and therapy. Pediatr Dermatol 4:185–188, 1987.
11. Misko ML, Terracina JR, Diven DG: The frequency of erythromycin-resistant Staphylococcus aureus in impetiginized dermatoses. Pediatr Dermatol 12:12–15, 1995.

12. Fitzpatrick TB, Johnson RA, Polano MK: Color Atlas and Synopsis of Clinical Dermatology. New York: McGraw-Hill, 1997.
13. Raz, Miron D, Colodner R, Staler Z, et al: A 1-year trial of nasal mupirocin in the prevention of recurrent staphylococcal colonization and skin infection. Arch Intern Med 156:1109–1112, 1996.
14. Doebbeling BN, Reagan DR, Pfaller MA, et al: Long-term efficacy of intranasal mupirocin ointment: A prospective cohort study of Staphylococcus aureus carriage. Arch Intern Med 154:1505–1508, 1994.
15. Sadick NS: Infectious diseases in dermatology: Current aspects of bacterial infections of the skin. Dermatol Clin 15:341–349, 1997.
16. Nesbitt LT: Treatment of tinea capitis. Int J Dermatol 39:261–262, 2000.
17. Bennett ML, Fleischer AB, Loveless JW: Oral griseofulvin (330–500 mg daily for 4–8 weeks) remains the treatment of choice for tinea capitis in children. Pediatr Dermatol 17:304–309, 2000.
18. Noble SL, Forbes RC, Stamm PL: Diagnosis and management of common tinea infections. Am Fam Phys 58:163–174, 177–178, 1998.
19. Hart R, Bell-Syer SEM, Crawford F, et al: Systematic review of topical treatments for fungal infections of the skin and nails of the feet. BMJ 319:79–82, 1999.
20. Weinstein A, Berman B: Topical treatment of common superficial tinea infections. Am Fam Phys 65:2095–2102, 2002.
21. Epocrates ID: Infectious Diseases. Accessed Sept. 22, 2002 at http://www.epocrates.com/.
22. Rodgers P, Bassler M: Treating onychomycosis. Am Fam Phys 63:663–672, 2001.
23. Dockrell DH, Kinghorn GR: Imiquimod and resiquimod as novel immunomodulators. J Antimicrob Chemotherapy 48:751–755, 2001.

Necrotizing Skin and Soft Tissue Infections

chapter 16

Henry M. Wu, M.D., D.T.M.&H.

Throughout the late 1980s and 1990s, outbreaks of necrotizing fasciitis caused by invasive group A streptococci raised public awareness about "flesh-eating bacteria."[1-3] While necrotizing fasciitis has been described throughout history,[2] increased public awareness of this uncommon but devastating infection quickly made it a "hot topic." Physicians must be familiar with this and other necrotizing soft tissue infections because of the urgent diagnosis and treatment that is necessary to control these aggressive and potentially lethal infections.

Types of Necrotizing Skin and Soft Tissue Infections

Necrotizing soft tissue infections can be classified by the tissue layer affected as well as the types of pathogens involved. Recalling soft tissue anatomy helps clarify the often-confusing nomenclature (Table 1). It should be noted, however, that progression of necrotizing soft tissue infections often leads to multiple levels of involvement.

Superficial Infections

Most superficial infections of the skin (e.g., erysipelas, impetigo, and cellulitis) are non-necrotizing and are described thoroughly in Chapter 15. Superficial necrotizing infections do exist and include gangrenous cellulitis of various causes, clostridial and nonclostridial anaerobic cellulitis, and several other syndromes.[4] They have patterns similar to their deep-tissue counterparts in regard to microbiology and general management principles, although these tend to cause less systemic toxicity.[4-6] This chapter focuses on necrotizing deep-tissue infections, since these are generally life-threatening and may be more difficult to recognize.

Necrotizing Fasciitis

Pathophysiology. In necrotizing fasciitis, fulminant bacterial infection of the subcutaneous tissue results in liquefactive necrosis of the superficial

TABLE 1. Anatomic Localization of Soft Tissue Infections*

Anatomic Tissues	Infectious Syndromes
Skin 　Epidermis 　Dermis	Erysipelas Impetigo Ecthyma Folliculitis, furunculosis, carbunculosis Cellulitis Gangrenous cellulitis[t] Anaerobic cellulitis[t]
Subcutaneous tissue 　Superficial fascia 　Subcutaneous fat 　Nerves, arteries, veins 　Deep fascia	Necrotizing fasciitis[t] Cellulitis Gangrenous cellulitis[t] Anaerobic cellulitis[t]
Muscle	Myositis/myonecrosis[t] Pyomyositis

*Necrotizing infections may secondarily affect other tissue layers.
[t]Necrotizing soft-tissue infections
Adapted from Green RJ, Dafoe DC, Raffin TA: Necrotizing fasciitis. Chest 110:219–229, 1996.

fascia, subcutaneous fat, and deep fascia.[2,6] Historic and modern terms referring to the infection and its subtypes include *hospital gangrene, phagedena, hemolytic streptococcal gangrene, progressive synergistic bacterial gangrene,* and many others.[2] Superficial skin initially remains intact as the necrosis extends along fascial planes in as little as a few hours.[6] The exudate is thin and often described as "dishwater pus."[2,6] Vascular thrombosis leads to necrosis of large areas of skin.[6]

Necrotizing fasciitis can affect any area of the body, but abdominal wall, extremities, and perineum are the most common.[2] The infection begins with the introduction of pathogens into the subcutaneous fascia. Possible routes include trauma, injections, cutaneous infections (including cellulitis, ulcers, abscesses, and varicella), insect bites, deep infections, or hematogenous spread from distant sites.[2,5] Inciting trauma may be minor and even unnoticed; some cases are idiopathic.[2,5]

Abdominal wall necrotizing fasciitis is usually a postoperative complication, particularly after fecal contamination of the abdominal cavity.[2] Abdominal wall infections have also occurred after gut perforation,[5] or secondary to other abdominal pathologies.[2] Fournier's gangrene typically refers to necrotizing fasciitis of the male genitalia and perineum, usually secondary to local infections (genitourinary, intra-abdominal, or perianal), trauma, or instrumentation.[2] Vulvar involvement in women has been described and has similar causes.[2] Head and neck cases are rare but particularly dangerous, given the possibility of spread along cervical fascial planes and involvement of major blood vessels and the mediastinum.[2]

Microbiology. Culture of microorganisms from infection sites reveals two major types of necrotizing fasciitis. Type I is polymicrobial, involving a mix of anaerobic and facultative bacteria, often including Enterobacteriaceae and non-group A streptococci.[2,5] Type II infections are caused by group A β-hemolytic streptococci (primarily *Streptococcus pyogenes*) alone or with staphylococci.[2,5] Increased virulence of some group A streptococcal strains may be related to exotoxins, surface proteins, and variable levels of immunity among hosts.[5,7,8]

Abdominal and perineal infections tend to be type I in nature and are typically caused by enteric pathogens.[2] Common bacteria include gram-negative enteric bacilli, enterococci, and anaerobic species, such as *Bacteroides* and *Clostridium* species.[2] Most studies have shown that necrotizing fasciitis of the extremities and idiopathic cases tend to be type II in etiology.[2] However, many observational studies may not have used rigorous anaerobic bacteria isolation methods, and one large case series described mostly polymicrobial infections predominated by anaerobes in any site.[9]

Marine *Vibrio* species, most notably *Vibrio vulnificus*, may cause necrotizing fasciitis following contact with seawater, fish, or shellfish.[2] Other causes include group B streptococci, *Pasturella multocida,* and *Candida* species.[2]

Risk Factors. Risk factors for necrotizing fasciitis are numerous and include diabetes mellitus, alcohol abuse, immunosuppression, intravenous drug abuse, peripheral vascular disease, malnutrition, and obesity.[2,5,6,9] However, young, otherwise healthy individuals can also be affected, particularly when the infection is caused by virulent strains of group A strepococci.[2,3] Some studies have linked prior nonsteroidal anti-inflammatory drug use to the development of necrotizing fasciitis.[2] Nonsteroidal anti-inflammatory drugs may attenuate inflammatory signs and delay diagnosis, or possibly affect host immune responses.[10] Therefore, some authors suggest caution or avoidance of these commonly used drugs for patients with soft tissue infections.[2,5]

Clinical Presentation. Patients usually present acutely with local signs of inflammation: redness, heat, swelling, and marked tenderness.[2,5] Margins may be indistinct.[2] Fever, tachycardia, tachypnea, and hypotension are also common signs.[2,5] In the earlier stages of infection, systemic toxicity and pain classically appear out of proportion to local findings.[5] The subcutaneous tissue may have a "wooden-hard" consistency on palpation,[3] and subcutaneous emphysema and crepitus may be present.[3,5] The usual disease course results in patches of blue-gray skin that progress to hemorrhagic cutaneous bullae and necrosis over

3 to 5 days.[2,5] Localized tenderness progresses to anesthesia secondary to sensory nerve destruction.[5,6] Circumferential involvement of a limb may lead to compartment syndrome and myonecrosis.[3] Septic shock ensues as exotoxins and bacteria are released into the blood.[2] Metastatic abscesses can occur in distant sites.[2,6]

In cases of infection due to group A streptococci, the presence of shock and organ failure completes the constellation of streptococcal toxic shock syndrome.[10] Among cases of streptococcal toxic shock syndrome, necrotizing fasciitis may be present in as many as 50%.[10]

Clostridial Myonecrosis

Pathophysiology, Microbiology, and Risk Factors. Clostridial myonecrosis refers to fulminant skeletal muscle infection caused by *Clostridium* species.[5] Commonly called gas gangrene, the infection has a prominent history as a complication of battlefield wounds. Prior to widespread use of antibiotics and improved surgical interventions, clostridial myonecrosis complicated as many as 5% of battlefield injuries in World War II.[5]

Clostridia are anaerobic, gram-positive rods found widely in the soil and as a colonizer of humans and animals.[6] Following inoculation, clostridia multiply in the anaerobic environment created by trauma, impaired blood supply, and foreign bodies.[5] Exotoxins appear to mediate a rapidly spreading myonecrosis, and extensive gas formation is classic.[5,6] *Clostridium perfringens* is the most common cause of clostridial myonecrosis, although other clostridia can also cause the infection.[5] As many as 60% to 85% of infections may additionally involve nonclostridial bacteria.[6]

Clostridial myonecrosis can be divided into three categories: post-traumatic, postoperative (nontraumatic), and spontaneous.[5] Causes of post-traumatic clostridial myonecrosis include compound fractures, other potentially contaminated injuries, burns, injections, and decubitus ulcers.[5] Procedures that may be complicated by postoperative clostridial myonecrosis include abdominal surgery, amputations, and other types of surgery.[5] Diabetes, advanced age, immunosuppression, chronic edema, and chronic debilitating illnesses have also been described as risk factors for clostridial myonecrosis.[5,6] Spontaneous clostridial myonecrosis is usually caused by *C. septicum* bacteremia, which is associated with lower gastrointestinal (particularly cecal) malignancies, diabetes, and neutropenic colitis.[5]

Clinical Presentation. Following the initial inoculation or traumatic event, an incubation period of 1 to 4 days is typical,[6] but a range of 1 hour to 6 weeks has been described.[5] Clostridial myonecrosis is classically characterized by a triad of severe pain, tachycardia out of proportion to fever, and crepitus on examination.[5] Early signs in postoperative cases include changes in wound appearance, pain, or onset of systemic toxicity.[5] Signs of progression include edema, bronze purplish or brown skin discoloration, mottling, and bullae with serosanguinous discharge.[5,6] Hypotension, shock, severe hemolysis, and acute renal failure may occur.[5,6]

General Approach and Differential Diagnosis

Since spread to adjacent tissues and progression to sepsis and death can occur in as little as a few hours,[2,5,6] a high index of suspicion is essential for necrotizing soft tissue infections. Delays in diagnosis and surgical débridement have been shown to increase mortality.[2,3,5,8,11] Although they may have different presentations, all types of necrotizing soft tissue infections have similar management principles, and any suspected case requires emergency surgical exploration and the initiation of adjunct treatment measures.[8]

It can be difficult to differentiate necrotizing soft tissue infections from non-necrotizing skin infections.[11] Because the deeper necrotizing infections do not initially affect the skin, symptoms and signs out of proportion to local findings are an early characteristic.[2,5,11] Crepitus, severe pain, and systemic toxicity are uncommon in cellulitis, and these findings should always raise suspicion for a deeper process.[5] Erysipelas usually manifests with well-demarcated borders, lymphangitis, lymphadenopathy, and minimal swelling, all of which are uncharacteristic of necrotizing fasciitis.[2,5,6] Other clues that suggest necrotizing fasciitis include firmness of the subcutaneous tissues beyond the area of skin involvement,[3] cutaneous anesthesia,[8] and cellulitis that does not respond to antibiotics in 24 to 48 hours.[3,11]

Recent history of trauma, surgery, or local infections should always raise the index of suspicion for a necrotizing infection. Patient risk factors such as diabetes mellitus, renal insufficiency, malnutrition, immunosupression, or history of intravenous drug use should also raise concern.[11] However, the absence of these conditions should never rule out the possibility of a necrotizing soft tissue infection.

Diagnostic Tests

A number of tests may be useful in the evaluation of a necrotizing soft tissue infection:

- *Laboratory tests* are generally nonspecific, and the leukocyte count may not be elevated.[5] Elevations in creatine phophokinase can reflect tissue necrosis.[8] Fat necrosis may lead to hypocalcemia.[5]
- *Blood culture* samples should always be collected, and they may reveal the causative pathogens in a significant number of cases.[5,9]

- *Rapid bedside procedures* that may assist in the diagnosis or management of necrotizing fasciitis include fine needle aspiration of the affected area,[11] frozen section biopsy,[5] measurements of muscle compartment pressure,[10] and probing along a fascial plane via a limited incision to assess for pathologic loss of resistance.[5,8]
- *Imaging* of the affected area can aid in determining the extent of involvement. *Plain radiographs* may reveal soft tissue gas, particularly in cases of clostridal myonecrosis.[5] However, gas may also be present in soft tissues secondary to a variety of traumatic and iatrogenic causes,[5] and the absence of gas on any study cannot rule out clostridial myonecrosis.[11] *Computed tomography* and *magnetic resonance imaging* show superior resolution of soft tissues.[12] These studies may help distinguish necrotizing soft tissue infections from cellulitis.[3,12] Computed tomography and magnetic resonance imaging may also evaluate the extent of infection, particularly in cases of cervical necrotizing fasciitis.[2] *Ultrasonography* can be particularly useful in differentiating Fournier's gangrene from other scrotal pathology.[2] Nevertheless, waiting for imaging results should never delay surgical consultation in cases that raise strong suspicion of a necrotizing soft tissue infection.[8]

Treatment Principles

Surgical Exploration and Débridement

As previously emphasized, early surgical intervention plays a central role in the diagnosis and management of necrotizing skin and soft tissue infections.[4–6] Surgical exploration of necrotizing fasciitis reveals dull gray fascia, thin brownish discharge, and a lack of resistance along fascial planes with blunt dissection.[6,8] In cases of clostridial myonecrosis, skeletal muscle necrosis is seen and gas is frequently encountered when entering the muscular compartment.[5]

Discharge and tissue samples should be collected and sent for Gram stain, cultures (aerobic and anaerobic), and susceptibility testing.[6] In necrotizing fasciitis, there is usually good correlation between Gram stain and culture results.[2] In suspected clostridial myonecrosis, Gram stain of wound discharge or tissue that reveals gram-positive rods without polymorphonuclear cells is diagnostic.[5] Culturing clostridia and other anaerobes from a wound may be difficult and requires special methods.[6,9]

All nonviable tissues must be excised until a healthy border is reached.[2,5] Wounds are left open in patients with necrotizing fasciitis as well as in cases of clostridial myonecrosis with significant soft tissue damage or contamination.[6] Repeat evaluations are necessary for patients with necrotizing fasciitis at 24-hour intervals and may also be necessary in cases of clostridial myonecrosis.[5,6] Multiple débridements or limb amputation may be required to control the infection.[2,5,6,9]

Antibiotics

Intravenous antibiotics should also be started early upon suspicion of a necrotizing soft tissue infection.[5] For necrotizing fasciitis, initial empiric therapy should cover streptococci, anaerobes, enteric gram-negative rods, and staphylococci.[5,8] Suggested regimens include combinations of a penicillin or cephalosporin, an aminoglycoside, and anaerobic coverage with either clindamycin or metronidazole.[2,3] Beta-lactamase inhibitor combinations (e.g., ampicillin/sulbactam) have also been suggested.[5,8] In nosocomial and some community-acquired settings, infection from methicillin-resistant *Staphylococcus aureus* is possible, and vancomycin may be considered.[3] Results of Gram stain, cultures, and susceptibility testing can assist in narrowing coverage.

High-dose penicillin is traditionally considered the drug of choice for treatment of group A streptococci, particularly due to *Streptococcus pyogenes* infections.[2] However, there are theoretical advantages of clindamycin, including its inhibition of bacterial toxin synthesis.[7] In experimental models of deep *S. pyogenes* infection, clindamycin has been shown to be superior.[7] For this reason, the addition of clindamycin to regimens has been suggested for any possible invasive streptococcal infection.[3,8,10]

Patients with suspected clostridial myonecrosis should be treated with high-dose intravenous penicillin.[6] Some sources also recommend the addition of clindamycin for similar reasons as in necrotizing fasciitis.[5] In penicillin-allergic patients, metronidazole has been combined with clindamycin.[5] Given that infections may be polymicrobial and the diagnosis of clostridial myonecrosis may initially be uncertain, broad-spectrum antibiotic coverage, as for necrotizing fasciitis, is prudent pending surgical exploration and microbiologic testing.

Other Treatment Modalities

Supportive measures such as fluid and electrolyte replacement, nutritional support, and intensive care are important adjunctive measures in these critically ill patients.[5,6] Ensuring that the patient has adequate tetanus immunity is also important with any cutaneous injury.[5]

Although controversial, hyperbaric oxygen (HBO) has been suggested as an adjunctive treatment for necrotizing soft tissue infections.[13] The theoretical benefits are strongest for clostridial myonecrosis, because HBO inhibits clostridial growth and the production of one of the exotoxins.[5] Limited experimental and clinical evidence supports adjunctive HBO in the treatment of clostridial myonecrosis[13]; however, no controlled trials have been performed.

There is less evidence supporting the use of HBO as an adjunctive treatment for necrotizing fasciitis,[13] and it should never be pursued prior to surgical débridement.[2] Some evidence supports the use of intravenous immunoglobulin for group A streptococcal necrotizing fasciitis and streptococcal toxic shock syndrome,[8,10,14] although there have been no prospective clinical trials.

Outcome

Following débridement and stabilization, intensive wound management is required. Closure of the site may require consultation of plastic surgeons.

Reported mortality rates for necrotizing fasciitis range widely, from as low as 9% to more than 70%.[5] The case-fatality rate for necrotizing fasciitis in the United States from 1989 to 1991 was 28%.[5] A similarly wide range of case-fatality rates has been described in various case series of clostridial myonecrosis.[5]

References

1. Nowak R: Flesh-eating bacteria: Not new, but still worrisome. Science 264:1665, 1994.
2. Green RJ, Dafoe DC, Raffin TA: Necrotizing fasciitis. Chest 110:219–229, 1996.
3. Stone DR, Gorbach SL: Necrotizing fasciitis: The changing spectrum. Dermatol Clin 15:213–220, 1997.
4. Swartz MN: Cellulitis and subcutaneous tissue infections. In: Mandell GL, Bennett JE, Dolin R, eds: Mandell, Douglas, and Bennett's Principles and Practice of Infectious Diseases, 5th ed. Philadelphia: Churchill Livingstone, 2000:1037–1057.
5. Chapnick EK, Abter EI: Necrotizing soft-tissue infections. Infect Dis Clin North Am 10:835–855, 1996.
6. Gonzalez MH: Necrotizing fasciitis and gangrene of the upper extremity. Hand Clin 14:635–645, 1998.
7. Stevens DL: Invasive group A streptococcal disease. Infect Agents Dis 5:157–166, 1996.
8. File TM, Tan JS, Dipersio JR: Group A streptococcal necrotizing fasciitis: Diagnosis and treating the "flesh-eating bacteria syndrome." Cleve Clin J Med 65:241–249, 1998.
9. Brook I, Frazier EH: Clinical and microbiological features of necrotizing fasciitis. J Clin Microbiol 33:2382–2387, 1995.
10. Bisno AL, Stevens DL: Streptococcal infections of skin and soft tissues. N Engl J Med 334:240–245, 1996.
11. Lille ST, Sato TT, Engrav LH, Foy H, Jurkovich GJ: Necrotizing soft tissue infections: Obstacles in diagnosis. J Am Coll Surg 182:7–11, 1996.
12. Struk DW, Munk PL, Lee MJ, et al: Imaging of soft tissue infections. Radiol Clin North Am 39:277–303, 2001.
13. Tibbles PM, Edelsberg JS: Hyperbaric-oxygen therapy. N Engl J Med 334:1642–1648, 1996.
14. Trent JT, Kirsner RS: Diagnosing necrotizing fasciitis. Adv Skin Wound Care 15:135–138, 2002.

Management of Dog, Cat, and Human Bites

chapter
17

Vincent Lo Re III, M.D.

A first glance, the inclusion of a chapter on the management of bites as a "hot topic" might seem strange. However, each year, several million Americans are bitten by animals, resulting in approximately 300,000 visits to emergency departments, 10,000 hospitalizations, and 20 deaths, mostly among young children.[1] Half of Americans at some time during their lives are bitten by a cat or a dog.[2]

A bite from a pet or even a human may send some people to seek medical attention. Prompt assessment and treatment can avert most problems. Wound management should address the physical trauma of a bite as well as the risk of infection, including tetanus and rabies. This chapter reviews the bacteriology of dog, cat, and human bite wounds, discusses the critical features of the initial evaluation, and provides recommended therapies. Tetanus and rabies prophylaxes are also addressed.

Dog Bites

The most common animal bite injuries in the United States are inflicted by dogs, accounting for approximately 70% to 93% of all bites.[3] Overall, 15% to 20% of dog-bite wounds become infected, and the greatest risk of infection occurs with puncture wounds, crush injuries, and hand wounds.[2] Infection of a dog bite usually manifests as localized cellulitis, but regional lymphadenopathy, lymphangitis, and fever may occur. Septic arthritis or osteomyelitis is common when the canine tooth penetrates a joint or bone.

Most infections that develop from dog bites are polymicrobial and involve both aerobic and anaerobic organisms (Table 1).[4] *Pasteurella* species (especially *Pasteurella canis*) are the most frequent isolates of dog bites.[5] Alpha-hemolytic streptococci and *Staphylococcus aureus* are also common isolates. Infection with *Capnocytophaga canimorsus,* a gram-negative rod, is rare but can occur in hosts compromised by immunosuppressive medications, asplenia, liver disease, renal failure, or

TABLE 1. Microorganisms Commonly Isolated from Bite Wounds		
	Aerobes	**Anaerobes**
Dogs and cats	Pasteurella multocida	Fusobacterium species
	Pasteurella canis (dogs)	Bacteroides species
	Alpha-hemolytic streptococci	Porphyromonas species
	Staphylococcus species	Prevotella species
	Neisseria species	Propionibacterium species
	Corynebacterium species	Peptostreptococcus species
Humans	Staphylococcus aureus	Fusobacterium nucleatum
	Eikenella corrodens	Peptostreptococcus species
	Haemophilus species	Prevotella species
	Alpha-hemolytic streptococci	Clostridium species

lymphoma.[2,3] The fatality rate is 30% and usually involves overwhelming sepsis, disseminated intravascular coagulation, and renal failure. The antibiotic of choice for *C. canimorsus* is penicillin.[4] The most frequently isolated anaerobes from dog bites include *Fusobacterium* species, *Bacteroides* species, *Porphyromonas* species, *Prevotella* species, and *Propionibacterium* species.[5]

Cat Bites

The infection rate of cat bites has been reported to exceed 50%.[2] Feline teeth are narrow and sharp and can more easily penetrate into bones and joints, increasing the risk of septic arthritis or osteomyelitis. *Pasteurella multocida* is the most common pathogen isolated from infected cat-bite wounds, occurring in approximately 50% of cases.[5] Rapidly developing cellulitis with fever and purulent discharge are the hallmarks of *P. multocida* infection.[3,6] It is often susceptible to penicillin, amoxicillin-clavulanate, doxycycline, or fluoroquinolones such as ciprofloxacin.[3] The microbiology of cat-bite wounds is otherwise similar to that for dog bites (see Table 1).

Human Bites

Human bites are generally more serious, owing to the bacteriology of the human oral flora and mechanisms of injury. The infection rate of human bites is estimated to be about 10%.[7] Most human bites occur during fights, but approximately 15% to 20% are associated with sexual activity ("love nips").[2]

Human bites consist of occlusional bites and clenched-fist injuries. A bite wound sustained when human teeth sink into skin is defined as occlusional. Clenched-fist injuries are more serious and occur when one person punches another in the mouth with a clenched fist. This can result in simple cellulitis or lead to septic arthritis or osteomyelitis by direct inoculation of bacteria into the third metacarpophalangeal joint space or bone. The force of the blow can sever a nerve or tendon or cause a fracture. Patients often ignore clenched-fist injuries until these become infected.

The majority of human-bite wounds demonstrate approximately five different microorganisms per wound, with three being anaerobes (see Table 1).[4] The most common infectious organisms isolated from human-bite wounds are *S. aureus, Eikenella corrodens, Haemophilus* species, and beta-lactamase producing oral anaerobes.[4,7] *E. corrodens,* a gram-negative rod, is part of the normal human oral flora. It is the most common organism isolated from clenched-fist injuries.[6] *E. corrodens* may be susceptible to penicillin, amoxicillin-clavulanate, doxycycline, or fluoroquinolones such as ciprofloxacin.[2,7]

Transmission of herpesvirus types 1 and 2, hepatitis B and C, and even syphilis has been documented with human bites.[4] The likelihood of transmission of human immunodeficiency virus (HIV) is very low but remains a possibility.

Principles of Management of Bite Wounds

History

The medical history is a critically important component of the initial evaluation of all bite wounds. Information that can help determine a patient's risk of wound infection includes the following:
- Circumstances of the injury (especially the time)
- Information about the biter
- Whether the animal was provoked or unprovoked
- Current location of the animal
- Patient's allergies
- Current medications
- Underlying medical illnesses
- Previous tetanus or rabies vaccinations

Factors that place a patient at higher risk for bite-wound infections are listed in Table 2.

Physical Examination

A thorough physical examination should include the following:
- Description of the location and extent of all wounds (diagrams are helpful)

TABLE 2.   Risk Factors for Bite Wound Infections[3,9]
Puncture wounds
Chronic alcoholism
Chronic edema of affected extremity
Crush injury
Diabetes mellitus
Immunocompromised state (organ transplant, human immunodeficiency virus, immuno-suppressive medications)
Liver dysfunction
Location on hand, foot, or face
Peripheral vascular disease
Proximity to prosthetic joint
Splenectomy
Treatment delay exceeding 12 hours

- Assessment of wound depth, including tendon, joint, or bone involvement
- Evaluation of neurovascular function
- Identification of any signs of infection (significant swelling and erythema around the wound, purulent discharge, fever, lymphadenopathy)

Consider photodocumentation in cases of disfigurement or cases that might involve litigation.

Cultures

Samples for a Gram stain and bacterial cultures should be obtained from any wound that appears infected or that has not responded to antimicrobial treatment. Both aerobic and anaerobic culture samples should be obtained from deep within the wound after removal of superficial crusts.[2,4,7] Cultures of bite wounds without clinical signs of infection are not necessary. Wounds examined more than 24 hours after the injury and without signs of infection also do not need to be cultured.[4] A Gram stain is not useful in predicting the risk of infection in clinically noninfected wounds and should not be routinely used in the evaluation of bite wounds.

Radiography

A radiograph of the affected area can be helpful in locating foreign bodies (teeth, for example) and for determining the presence of a fracture.[8,9] Radiographs may also be important at baseline when a wound is near a joint or bone.

Irrigation and Débridement

All wounds should be irrigated with copious volumes of normal saline (minimum of 150 mL), since this reduces the bacterial inoculum in the wound.[2,6] Irrigation can be performed with a 20 mL to 50 mL syringe and an 18- to 20-gauge angiocatheter.

Devitalized tissue, including eschars, should be cautiously débrided to expose and assess the underlying tissue. An evaluation for potential surgical intervention should be made.

Wound Closure

The approach to closure of bite wounds remains controversial. Deep puncture wounds, bites to the legs or arms (especially the hands), wounds examined more than 24 hours after a bite, human bites, and clinically infected wounds should not be sutured.[4,7] Delayed primary closure can be performed 3 to 5 days after the bite if no sign of infection is present.[10] Bites to the face and head are often closed by a plastic surgeon to avoid scarring. Good results are likely due to the rich blood supply to the area and lack of edema.

Immobilization and Elevation

Elevation of the injured area is an essential component of therapy and should be continued for several days until edema has largely resolved. A 3- to 5-day period of immobility using a plaster splint in the position of function may be helpful in the treatment of hand wounds.[10]

Antimicrobial Therapy

The use of prophylactic antibiotics when no obvious clinical signs of infection are present is recommended for wounds that have a high risk of infection (see Table 2), such as deep punctures (particularly by cats), those that require surgical repair, and those involving the hands.[10,11] Wound characteristics, host factors, and anticipated degree of compliance should be considered in all treatment decisions. The chosen antibiotic should cover the normal aerobic and anaerobic flora of the biter, the skin flora of the victim, and possible environmental contaminants. The patient's history of drug allergies, medication interactions, and relative contraindications should also influence this choice. The duration of oral prophylactic antibiotic treatment ranges from 3 to 5 days.[8]

Antibiotics should be used to treat any overtly infected bite wound. The duration of therapy depends on the specific features of the infection, including location and severity. Simple cellulitis typically requires a total course of 14 days, whereas septic arthritis and osteomyelitis require longer courses.[2]

Amoxicillin-clavulanate will cover most bite pathogens.[2,8,11] Doxycycline is suggested for patients who are allergic to penicillin but is contraindicated in children and pregnant women.[10] Fluoroquinolones (ciprofloxacin, levofloxacin) have also been used in adult patients allergic to penicillin, but their inadequate spectrum against anaerobes requires the addition of further coverage with metronidazole or clindamycin. Intramuscular ceftriaxone may be useful when the degree of patient compliance is questionable or when rapid achievement of high degree of serum levels is desired.[10] Since *Pasteurella multocida* is generally resistant to first-generation cephalosporins and erythromycin, these antibiotics cannot be recommended. The recommended antimicrobial treatments with adult dosages are listed in Table 3.

Decision for Inpatient Therapy

Most patients with infected bite wounds can be treated on an outpatient basis. Indications for inpatient treatment of bite wounds are listed in Table 4. Consultation with an infectious diseases specialist or an orthopedic surgeon may be necessary.

Tetanus

Tetanus infection remains a risk of bite wounds. The tetanus status of all patients with a bite wound should be determined during the history. If a tetanus booster has not been received in the last 5 years, tetanus toxoid (0.5 mL subcutaneously or intramuscularly) should be administered to the patient.[11] Patients who have never been fully immunized may require a primary immunization series (three doses given 1 month apart) as well as tetanus immune globulin (250 to 500 U intramuscularly, depending on the severity of the wound).

Rabies

One of the most feared complications of animal-bite wounds is infection with rabies. Although the dog is the major animal reservoir for rabies worldwide, the principal wildlife vectors in the United States are

TABLE 3. Antimicrobial Therapies for Bite Wounds (Adult Dosages)	
Oral Agents	**Parenteral Agents**
Amoxicillin-clavulanate (Augmentin) 875 mg twice daily	Ampicillin-sulbactam (Unasyn) 1.5–3.0 g every 6 hours
Amoxicillin-clavulanate (Augmentin) 500 mg three times daily	Cefoxitin (Mefoxin) 1–2 g every 4 to 8 hours
Doxycycline (Vibramycin) 100 mg twice daily	Doxycycline (Vibramycin) 100 mg every 12 hours
Levofloxacin (Levaquin) 500 mg daily *or* ciprofloxacin (Cipro) 500 mg twice daily *plus*	Levofloxacin (Levaquin) 500 mg daily *or* ciprofloxacin (Cipro) 500 g every 12 hours *plus*
Metronidazole (Flagyl) 500 mg every 12 hours *or* clindamycin (Cleocin) 300 mg every 6 hours	Metronidazole (Flagyl) 500 mg every 12 hours *or* clindamycin (Cleocin) 300 mg every 6 hours

TABLE 4.	Indications for Inpatient Treatment of Bite Wounds
	Severe cellulitis
	Systemic signs of infection
	Bone, joint, tendon, or nerve involvement
	Failure of appropriate oral antibiotic therapy
	Poor patient compliance

raccoons, skunks, foxes, and bats.[12,13] An exposure to rabies is defined as an animal bite or contamination of an open wound or mucous membrane with saliva or infected tissue. Local health departments should be contacted regarding rabies prevalence among wild animals.

Rabies is caused by a highly neurotropic RNA virus. A bite from a rabid animal may inoculate the surrounding soft tissue with rabies virus. The incubation period varies from approximately 5 days to 1 year, although the usual period varies from 20 to 60 days.[14] Usually, the virus is first amplified in adjacent skeletal muscle cells near the site of inoculation. Once the concentration of virus is sufficient, it can directly enter peripheral nerves (unmyelinated sensory and motor terminals) and spread by retrograde axoplasmic flow until it reaches the spinal cord, causing pain at the wound site.[13] At this point, the virus is sequestered from the immune system and can no longer be halted by vaccination. After the virus has reached the spinal cord, it disseminates to the central nervous system and causes rapidly progressive encephalitis. It then spreads throughout the body along peripheral nerves, including those of the salivary glands, where it is shed. Death occurs by respiratory collapse, and infection is thought to be 100% fatal.

When exposure to rabies is confirmed or a high risk identified (particularly in unprovoked animal attacks), rabies prophylaxis must be initiated promptly. Prophylactic therapy after exposure includes local wound care, passive immunization with human rabies immunoglobulin (HRIG), and vaccination. HRIG should be administered at the started of antirabies prophylaxis (day 0) as a single 20 IU/kg dose, half infiltrated around the site of exposure and the other half given intramuscularly.[12] Three vaccines are available in the United States: human diploid cell vaccine (HDCV), rabies vaccine adsorbed (RVA), and purified chick embryo cell vaccine (PCEC). All three types of rabies vaccine are considered equally safe and efficacious.[12] HDCV, RVA, and PCEC should be administered intramuscularly in a series of five 1.0 mL injections given on days 0, 3, 7, 21, and 28.[12] The deltoid muscle of adults or the anterolateral thigh of small children are recommended. The gluteal region has been associated with treatment failures and is not advised. Vaccine induces an active immune response within 7 to 10 days, and immunity persists for approximately 2 years.[9] Previously vaccinated patients do not need HRIG but should receive two doses of rabies vaccination on days 0 and 3.

Depending on the type of bite, animals should either be observed for erratic behavior for a 5- to 10-day period or euthanized at once to determine whether rabies virus is present. Examination of the animal's brain tissue is the only reliable method of diagnosis. Healthy-appearing cats and dogs can be quarantined for 10 days and euthanized if signs of illness appear.

Follow-up

Before discharge from a physician's care, patients should be told to return if pain, swelling, or functional status worsen. In cases managed on an outpatient basis, clinical follow-up should occur within 24 to 48 hours to assess the status of the wound. Additional follow-up visits may be necessary.

References

1. Weiss HB, Friedman DI, Coben JH: Incidence of dog bite injuries treated in emergency departments. JAMA 2798:51–53, 1998.
2. Goldstein EJC: Bite wounds and infection. Clin Infect Dis 14:633–640, 1992.
3. Weber DJ, Hansen AR: Infections resulting from animal bites. Infect Dis Clin North Am 5:663–680, 1991.
4. Griego RD, Rosen T, Orengo IF, Wolf JE: Dog, cat, and human bites: A review. J Am Acad Dermatol 33:1019–1029, 1995.
5. Talan DA, Citron DM, Abrahamian FM, Moran GJ: Bacteriologic analysis of infected dog and cat bites. N Engl J Med 340:85–92, 1999.
6. Kelleher AT, Gordon SM: Management of bite wounds and infection in primary care. Cleveland Clin J Med 64:137–141, 1997.
7. Bunzli WF, Wright DH, Hoang AT, et al: Current management of human bites. Pharmacotherapy 18:227–234, 1998.
8. Goldstein EJC: Bites. In: Mandell GL, Bennett JE, Dolin R, eds. Mandell, Douglas, and Bennett's Principles and Practice of Infectious Diseases, 5th ed. Philadelphia: Churchill Livingstone, 2000:3202–3206.
9. Presutti RJ: Bite wounds: Early treatment and prophylaxis against infectious complications. Postgrad Med 101:243–254, 1997.
10. Lewis KT, Stiles M: Management of cat and dog bites. Am Fam Phys 52:479–490.
11. Fleisher GR: The management of bite wounds [editorial]. N Engl J Med 340:138–140, 1999.
12. Anonymous: Human rabies prevention—United States, 1999: Recommendations of the Advisory Committee on Immunization Practices (ACIP). MMWR Morbid Mortal Wkly Rep 48(RR-1):1–23, 1999.
13. Fishbein DB, Robinson LE: Rabies. N Engl J Med 329:1632–1638, 1993.
14. Whitley RJ, Gnann JW: Viral encephalitis: Familiar infections and emerging pathogens. Lancet 359:507–514, 2002.

Osteomyelitis

Henry M. Wu, M.D., D.T.M.&H.

chapter

18

Osteomyelitis is the inflammation of the bone and marrow, typically caused by infection.[1] Despite much study on adult osteomyelitis, the wide range of presentations and the complex diagnostic and management issues have made this a "hot topic" with many unanswered questions.

Pathophysiology

The origin of infection can be used to categorize osteomyelitis. The route of infection may be (1) hematogenous, (2) contiguous from an adjacent site of infection, or (3) secondary to direct inoculation.[1–3]

Osteomyelitis can also be described as acute or chronic. Acute osteomyelitis implies a newly recognized infection.[4] Chronic osteomyelitis suggests relapsing or untreated disease,[4] or the presence of inert substrate for bacterial attachment that makes the infection refractory to antibiotics alone.[2] Possible inert substrates include sequestrum, defined as necrotic bone resulting from ischemia caused by suppurative build-up, as well as prosthetic devices and other foreign bodies.[1] Other pathologic findings of chronic osteomyelitis may include draining sinuses and formation of reactive bone, called *involcrum*.[1]

Microbiology

Familiarity with the common pathogens in different types of osteomyelitis is important to direct empiric antibiotic therapy when culture results are not yet available. In approximately 50% of cases, no organism is isolated,[1] and treatment must be directed against anticipated pathogens.

Among most types of osteomyelitis, *Staphylococcus aureus* (methicillin-susceptible or -resistant) is the microorganism most frequently isolated.[4] Other types of bacteria, as well as fungi, have been associated with specific patient populations or clinical syndromes (Table 1). Infections associated with prosthetic joints are typically caused by *S. aureus* or coagulase-

TABLE 1. Microorganisms (Other than *Staphylococcus aureus*) Commonly Associated with Osteomyelitis of Various Clinical Scenarios

Clinical Scenario	Microorganisms
Foreign-body associated	Coagulase-negative staphylococci Propionibacterium
Nosocomial infections	Enterobacteriaceae *Pseudomonas aeruginosa*
Diabetic foot osteomyelitis[5]	Polymicrobial: 　Aerobic gram-positive cocci 　Aerobic gram-negative bacilli 　Anaerobes
Hemodialysis related[3]	*Staphylococcus epidermidis*
Intravenous drug abuse related[3]	*S. epidermidis* Gram-negative bacilli *Candida* spp.
Human immunodeficiency virus infection	*Bartonella henselae*
Immunocompromised hosts	Aspergillus *Mycobacterium avium* complex *Candida albicans*
Sickle cell disease related	*Salmonella* species *Streptococcus pneumoniae*

Adapted from Lew DP, Waldvogel FA: Osteomyelitis. N Engl J Med 336:999–1007, 1997.

negative staphylococci.[4] Osteomyelitis due to diabetic foot infections is often polymicrobial, with aerobic and anaerobic bacteria.[5] Osteomyelitis in intravenous drug abusers is commonly associated with staphylococci, gram-negative rods, or *Candida* species.[3] *Mycobacterium tuberculosis* may cause osteomyelitis and typically affects the axial skeleton in adults (Pott's disease).[3] Pathogens related to specific exposures such as bites or animal contact, as well as the endemic mycoses (for example, blastomycosis and coccidioidomycosis) may also cause osteomyelitis in exposed individuals.[4]

Clinical Presentation and Syndromes

In general, patients may present with systemic symptoms of infection along with local signs of inflammation. However, in the chronic spectrum of osteomyelitis secondary to any cause, systemic symptoms such as fevers may be minimal, and local pain or a discharging sinus tract may be prominent features.[3]

Hematogenous osteomyelitis, most common in children and the elderly, may manifest acutely or chronically with fevers, chills, malaise, and localized pain and swelling.[3,4] In adults, hematogenous infection typically affects the vertebrae, sternoclavicular joint, sacroiliac joint, and symphysis pubis.[2] In vertebral osteomyelitis, the lumbar spine is affected in 45% of cases, while the thoracic and cervical spines represent 35% and 30% of cases, respectively.[3] Patients usually present with localized pain that may progress slowly over weeks to months, and fever may be absent in 50% of patients.[3] Peripheral neurologic findings can be found in 6% to 15% of patients.[3] Prosthetic hardware and sites of previous trauma are also at risk of being hematogenously seeded.[2] Patients with prosthesis-associated osteomyelitis of any cause may present without fever; localized pain and evidence of mechanical loosening may be the main findings.[4]

Osteomyelitis due to direct inoculation of microorganisms can result from surgical procedures, trauma, or local soft tissue infection. Infections usually appear within 1 month of inoculation, and typical symptoms include low-grade fever, pain, and drainage.[3] Osteomyelitis following surgery may appear several months after the procedure.[4] Decubitus ulcers may also result in osteomyelitis.[2]

Patients with peripheral vascular disease with or without diabetes frequently develop osteomyelitis in the foot, usually secondary to minor trauma.[3–5] The infection may be insididous, and most patients with diabetic foot osteomyelitis present in the chronic phase.[5] Diabetic peripheral neuropathy may result in the absence of pain, and contiguous soft tissue infection may make diagnosis difficult.[3,5] On average, among studied series of diabetic patients presenting with foot infections, evidence of osteomyelitis can be found in one third.[5] Vascular insufficiency and decreased immunity in diabetics may result in poor healing conditions,[5] and recurrence after treatment is common.[3]

Evaluation of the Patient with Osteomyelitis

History and Physical Examination

Symptoms and signs elicited on history taking and physical examination may not be specific for osteomyelitis. In the case of diabetic foot infections, the distinction between osteomyelitis and other pathologic conditions is particularly difficult given the high prevalence of soft tissue infections and neuropathic osteoarthropathy.[5] Any diabetic foot infection that has been present for more than 1 or 2 weeks should be considered at high risk for osteomyelitis.[5] The finding of visibly exposed bone or bone that can be probed in a diabetic foot infection has been found in one study to have a positive predictive value of 89% for underlying osteomyelitis.[5]

Microbiologic Cultures and Laboratory Tests

Histopathologic examination and microbiologic cultures (aerobic and anaerobic) of bone samples remain the gold standards for osteomyelitis diagnosis.[2,4] Identification of the pathogenic microorganism is extremely important to direct antibiotic treatment.[3] Blood culture samples should be drawn when hematogenous osteomyelitis is suspected, and a positive culture may make biopsy unnecessary if radiologic evidence is clear.[3,4] Bone sampling can be done by needle biopsy or as an open procedure, often in conjunction with surgical débridement.[5] Studies have shown that cultures taken from sinus tracts are unreliable, except perhaps when *S. aureus* is isolated.[2,3] In the case of diabetic foot infections, soft-tissue cultures have not proven to be reliably predictive of concurrent bone cultures.[5]

Other tests include blood leukocyte counts and nonspecific markers of inflammation, such as the erythrocyte sedimentation rate (ESR) and the C-reactive protein (CRP) level. These tests are neither sensitive nor specific but may be helpful diagnostically or be used to assess response to treatment when initially elevated.[2,3]

Imaging of Osteomyelitis

Many radiologic modalities are available for bone imaging, and no widely supported algorithm is available for the clinician in choosing studies to diagnose osteomyelitis. However, imaging plays an important role in osteomyelitis management. In addition to diagnosis, imaging may assist in characterizing a lesion for interventions such as biopsy or surgical débridement.[6] Furthermore, imaging may help rule out other conditions in the differential diagnosis of osteomyelitis such as soft tissue infections, malignancy, or arthropathy.

Plain Film Radiography. Conventional radiography is usually recommended as an initial study.[2,4,6] Although conventional radiographic findings may be normal in the first 10 to 21 days of an infection, early findings include soft tissue swelling and localized osteoporosis.[6] Subsequent findings may include cortical lucencies, periostitis, involcrum formation, and pathologic fractures.[6] Early periosteal reaction may be seen in cases with contiguous sources of infection.[6] Characteristic findings on a conventional radiograph in a patient with typical signs and symptoms of osteomyelitis may lead to a probable diagnosis.[5] However, the low sensitivity and specificity of radiography limits its usefulness as a single modality in the imaging of osteomyelitis. In the case of diabetic foot osteomyelitis, a mean sensitivity of 60% and specificity of 66% have been reported.[5]

Bone Scanning. There are several radionuclide scintigraphic techniques in use to image osteomyelitis. Bone scanning with technetium (Tc) 99m disphosphonates are most commonly used. ^{99m}Tc tracers localize to areas of increased vascularity and bone formation activity. In addition to osteomyelitis, other processes that can lead to a positive scan include sterile trauma, post-surgical changes, tumors, and degenerative joint disease.[5,7] Studies have shown a wide range of sensitivity and specificity for osteomyelitis, averaging 86% and 45%, respectively, in the setting of the diabetic foot.[5] Other modalities include indium-111 leukocyte scintigraphy and gallium-67 scanning. They appear to be more specific than ^{99m}Tc scans,[2] and some studies suggest that either test combined with ^{99m}Tc scintigraphy may achieve higher specificities.[7,8] An inherent weakness of any type of scintigraphy is the relatively poor spatial resolution.[7] Positron emission tomography is a newer modality showing promise in higher image resolution.[9]

Computed Tomography/Magnetic Resonance Imaging. Computed tomography (CT) and magnetic resonance imaging (MRI) are also used to diagnose osteomyelitis. CT can show detailed cortical structure, soft tissue extension, intraosseous gas, and sequestra.[6] This is particularly useful in chronic osteomyelitis management, as characterization of sequestra is necessary for definitive surgical débridement.[6] MRI provides superior soft tissue visualization[6] and has further advantages over CT in its ability to identify early bone marrow changes in osteomyelitis.[6,7] Reported sensitivity and specificity ranges from 60% to 100% and 50% to 90%, respectively.[6–8] Other conditions that may have MRI bone marrow findings similar to those of osteomyelitis include contusions, healing fractures, osteonecrosis, and metastases.[6] MRI is considered the best imaging for suspected spinal osteomyelitis.[2] Although some authors believe MRI to be the best single modality for diagnosing osteomyelitis, expense considerations have made its routine role unclear.[2,5]

Choosing an Imaging Modality. Given the many imaging modalities available, the clinician is often faced with the difficult decision of which test to use. The decision is ultimately based on multiple factors, including local availability, urgency of diagnosis, cost, and need for detailed spatial resolution. Patient factors such as the likelihood of diagnoses other than osteomyelitis and individual preference should be considered. For example, performing more than one scintigraphic test can be more expensive than MRI, provides less spatial resolution, and may take as long as 3 days for completion.[7,8] When interpreting results, clinicians should carefully consider the test's potential diagnostic strengths and weaknesses so that guided decisions can be made about subsequent management or additional diagnostic studies.

Treatment

Parenteral Antibiotic Therapy

Although parenteral antibiotic therapy plays a key role in treatment, there are few controlled trials comparing regimens or lengths of treatment in osteomyelitis. A review in 1996 found only five prospective, comparative trials of treatment regimens, with a total of 154 patients, in the literature.[2] None of the studies could demonstrate the superiority of any regimen over another. Well-controlled trials are difficult to perform because of the variety of clinical scenarios, the need for long-term follow-up, and the effect surgical débridement may have on the success of treatment.[2] Furthermore, the results of any trial must be carefully evaluated in light of current and local bacterial resistance patterns.

Bone culture and sensitivity test results should guide the choice of antibiotic. In a patient who is clinically stable, antibiotics may be delayed for 24 to 48 hours prior to biopsy to increase the diagnostic yield of cultures.[3,11] When biopsy is not possible or treatment must be started before culture results are available, empiric regimens can be used. While some antibiotics have excellent bone penetration, particularly the fluoroquinolones[10] and clindamycin,[3] experts have concluded that most antibiotics achieve concentrations in bone similar to that in serum.[5]

For cases in which *S. aureus* is the most likely pathogen, antistaphylococcal agents such as nafcillin, cefazolin, or clindamycin may be considered.[4] Vancomycin may be considered for suspected methicillin-resistant coagulase-positive or negative staphylococci. In the case of osteomyelitis of the foot due to diabetes or vascular insufficiency, a single or combination regimen may be considered to cover mixed infections of aerobic and anaerobic bacteria. Examples include ampicillin-sulbactam, imipenem-cilastin, or the combination of a fluoroquinolone and clindamycin.[2,5] When results of bacterial susceptibility testing are available, the regimen should be adjusted accordingly.

Traditional guidelines usually recommend parenteral antibiotics for a total of 4 to 6 weeks, and if surgical intervention is performed, the treatment course should extend from the last débridement procedure.[2–4] Treatment for less than 4 weeks has been associated with an increased risk of failure.[10] Suitable patients can use long-term intravenous catheters to complete parenteral treatment courses as outpatients.[3] When infected bone is completely removed, some experts recommend a 2-week short course of parenteral antibiotics, primarily to treat the soft tissue infection.[3,5] For vertebral osteomyelitis, 8 weeks of antibiotic treatment is considered optimal.[10]

Oral Antibiotic Therapy

Oral antibiotics with excellent bioavailability have potential use in managing osteomyelitis, and benefits include reduction in overall treatment cost and complications related to intravenous catheters.[11,12] Some trials of oral fluoroquinolone therapy suggest similar efficacy with parenteral regimens, particularly when the pathogen is a gram-negative bacillus.[11–13] However, oral fluoroquinolones appear less successful against *S. aureus*[10,13] and *Pseudomonas aeruginosa*.[13] Other oral antibiotics with good bioavailability that have been considered for osteomyelitis include clindamycin,[14] co-trimoxazole,[12] and some beta-lactams.[11,12]

Some authors suggest switching to oral antibiotics after an initial 2 weeks of parenteral treatment.[3,10] A drawback of oral treatment may be the potential for decreased compliance as compared with parenteral treatment.[2,10] Close follow-up is recommended.[3] Nevertheless, there are few controlled trials comparing oral and parenteral treatments for most clinical situations.

Surgical Débridement

In addition to antibiotics, definitive treatment of osteomyelitis often requires drainage of collections and removal of any nonvital substrate such as sequestra or prosthetic devices.[2,5] Bacteria adherent to prosthetic materials typically resist sterilization.[2,4] Débrided bone should be sent for pathologic and microbiologic study. Vertebral osteomyelitis usually does not require surgical therapy unless there is extension of infection (e.g., paravertebral or epidural abscess), failure of antibiotic therapy, or structural instability.[3]

Following débridement, surgical revascularization may be necessary in cases associated with vascular insufficiency.[2,4,5] Grafting of bone, muscle, or skin may also be a method of revascularization and support.[4] In refractory cases, amputation may be the only option for definitive cure;[2,4,5] however, definitive treatment may result in morbidity worse than the disease itself, and chronic suppressive antibiotics may also be considered.[2,3]

Other treatment options include local use of antibiotic-impregnated beads or prosthetic joint cement. These have been studied only in the context of prosthetic joint osteomyelitis, and data are lacking for general use.[2,4] Hyperbaric oxygen has been suggested as an adjunctive treatment for chronic osteomyelitis, but there are limited data at this time to support its routine use.[2,3]

Complications

Treatment failures are not unusual, and relapses may occur, sometimes years later.[2] Complications of chronic osteomyelitis include sinus tract formation, squamous cell carcinoma arising from the tract, pathologic fractures, secondary amyloidosis, endocarditis, sepsis, and, rarely, osteosarcoma.[1] In the case of diabetic foot infections, retrospective studies have shown an amputation rate averaging about 40% over 1 to 3 years and a 2-year mortality rate of 35% to 50%.[5]

References

1. Rosenberg A: Bones, joints, and soft tissue tumors. In: Cotran RS, Kumar V, Collins T, eds: Robbins Pathologic Basis of Disease, 6th ed. Philadelphia: W.B. Saunders, 1999:1215–1268.
2. Haas DW, McAndrew MP: Bacterial osteomyelitis in adults: Evolving considerations in diagnosis and treatment. Am J Med 101:550–561, 1996.
3. Mader JT, Calhoun J: Osteomyelitis. In: Mandell GL, Bennett JE, Dolin R, eds: Mandell, Douglas, and Bennett's Principles and Practice of Infectious Diseases, 5th ed. Philadelphia: Churchill Livingstone, 2000:1182–1196.
4. Lew DP, Waldvogel FA: Osteomyelitis. N Engl J Med 336:999–1007, 1997.
5. Lipsky BA: Osteomyelitis of the foot in diabetic patients. Clin Infect Dis 25:1318–1326, 1997.
6. Tehranzadeh J, Wong E, Wang F, Sadighpour M: Imaging of osteomyelitis in the mature skeleton. Radiol Clin North Am 39:223–250, 2001.
7. Boutin RD, Brossmann J, Sartoris DJ, et al: Update on imaging of orthopedic infections. Orthop Clin North Am 29:41–66, 1998.
8. Morrison WB, Schweitzer ME, Wapner KL, et al: Osteomyelitis in feet of diabetics: Clinical accuracy, surgical utility, and cost-effectiveness of MR imaging. Radiology 196:557–564, 1995.
9. De Winter F, Vogelaers D, Gemmel F, Dierckx RA: Promising role of 18-F-fluoro-D-deoxyglucose positron emission tomography in clinical infectious diseases. Eur J Clin Microbiol Infect Dis 21:247–257, 2002.
10. Rissing JP: Antimicrobial therapy for chronic osteomyelitis in adults: Role of the quinolones. Clin Infect Dis 25:1327–1333, 1997.
11. Gentry LO: Oral antimicrobial therapy for osteomyelitis. Ann Intern Med 114:986–987, 1991.
12. MacGregor RR, Graziani AL: Oral administration of antibiotics: A rational alternative to the parenteral route. Clin Infect Dis 24:457–467, 1997.
13. Lew DP, Waldvogel FA: Quinolones and osteomyelitis: State-of-the-art. Drugs 49(Suppl 2):100–111, 1995.
14. Glatt AE: Osteomyelitis [letter]. N Engl J Med 337:428–429, 1997.

Infectious Arthritis

Serena Cardillo, M.D.

chapter

19

Septic arthritis is defined as an inflammatory reaction within the joint space in response to the presence of a microorganism.[1] Synovial tissue is particularly vulnerable to infection in the setting of systemic bacteremia, given its vascularity and lack of a basement membrane. Thus, a pathogen may be introduced into the joint via hematogenous spread from a distant site. Direct introduction of bacteria into the joint space can also occur in the setting of trauma or procedures such as intra-articular injections, arthrocentesis, or arthroscopy.[2]

This chapter discusses the epidemiology, causes, and clinical presentation of infectious arthritis. The approach to the diagnosis is presented, with particular focus on synovial fluid analysis, and options for empiric treatment are reviewed.

Epidemiology

In the general population, an estimated 2 to 5 per 100,000 new cases of infectious arthritis have been diagnosed annually.[1] The incidence is higher among patients with rheumatoid arthritis (28 to 38 per 100,000 per year) and those with prosthetic joints (40 to 68 per 100,000 per year).[2] Predisposing host factors[1,3,4] to septic arthritis typically include the following:

- Malignancy
- Diabetes
- Immunosuppressive therapy
- Preexisting arthritis, with or without a history of intra-articular injections
- Intravenous drug use
- Extra-articular infections
- Presence of a prosthetic joint

For patients without chronic arthritis, trauma often precedes infection.[3]

193

Causes of Infectious Arthritis

There are a number of causes of infectious arthritis (Table 1). Gram-positive aerobes are implicated in the majority of cases of infectious arthritis and are seen in an estimated 70% to 80% of patients.[4,5] *Staphylococcus aureus* is the most common pathogen in this group and is responsible for about 60% of infections in the joint space.[1-5] The organism can also cause an acute septic bursitis following trauma. Streptococcal infections are also common and may be due to group A β-hemolytic streptococci as well as groups B, C, and G streptococci.

TABLE 1. Common Causes of Arthritis	
Infectious	**Noninfectious**
Bacteria	**Crystalline Diseases**
Gram-positive	Gout
Staphylococcus aureus	Pseudogout
Streptococci (groups A, B, C, G)	**Hemarthrosis**
Coagulase-negative staphylococci*	Trauma
Enterococcus species*	Anticoagulation
Gram-negative	Clotting disorder
Neisseria gonorrhoeae	**Malignancy**
Pseudomonas aeruginosa	**Rheumatic Diseases**
Brucella species	Rheumatoid arthritis
Pasteurella multocida	Spondyloarthropathy
Mycobacteria	Systemic lupus erythematosus
Mycobacterium tuberculosis	Osteoarthritis
Mycobacterium kansasii	**Trauma**
Mycobacterium marinum	
Fungi	
Coccidioides immitis	
Blastomyces dermatitidis	
Sporothrix schenckii	
Candida albicans	
Viruses	
Rubella	
Mumps	
Parvovirus B19	
Hepatitis B	
Chikungunya	
O'nyong-nyong fever	
Spirochete	
Borrelia burgdorferi	

*May be implicated in prosthetic joint infections
Adapted from Towheed TE, Hochberg MC: Acute monoarthritis: A practical approach to assessment and treatment. Am Fam Phys 54:2239–2243, 1996; Baker DG, Schumacher HR: Acute monoarthritis. N Engl J Med 329:1013–1020, 1993.

Gram-negative bacilli are responsible for about 9% to 20% of cases of infectious arthritis.[1,4,5] These infections typically occur in the elderly and in patients with comorbid conditions such as immunocompromised states or chronic arthritis. *Pseudomonas aeruginosa* is often the underlying cause in intravenous drug users with sternoclavicular or sacroiliac infections.[3] *Brucella* can also cause arthritis of the sacroiliac joint in patients exposed to unpasteurized dairy products. *Pasteurella multocida* should be considered in patients who present with an animal bite to a joint.

Neisseria gonorrhoeae remains the predominant cause in adults younger than 30 years of age.[3] Disseminated gonococcal infection often manifests as a triad of polyarthritis, dermatitis (vesiculopustular skin lesions), and tenosynovitis. Synovial cultures yield the diagnosis in less than 50% of patients.[1,3] *N. gonorrhoeae* can be recovered from pharyngeal, rectal, urethral, or cervical cultures. Gonococcal infection can also result in a monoarticular purulent arthritis without skin involvement. Synovial cultures are more often positive in these cases [1]

Chronic monoarticular arthritis of the large joints, most commonly the knee, can be present in the later stages of Lyme disease. The organism, *Borrelia burgdoferi*, is rarely detected in synovial fluid, and the diagnosis is made through serologic testing.[3]

Mycobacterial infections can manifest as a more indolent and progressive monoarthritis. Tendon sheaths can be involved as well, particularly in infections with atypical mycobacteria.[1,3,6] Potential organisms include *Mycobacterium tuberculosis, Mycobacterium kansasii,* and *Mycobacterium marinum.* Diagnosis is primarily made through culture of the synovial tissue.

Chronic monoarthritis can occasionally be caused by fungal organisms, usually in immunocompromised patients. Disseminated coccidioidomycosis, blastomycosis, and sporotrichosis (particularly in people exposed to soil) have all been reported. Candidal infections may also occur, typically via hematogenous seeding, and are more acute in onset.[1,3,7]

Arthritis can be a significant feature of a number of viral illnesses. Polyarthritis can occur in patients with infection with mumps and parvovirus B19. It has also been reported during the preicteric period in patients with hepatitis B. Infections with rarer arthropod-borne alpha viruses endemic to East Africa, such as Chikungunya and O'nyong-nyong fever, are abrupt and can cause severe pain in large joints.[1,3]

Clinical Presentation

Ninety percent of patients with infectious arthritis present with pain and limited range of motion in one joint. Polyarticular arthritis is seen in about 10% of patients, often in the setting of underlying rheumatoid arthritis.[1,3,4] The knee is most commonly involved in acute bacterial arthritis, followed by the hip and the shoulder.[3] Wrists, ankles, and elbows are infrequently affected. Interphalangeal joint involvement is seen in cases of gonococcal infection. Intravenous drug users are more disposed to develop sacroiliac or sternoclavicular infections.

Joint tenderness and swelling secondary to the presence of an effusion are common clinical features. Patients may be unable to bear weight on the affected joint. Systemic symptoms may include mild fever, chills, and malaise. These symptoms may help to distinguish between underlying infection and inflammatory states such as gout. A complete differential diagnosis including both infectious and noninfectious causes, such as crystalline disease, hemarthrosis, tumor, and rheumatic diseases, should be explored when evaluating these patients (see Table 1).[4,8]

Thus, the history and physical examination of a patient with a potentially infected joint should focus on the following:

History

- Joints involved
- Duration of symptoms including pain, swelling, and erythema
- Systemic complaints including fever, chills, malaise, rash
- Risk factors (comorbid illnesses, immunosuppressive therapy)
- Recent travel history
- Social history (sexual activity, intravenous drug use)

Physical Examination

- Number of involved joints
- Soft tissue swelling
- Warmth over the joint
- Presence of an effusion
- Inability to bear weight on affected joint
- Skin findings (vesicopustular lesions)

Laboratory Studies

The most valuable study in the evaluation of acute monoarthritis is synovial fluid analysis. Examination of the fluid can distinguish between noninflammatory, inflammatory, and infectious effusions. Fluid should be sent for total leukocyte count with differential, Gram stain, and culture (both aerobic and anaerobic) as well as crystal analysis with polarized light microscopy. It should be noted, however, that the presence of either uric acid or calcium pyrophosphate crystals does not necessarily exclude the possibility of infection. Protein and glucose are not useful clinical indicators of infection. While both elevated protein and decreased glucose levels are common in infectious arthritis, these measurements are not specific.[1,9]

In septic arthritis, the synovial fluid is purulent in about 80% to 90% of cases.[3] The leukocyte count is usually greater than 50,000 cells/mm^3 with predominant (greater than 75%) polymorphonuclear cells.[1,3,8,10] Fluid taken from patients with rheumatoid arthritis or crystalline disease can also contain a significant amount of neutrophils in the absence of infection. Meanwhile, in infected patients with cancer or a history of intravenous drug use or steroid use, the total leukocyte count may not exceed 50,000 cells/mm^3 (Table 2).[1,3]

Additional studies that may be helpful, include rheumatoid factor and antinuclear antibody measurements. Erythrocyte sedimentation rate and C-reactive protein are usually elevated and can be useful in following the progression of treatment. A complete blood cell count is not often useful in adults, who typically have little to no rise in peripheral blood leukocyte count.[1] If gonococcal infection is suspected, pharyngeal, rectal, and urethral or cervical cultures should be obtained. For patients with chronic monoarthritis, in whom there is a persistent effusion or an underlying immunocompromised state, synovial tissue should be sent for mycobacterial and fungal cultures. Peripheral blood cultures are positive in about one third of patients, particularly in those with polyarticular involvement or infection at extra-articular sites.[3]

Imaging Studies

Radiographic studies may be useful in the evaluation of an acute monoarthritis. Plain radiographs are useful in the setting of trauma and can confirm the presence of a fracture. Periarticular soft tissue swelling is the most common abnormality seen.[2] Joint space widening can be seen in the early stages of septic arthritis, whereas narrowing of the

TABLE 2. Interpretation of Synovial Fluid Leukocyte Counts	
Synovial Fluid Cell Count, cells/mm^3	**Interpretation**
<200	Normal
<2000	Noninflammatory
2000–20,000	Mild inflammation
20,000–50,000	Moderate inflammation; possibly septic arthritis
>50,000	Severe inflammation; possibly septic arthritis
>100,000	Septic arthritis

Adapted from Towheed TE, Hochberg MC: Acute monoarthritis: A practical approach to assessment and treatment. Am Fam Phys 54:2239–2243, 1996; Baker DG, Schumacher HR: Acute monoarthritis. N Engl J Med 329:1013–1020, 1993.

space due to cartilage destruction is seen later in the course.[3] Computed tomography or magnetic resonance imaging can be helpful in the diagnosis of periarticular osteomyelitis. Three-phase bone scan is used in evaluating infection of the sacroiliac joint or for diagnosing concurrent joint infections in patients with osteomyelitis.[3]

Treatment

Septic arthritis is classified as a "rheumatologic emergency" warranting hospital admission and the initiation of parenteral antibiotics to prevent permanent damage to the joint.[8] After obtaining synovial fluid and peripheral blood for cultures, empiric antibiotics should be started. The choice of empiric antibiotic therapy is initially based on Gram stain, age, history of sexual activity, and synovial fluid culture results.[1] Once a specific pathogen is identified, the empiric antibiotic regimen can be suitably narrowed (Table 3).

For treatment of *S. aureus* infection, a parenteral beta-lactam, such as nafcillin (typically 2 g intravenously every 4 hours) or cefazolin (500 mg in-

TABLE 3.	Treatment of Common Causes of Infectious Arthritis		
Cause	**Drug**	**Dosage**	**Duration**
Staphylococcus aureus	**Nafcillin** Alternatives: Cefazolin Vancomycin (for MRSA/beta-lactam allergy)	**2 g IV every 4 hours** 500 mg IV every 8 hours 1 g IV every 12 hours	3 weeks
Streptococci	**Penicillin G** Alternatives: Cefazolin, Vancomycin	**12–18 million units/day** divided into q4-hour doses	2 weeks
Neisseria gonorrhoeae	**Ceftriaxone** *then* Cefixime *or* Ciprofloxacin *plus* Doxycycline	**1 g IV every 24 hours for** 48 hours beyond symptom resolution *then* 400 mg PO twice daily 500 mg PO twice daily *plus* 100 mg PO twice daily	7 to 10 days
Gram-negative rods*	**Levofloxacin** *or* Cefepime	**500 mg IV daily** 2 g IV every 12 hours	3 weeks

* Final antibiotic regimen depends on culture susceptibility results.
Adapted from Smith JW, Hasan MS: Infectious arthritis. In: Mandell GL, Bennett JE, Dolin R, eds: Mandell, Douglas, and Bennett's Principles and Practice of Infectious Diseases, 5th ed. Philadelphia: Churchill Livingstone, 2000:1175–1182; and Smith JW, Piercy EA: Infectious arthritis. Clin Infect Dis 20:225–231, 1995.

travenously every 8 hours) is recommended. If the patient is penicillin-allergic or at risk for infection with methicillin-resistant *S. aureus,* vancomycin should be substituted (1 g intravenously every 12 hours). The recommended total duration of treatment for *S. aureus* septic arthritis is 3 weeks.[1,3]

Streptococcal infections should be treated with intravenous penicillin (12 to 18 million units/day administered every 4 hours). Alternative antibiotics include vancomycin and cefazolin. The recommended treatment course for streptococcal septic arthritis is 2 weeks.[1,3]

For gonococcal septic arthritis, the initial drug of choice is ceftriaxone (1 g intravenously every 24 hours). Response to treatment is typically rapid, and parenteral administration should continue until 48 hours after symptom resolution. Oral medications, including cefixime (400 mg twice daily) or ciprofloxacin (500 mg twice daily), can then be initiated to complete a total course of 7 to 10 days. Doxycycline (100 mg twice daily) should also be given to treat presumed chlamydial coinfection.[1–3]

For some patients, the initial Gram stain may not be helpful in directing the course of therapy, and broad antimicrobial coverage must be initiated. Treatment for infection with gram-negative rods consists of 3 weeks of a parenteral antibiotic chosen according to culture susceptibility results. In cases in which the initial Gram stain is negative, broad coverage with ceftriaxone for gonococci, streptococci, and staphylococci can be started and altered based on culture results.[1,3] Patients in whom tissue culture confirms mycobacterial or fungal infection should be referred to an infectious disease specialist for initiation of the appropriate course of therapy.

Repeated needle aspiration of the affected joint may be necessary for any fluid reaccumulation within the first week of treatment. If the patient fails to clinically respond to antimicrobial therapy and repeated aspiration, surgical drainage may be required. Infections of the hip and shoulder typically require open drainage.

Septic Arthritis in the Prosthetic Joint

Prosthetic joint infections are very common in the first 2 years after implantation of the prosthesis. Reported postoperative incidence is around 6.5 per 1000 within in the first year and 3.2 per 1000 in the second year.[2] Risk factors for infection are the same as those previously mentioned for septic arthritis of a native joint but also include prior joint surgery and perioperative wound complications. Infectious organisms can be introduced directly into the wound or via airborne contamination during the procedure itself. Infection can also occur in the setting of postoperative bacteremia through hematogenous spread.[2] Clinical presentation can vary from acute infectious arthritis to chronic pain due to prosthesis failure. Patients often complain of limited range of motion in the affected joint.

The most common organisms implicated in prosthetic joint infections are coagulase-negative staphylococci (25% of patients), followed by *S. aureus,* gram-negative bacilli, streptococci, anaerobes, and *Enterococcus* species.[1,2] Polymicrobial infection is also commonly seen. These organisms can be isolated through culture of preoperative synovial fluid aspirate or intraoperative tissue. Additional diagnostic studies include erythrocyte sedimentation rate, complete blood cell count, C-reactive protein, and imaging through the use of plain radiographs, bone scan, MRI, or CT.

The choice of antibiotics is based on culture results. Vancomycin is the drug of choice for coagulase-negative staphylococcal infections, whereas nafcillin or cefazolin can be used to treat joint infections caused by *S. aureus.* Patients with gram-negative bacilli isolated on culture should be given a beta-lactam such as piperacillin, which can be combined with gentamicin.[1]

Eradication of infection can be achieved in the majority of patients through removal of the prosthesis combined with 4 to 6 weeks of intravenous antibiotic therapy directed at the appropriate pathogen. While reimplantation of a new prosthesis can be performed during the initial extraction, improved outcomes have been demonstrated with a two-stage procedure in which reimplantation follows the completion of a 6-week antibiotic course.[1,2]

Chronic antibiotic suppression is used in select patients for whom prosthesis removal is not performed. Lifelong oral antibiotics can be given with some success to compliant patients in whom surgical removal is contraindicated. For these patients, one must demonstrate that the prosthesis is not loose and that the causative organism is of low virulence and is sensitive to oral antibiotics. This form of therapy may place patients at risk for developing antimicrobial resistance as well as extension of the infection beyond the joint space.[1,2]

References

1.   Smith JW, Hasan MS: Infectious arthritis. In: Mandell GL, Bennett JE, Dolin R, eds: Mandell, Douglas, and Bennett's Principles and Practice of Infectious Diseases, 5th ed. Philadelphia: Churchill Livingstone, 2000:1175–1182.
2.   Osmon DR, Steckelberg JM: Osteomyelitis, infectious arthritis and prosthetic joint infections. In: Wilson WR, Sande MA, eds: Current Diagnosis and Treatment in Infectious Diseases. New York: McGraw Hill, 2001:191–202.
3.   Smith JW, Piercy EA: Infectious arthritis. Clin Infect Dis 20:225–231, 1995.
4.   Baker DG, Schumacher HR: Acute monoarthritis. N Engl J Med 329:1013–1020.
5.   Pioro MH, Mandell BF: Septic arthritis. Rheum Dis Clin North Am 23:239–258, 1997.
6.   Sutker WL, Lankford LL, Tompset R: Granulomatous synovitis: The role of atypical mycobacteria. Rev Infect Dis 1:729–735, 1979.

7. Cuellar ML, Silviera LH, Espinoza LR: Fungal arthritis. Ann Rheum Dis 51:690–697, 1992.

8. Towheed TE, Hochberg MC: Acute monoarthritis: A practical approach to assessment and treatment. Am Fam Phys 54: 2239–2243, 1996.

9. Shemerling RH, Delbanco TL, Tosetson ANA, et al: Synovial fluid tests. JAMA 264: 1009–1014, 1990.

10. Hasselbacher P: Arthrocentesis, synovial fluid analysis, and synovial biopsy. In: Klippel JH, Weyand CM, Wortmann RL, eds: Primer on the rheumatic diseases. Atlanta: Arthritis Foundation, 1997:98–104.

Recognition and Diagnosis of Human Immunodeficiency Virus Infection

chapter 20

*Todd D. Barton, M.D., and
Janet M. Hines, M.D.*

The human immunodeficiency virus (HIV) epidemic in the United States has entered its third decade, and with the passage of time, new challenges have arisen for the medical community. Whereas the first decade of the epidemic was marked by careful study of viral biology and the opportunistic infections that complicate advanced HIV infection, the second decade offered an explosion of antiretroviral treatment options and new hope for long-term control of the virus. But this new optimism is tempered by the ongoing recognition that many HIV-infected patients still present late in the illness, often with serious opportunistic infections or late complications of disease that are only partially reversible (e.g., peripheral neuropathy, nephropathy). Therefore, the third decade of the American HIV epidemic opens with an important challenge that will largely fall to primary care physicians: the identification of all patients infected with HIV. The Centers for Disease Control and Prevention (CDC) estimate that up to 280,000 HIV-infected people in the United States are unaware of their diagnosis.[1] Unless they are identified, these patients—and some portion of the 40,000 patients newly infected each year[2]—will continue to suffer the consequences of advanced HIV infection while simultaneously (and unknowingly) propagating the spread of the virus and the continuation of the deadliest epidemic in more than 80 years.

In this chapter, we offer a focused discussion of important issues relating to the recognition and diagnosis of HIV infection. We begin by reviewing risk behaviors that increase the probability of HIV infection and summarize the available data on populations known to have high prevalences of HIV infection. We then discuss the signs and symptoms associated with primary HIV infection and conclude with a brief discussion of HIV testing.

Persons at Increased Risk for HIV Infection

Infection with HIV is more likely to be found in individuals with certain risk behaviors, which will be discussed. However, these behaviors are exactly the ones that patients are least likely to report to their care provider. Reasons for nondisclosure can include either a new relationship with a provider or a desire to please a provider with whom the patient has had a long-term relationship. The absence of risk factors, therefore, should not be a reason *not* to consider testing a patient for HIV infection.

Although taking an agnostic approach to the role of risk factors in screening will allow more patients to be screened, it does not allow the provider to discuss in detail risk reduction. Many patients will be grateful that their provider has opened the door for a meaningful discussion of such behaviors, and the efficacy of the provider-patient relationship is intensified. As such, the risk behaviors are discussed below.

One additional note is that individuals in high-risk groups who continue to engage in high-risk behavior may avoid attempts to change their behavior. The reality of an HIV test can be threatening to them, and they may report that they have undergone testing elsewhere. Verification of such testing is necessary. The patient should be asked to provide a copy of the results, and if no copy can be produced, then repeat testing should be offered.

Risk Groups

A summary of common indications for HIV testing is given in Table 1. Most patients with unrecognized HIV infection are asymptomatic, and therefore primary care providers must be keenly aware of risk behaviors and high-risk populations to target HIV testing to the groups in whom it is most needed. Recent studies have consistently shown that at least half of patients at highest risk for HIV perceive themselves to be at low risk,[3,4] and most have never been tested.[3,6]

Unprotected Sex and Sharing of Needles. The most important behaviors conferring increased risk of HIV infection are unprotected vaginal, anal, or oral sex (including heterosexual sex) and the sharing of needles for intravenous drug use.

An HIV infection can only be acquired through person-to-person transmission of infected blood, semen, or vaginal fluid. Therefore, the first step in assessing any patient's risk of HIV infection is directed questioning about any of the above behaviors. Patients with a history of multiple sexual partners or a single reported episode of intravenous drug use are at high risk for HIV infection. In addition, patients who engage in substance abuse of any kind (including noninjection drugs) or trading sex for money or drugs are at high risk for HIV infection. The CDC does not

TABLE 1. Who Should Be Tested for HIV Infection?

High-Risk Populations
  Men who have sex with men
  Persons with multiple sex partners
  Persons who give or have been given money or drugs for sex
  Intravenous drug users
  Persons who have had sex with any partner at risk for or known to have HIV infection
  Patients from regions of high prevalence (e.g., sub-Saharan Africa, Haiti, southeast Asia)

Associated Diagnoses
  Chronic viral hepatitis (B or C)
  Tuberculosis
  Herpes zoster in a patient younger than 50 years
  Severe or new-onset psoriasis or seborrheic dermatitis
  Any sexually transmitted disease, including
    Gonorrhea
    Chlamydia
    Human papillomavirus infection/cervical dysplasia
    Syphilis
    Genital herpes simplex
    Trichomoniasis
  Pregnancy
  Major psychiatric illness
  Injection or noninjection substance abuse
  Other opportunistic infections (e.g., *Pneumocystis* pneumonia, cryptococcosis)
  Molluscum contagiosum

Clinical Syndromes
  Signs or symptoms consistent with primary HIV infection (see Table 2)
  Persistent generalized lymphadenopathy
  Oral candidiasis
  Recurrent vaginal candidiasis
  Recurrent or refractory oral ulcers
  Unexplained weight loss

Adapted from Fennema H, van den Hoek A, van der Heijden J, et al: Regional differences in HIV testing among European patients with sexually transmitted diseases: Trends in the history of HIV testing and knowledge of current serostatus. AIDS 14:1993–2001, 2000; and Kasten MJ: Human immunodeficiency virus: The initial physician-patient encounter. Mayo Clin Proc 77:957–963, 2002.

keep statistics on the prevalence of cocaine or crack use among those infected with HIV, so the magnitude of this risk factor is possibly underemphasized.

Male Homosexual Contact. Almost half of the HIV-infected patients in the United States are men having sex with men (MSM).[7] Similarly, an estimated 42% of new HIV infections will occur in this risk group.[2]

While patients in this risk group no longer account for the majority of HIV cases, it is important to note that MSM are still dramatically overrepresented in both known and new HIV cases. In some urban populations, the seroprevalence of HIV in MSM has been reported as high as

16%.[3] Additionally, the subpopulation of MSM whose prevalence is increasing the fastest is adolescents and young adults, perhaps because they have not seen friends die of AIDS like older generations of MSM have. Some may foster feelings of immortality common to their age group. For these reasons, all MSM should be offered HIV testing at least once. Patients with ongoing risk behaviors should be considered for annual or even semiannual testing.

Heterosexual Contact. About 16% of all currently HIV-infected patients acquired the infection through heterosexual contact.[7] However, *one third* of new infections will occur in this risk group.[2]

Physicians have been slow to recognize the increasing numbers of patients, particularly women, who acquire HIV infection through heterosexual contact. One survey of patients infected through heterosexual contact showed that only 1.3% had been tested primarily because they were perceived to be in a high-risk group.[8] Therefore, the percentage of newly infected patients in this group continues to rise. Any patient with two or more heterosexual partners (at any time) or a history of unprotected sex with a single partner is at higher risk of HIV infection. This applies to both men and women, although viral transmission is more efficient from men to women than from women to men.

Racial Minority. The majority of new infections and the majority of established HIV infections are in members of minority racial groups.[2,7]

Infection with HIV occurs in members of all racial groups, but it is important to note that minorities, and black Americans in particular, account for the majority of patients with HIV infection. The CDC estimates that more than one half of new HIV infections occur in blacks, and that an additional 19% occur in Hispanic Americans.[2] Similarly, approximately two of every three persons living with HIV infection in the United States are black or Hispanic.[7] Although race and ethnicity are not independent risk factors for HIV infection, providers must be aware that members of these groups are statistically more likely to have HIV infection.

Associated Diagnoses

Questions about risk behaviors are the most direct way to gauge a patient's risk of HIV infection. However, it is also important to be aware of diseases that are acquired through similar risk behaviors—the presence of any one of these diseases (summarized in Table 1) significantly increases a patient's risk of testing positive for HIV infection.

Other Sexually Transmitted Disease. The diagnosis of any sexually transmitted disease markedly raises the likelihood of HIV infection.[6,9]

Not all sexually transmitted diseases (STDs) require the passage of infected body fluids from person to person for disease transmission (e.g., herpes simplex, syphilis), and therefore not all patients with STDs engage in risk behaviors that increase the likelihood of acquiring HIV infection. However, multiple studies have consistently shown marked increases in HIV seroprevalence among patients seeking treatment for other STDs. Certain STDs (e.g., gonorrhea) may be more associated with HIV than others,[9] but in general, approximately 5% to 10% of patients with other STDs are HIV-infected.[6,9] Unfortunately, studies also show that one half to two thirds of patients presenting for STD care have never been tested for HIV.[3,5,6] Any STD diagnosis must prompt a recommendation for HIV testing.

Hepatitis. Patients with acute or chronic hepatitis B or C infections should be tested for HIV infection.

Chronic liver disease has become a major cause of morbidity and mortality in HIV-infected patients. Hepatitis B infection can be acquired either through sexual transmission or through exposure to contaminated blood. Hepatitis C infection is predominantly spread through blood exposure, most often in the setting of shared needles during intravenous drug use. Since the modes of acquisition of these infections are also risk factors for HIV infection, all patients with chronic viral hepatitis and patients with acute hepatitis B should be tested for HIV.

Psychiatric Illness. The prevalence of HIV infection in patients with severe psychiatric illnesses, including noninjection substance abuse, may be as high as 5% to 8%.[10]

One review of seroprevalence studies demonstrated an aggregate seroprevalence of 8.5% in samples from mentally ill patients in New York City, but a 5.6% seroprevalence in smaller cities in the eastern United States. A later statewide seroprevalence survey from North Carolina found that 1.6% of patients admitted to state mental hospitals were HIV-infected.[11] While this last number is significantly lower than those from urban centers, it still represents a fourfold increased risk over the United States population as a whole. Furthermore, it is worth noting that many patients with severe mental illness are chronically cared for in settings where HIV testing should be readily available.

As mentioned earlier, noninjection substance abuse (e.g., alcoholism or inhalational or crack cocaine use) has consistently been found to be a risk factor for HIV infection, presumably through the effect of intoxication on a patient's ability to make sound decisions regarding risk behaviors. Although injection drug use is probably a more significant risk factor, noninjection substance abuse is much more prevalent and likely drives a large number of the new HIV infections each year. Patients with active or past noninjection substance abuse are at higher risk for HIV infection.

Pregnancy. All pregnant women should be tested for HIV infection.

Babies born to HIV-infected mothers have a 25% chance of acquiring the infection in the perinatal period if the mother is not treated. However, with the advent of highly active antiretroviral therapy, it is estimated that the risk of transmission can be lowered to less than 2%.[12] Unfortunately, a recently released report from CDC shows that only about half of pregnant women had documented HIV tests.[12] It is precisely the process of offering HIV testing only to those women in perceived risk groups that limits the scope of testing. Because the risk-to-benefit ratio of preventing perinatal transmission so strongly favors testing, all pregnant women should be strongly encouraged to be tested. One issue that prevents an appropriately counseled woman from accepting the test may relate to domestic violence, so inquiring about its presence should be a part of counseling in such situations. A more thorough discussion of issues pertaining to HIV testing of pregnant women can be found elsewhere.[13]

Symptomatic Patients

Although the vast majority of patients with undiagnosed HIV infection are asymptomatic, several studies have shown that about half of new HIV diagnoses are made in the setting of symptomatic disease.[5,8] It is not the goal of this chapter to present a review of opportunistic infections, some of which (e.g., *Pneumocystis* pneumonia) are well-known to many U.S. physicians. However, providers should be familiar with symptoms commonly caused by chronic HIV infection, including the following:

- Persistent generalized lymphadenopathy
- Oral candidiasis without recent use of inhaled steroids or systemic antibiotics
- Recurrent vaginal candidiasis
- Recurrent or refractory oral ulcers
- Unexplained weight loss
- Signs or symptoms consistent with primary HIV infection (see next section)

Although each of these syndromes is most likely not due to HIV infection, patients with any of these clinical findings should be offered HIV testing as part of the work-up for their illnesses, particularly when risk factors for HIV infection are identified.

Primary HIV Infection

Until now, the mainstay of HIV testing and surveillance efforts has been the testing of patients at increased risk for chronic HIV infection, as described in the previous section. However, an increasing focus of attention is the recognition and diagnosis of primary HIV infection. Up to 90% of patients experience some symptoms at the time of initial infection with HIV,[14–22] but the diagnosis is missed in the overwhelming majority of cases. This has important prognostic implications for the patient and the population as a whole, as a diagnosis of primary HIV infection could

- Prompt early antiretroviral treatment, which may
  - Delay the onset of symptomatic acquired immune deficiency syndrome
  - Decrease future viral load "set point," or the maximum viral load that a patient may achieve off of antiretroviral therapy
  - Preserve, to some extent, native immunity against HIV
- Identify HIV-infected patients up to 10 to 15 years before they would otherwise be diagnosed, which may
  - Limit the epidemic spread of the virus
  - Allow for retrospective identification of patients likely to have transmitted the infection

Furthermore, recent studies suggest that obtaining an HIV genotype in recently infected patients has a significant yield for discovery of resistant viral populations,[24] which could have an important impact on choice of antiretroviral treatment regimen and chance of success.

One of the major barriers to diagnosis of primary HIV infection is the nonspecific nature of the clinical presentation: it can look like mononucleosis, influenza, or other nonspecific viral illnesses. In many cases, careful scrutiny will reveal symptoms not typical of these illnesses, but in most the provider must have a high index of suspicion in order to offer HIV testing. Symptoms commonly found in documented cases of primary HIV infection are presented in Table 2.

TABLE 2. Symptoms, Signs, and Laboratory Abnormalities Associated with Primary HIV Infection

Finding	% of Patients (range)
Fever	80 (53–95)
Malaise or fatigue	75 (66–90)
Pharyngitis	55 (43–70)
Rash	55 (35–80)
Headache	55 (32–70)
Myalgias or arthralgias	50 (28–60)
Night sweats	40 (22–51)
Anorexia or weight loss	40 (21–68)
Nausea, vomiting, or diarrhea	35 (24–50)
Oral ulcers	30 (8–43)
Anogenital ulcers	5 (2–15)
Lymphadenopathy	50 (38–70)
Thrombocytopenia	45
Leukopenia	40
Transaminitis	21

Data from Vanhems et al,[15] Vanhems and Beaulieu,[16] Daar et al,[17] Hecht et al,[18] Perlmutter et al,[21] and Schacker.[22]

The most common presenting symptoms of primary HIV infection are fever, maculopapular rash, and pharyngitis or oral ulcers. Fever is present in approximately 80% of primary HIV infection cases, and rash, oropharyngeal disease, myalgias or arthralgias, and fatigue are present in approximately 60% of cases.[14–22] As mentioned earlier, these symptoms are common to a number of other illnesses, and providers should consider primary HIV infection in the differential diagnosis of syndromes such as infectious mononucleosis (particularly heterophile-negative) or streptococcal pharyngitis (particularly when rapid streptococcal testing or culture findings are negative). Table 3 reviews the differential diagnosis of primary HIV infection.

In high-risk populations, some of the more common symptoms of primary HIV infection (e.g., fever, rash, malaise) have positive predictive values of 25% to 35%.[15,17,18] Combining any two of these symptoms (e.g., fever and rash) increases the positive predictive value of the clinical syndrome to 50%. However, these numbers should be applied with caution—they may be applicable in high-risk populations, but in wider use, the positive predictive value of any symptomatic diagnosis alone will fall dramatically as patients at lower risk are included. Nevertheless, given the value of identification of primary HIV infection and the relative infrequency of false-positive HIV test results, providers should strongly consider testing for primary HIV infection when patients have analogous clinical syndromes with no known cause.

TABLE 3. Differential Diagnosis of Primary HIV Infection	
Infectious	**Noninfectious**

Bacterial
  Streptococcal pharyngitis
  Secondary syphilis
  Rickettsial infection (e.g., Rocky Mountain
  Spotted Fever)
	Collagen vascular disease (e.g., systemic
	  lupus erythematosus)
	
	Drug reaction
	
	Fever of unknown origin

Viral
  Infectious mononucleosis
  Viral (e.g., coxsackie) pharyngitis
  Aseptic (e.g., enteroviral) meningitis
  Influenza	

Parasitic Primary toxoplasmosis	
Fever of unknown origin	

Adapted from Perlmutter BL, Glaser JB, Oyugi SO: How to recognize and treat acute HIV syndrome. Am Fam Phys 60:535–546, 1999; and Schacker T: Primary HIV infection: Early diagnosis and treatment are critical to outcome. Postgrad Med 102:143–151, 1997.

HIV Testing

Mechanics of HIV Testing and Counseling

Testing for HIV requires informed consent, as though it were an invasive procedure. The history of this requirement is complex, but ultimately the HIV test is treated differently from other diagnostic tests because of the potential implications for job or housing discrimination. All too commonly, the fact that this test is set apart from others minimizes the likelihood that it will be offered by providers.

If the following recommendations are adhered to, then the counseling and testing can proceed legally in all states. Proper HIV test counseling should include the following:

- A discussion of what HIV is, how it is transmitted, and how to minimize the risk of transmission
- A discussion of the fact that the test results are confidential, and can only be shared with other medical personnel who have a need to know. They cannot legally be shared with anyone else without the patient's expressed written consent. Referral for anonymous testing can be offered as an option as well.
- A discussion of the meanings of positive or negative results (i.e., implications for the patient's health and for transmission to others).
- A discussion of the meaning that the test has for the patient—whether he or she has sufficient support to adjust to bad news, should it occur.
- Thorough counseling for risk reduction.
- Arranging a time for sharing of results and post-test counseling.

The more detailed the information provided to the patient is, the more likely it is that the counseling session will be useful to the patient. Trained HIV counselors cannot be present at all practice sites, so it remains prudent for all providers to refer to the CDC guidelines on counseling and testing, published in 2001 in the Morbidity and Mortality Weekly Report.[25]

Types of HIV Tests

The detailed test characteristics of each available HIV test are beyond the scope of this review. However, care providers must have a basic familiarity with each of the available test types and knowledge of when to use them in order to select the appropriate test and provide an accurate interpretation for the patient. Consultation with an expert is strongly recommended when care providers require assistance with either the choice or the interpretation of HIV testing.

Screening Tests. Screening tests for chronic HIV infection are commonly enzyme-linked immunosorbent assays (ELISAs). These tests are highly sensitive assays, positive in more than 99% of chronically infected patients.

These tests are most commonly run on serum in a hospital or laboratory setting, but home kits are available that offer anonymous testing through oral secretions, urine, or a dried blood spot. All have similar test characteristics.[25] Later generation tests are able to accurately detect all strains of HIV-1, and false-positive test results, once feared, have become rare. However, given the history of higher rates of false-positive results and the significance of a true-positive result, confirmatory testing must always be sought if a screening ELISA is positive.

The most common reason for a falsely negative ELISA is the so-called "window period" after new infection. Since ELISA tests measure the host's antibody response, which can take weeks to months to evolve, patients with primary HIV infection may test negative with this test modality. Older and less sensitive assays could take up to 6 months to become positive, but later generation tests are essentially universally positive within 3 months. In fact, recent data suggest that the vast majority of patients become ELISA-positive only 1 month after infection.[26] Although false-negative results are otherwise rare, this possibility should be entertained in high-risk patients with hypogammaglobulinemia, and alternative testing may be considered.

Occasionally a provider may encounter an "indeterminate" ELISA result, and this must not be misconstrued as negative. In fact, many indeterminate results are from patients evolving primary infection, and, as reviewed, it is especially important to identify these patients. All indeterminate ELISA tests should be repeated at least once.

Confirmatory Testing. Confirmatory testing is usually done through Western blot testing. These tests are very specific, making false-positive results extremely unlikely.

A positive ELISA followed by a positive Western blot confirms the diagnosis of chronic HIV infection. Upon reporting these results to patients, physicians commonly encounter denial. It may be reasonable in limited circumstances to offer repeat testing to a patient who believes his or her test to be falsely positive, but the provider should pursue other testing (e.g., CD4 count, hepatitis testing, complete blood cell count) assuming that the repeat test finding will also be positive.

Western blot tests should not be used for screening, as their sensitivity is unacceptably low. Circumstances in which an ELISA may not be optimal for screening should prompt consultation with a specialist, not the use of Western blot testing as an alternative.

Viral Load Assays. HIV viral load assays should not be used for the diagnosis of chronic HIV infection but may be very useful for the diagnosis of primary HIV infection if results are interpreted properly.

Viral load testing has become a critical component in the management of chronically HIV-infected patients, as the results may be used to forecast a decrement in CD4 cells or guide antiretroviral therapy. These tests are based either on polymerase chain reaction or on DNA polymerization techniques and measure the number of copies of HIV nucleic acid in a patient's serum.

During primary HIV infection, viral loads are often exceptionally high, almost universally greater than 100,000 copies per milliliter. Since (as noted earlier) ELISA testing may not yet be positive, viral load testing should be performed in patients with suspected primary HIV. However, the results of such testing must be interpreted with caution. Low positive results (less than 10,000 copies per milliliter) are usually not indicative of primary infection and may represent false-positive results for any HIV infection.[27] Therefore, in the case any low positive result, testing should be repeated before the results are used to diagnose acute or chronic infection. It is unclear how to interpret results between 10,000 and 100,000 copies per milliliter when testing for primary HIV infection; consultation with a specialist is advised.

Cell Subset Analysis. T cell subset analysis should never be used to diagnose HIV infection.

Most providers are familiar with the decline in CD4 cells that is the hallmark of chronic HIV infection. However, the CD4 cell count can fluctuate in normal populations and can be very low in HIV-negative patients who are acutely ill or treated with corticosteroids. Therefore, although leukopenia and low CD4 cell count are common in patients with chronic HIV infection and may prompt consideration for HIV testing, these measures should never be used as adjunctive HIV tests.

References

1. Centers for Disease Control and Prevention: Diagnosis and reporting of HIV and AIDS in states with HIV/AIDS surveillance—United States, 1994–2000. MMWR Morbid Mortal Wkly Rep 51:595–598, 2002.
2. Centers for Disease Control and Prevention: A glance at the HIV epidemic. http://www.cdc.gov/nchstp/od/news/At-a-Glance.pdf. Accessed November 18, 2002.
3. Centers for Disease Control and Prevention: Unrecognized HIV infection, risk behaviors, and perceptions of risk among young black men who have sex with men—six U.S. cities, 1994–1998. MMWR Morbid Mortal Wkly Rep 51:733–736, 2002.
4. Barry SM, Lloyd-Owen SJ, Cozzi-Lepri A, et al: The changing demographics of new HIV diagnoses at a London centre from 1994 to 2000. HIV Med 3:129–134, 2002.
5. Valdisserri RO, Holtgrave DR, West GR: Promoting early HIV diagnosis and entry into care. AIDS 13:2317–2330, 1999.
6. Fennema H, van den Hoek A, van der Heijden J, et al: Regional differences in HIV testing among European patients with sexually transmitted diseases: Trends in the history of HIV testing and knowledge of current serostatus. AIDS 14:1993–2001, 2000.

7. Centers for Disease Control and Prevention: HIV/AIDS surveillance report. 13:5, 2001.

8. Wortley PM, Chu SY, Diaz T, et al: HIV testing patterns: Where, why, and when were persons with AIDS tested for HIV. AIDS 9:487–492, 1995.

9. Torian LV, Makki HA, Menzies IB, et al: High HIV seroprevalence associated with gonorrhea: New York City Department of Health, sexually transmitted disease clinics, 1990–1997. AIDS 14:189–195, 2000.

10. Cournos F, McKinnon K: HIV seroprevalence among people with severe mental illness in the United States: A critical review. Clin Psychol Rev 17:259–269, 1997.

11. Kirkland KB, Meriwether RA, MacKenzie WR, et al: Clinician judgment as a tool for targeting HIV counseling and testing in North Carolina state mental hospitals, 1994. AIDS Patient Care STDs 13:473–479, 1999.

12. Centers for Disease Control and Prevention: HIV testing among pregnant women—United States and Canada, 1998–2001. MMWR Morbid Mortal Wkly Rep 51:1013–1016, 2002.

13. Institute of Medicine: Reducing the odds: Preventing perinatal transmission of HIV in the United States. Washington, DC: National Academy Press, 1998.

14. Vanhems P, Lecomte C, Fabry J: Primary HIV-1 infection: Diagnosis and prognostic impact. AIDS Patient Care STDs 12:751–758, 1998.

15. Vanhems P, Dassa C, Lambert J, et al: Comprehensive classification of symptoms and signs reported among 218 patients with acute HIV-1 infection. J Acquir Immune Defic Syndr 21:99–106, 1999.

16. Vanhems P, Beaulieu R: Primary infection by type 1 human immunodeficiency virus: Diagnosis and prognosis. Postgrad Med J 73:403–408, 1997.

17. Daar ES, Little S, Pitt J, et al: Diagnosis of primary HIV-1 infection. Ann Intern Med 134:25–29, 2001.

18. Hecht FM, Busch MP, Rawal B, et al: Use of laboratory tests and clinical symptoms for identification of primary HIV infection. AIDS 16:1119–1129, 2002.

19. Yu K, Daar ES: Primary HIV infection: Current trends in transmission, testing, and treatment. Postgrad Med 107:114–122, 2000.

20. Flanigan T, Tashima KT: Diagnosis of acute HIV infection: It's time to get moving! Ann Intern Med 134:75–77, 2001.

21. Perlmutter BL, Glaser JB, Oyugi SO: How to recognize and treat acute HIV syndrome. Am Fam Phys 60:535–546, 1999.

22. Schacker T: Primary HIV infection: Early diagnosis and treatment are critical to outcome. Postgrad Med 102:143–151, 1997.

23. Kasten MJ: Human immunodeficiency virus: The initial physician-patient encounter. Mayo Clin Proc 77:957–963, 2002.

24. Little SJ, Holte S, Routy J, et al: Antiretroviral drug resistance among patients recently infected with HIV. N Engl J Med 347:385–394, 2002.

25. Centers for Disease Control and Prevention: Revised guidelines for HIV counseling, testing, and referral and revised recommendations for HIV screening of pregnant women. MMWR Morbid Mortal Wkly Rep 50:6–32, 2001.

26. Lindback S, Thorstensson R, Karlsson AC, et al: Diagnosis of primary HIV-1 infection and duration of follow-up after HIV exposure. AIDS 14:2333–2339, 2000.

27. Rich JD, Merriman NA, Mylonakis E, et al: Misdiagnosis of HIV infection by HIV-1 plasma viral load testing: A case series. Ann Intern Med 130:37–39, 1999.

Urinary Tract Infections

Barry E. Kenneally, M.D.

chapter

21

Urinary tract infections (UTIs) have long been a "hot topic" in primary care. UTI is described by some practioners as the most common bacterial infection. In the United States, UTI accounts for more than 7 million outpatient office visits per year as well as 1 million emergency room visits.[1] Nosocomial UTI also accounts for an estimated 1 million extra hospital days per year, often by causing gram-negative bacteremia.[1] UTI encompasses a number of diagnoses, including cystitis, pyelonephritis, and prostatitis. This chapter provides an overview of the more common presentations of UTI.

Acute Uncomplicated Cystitis

Cystitis is an inflammatory process of the bladder that is nearly always due to a bacterial infection. *Acute uncomplicated cystitis* can be defined as cystitis in a healthy, young, nonpregnant woman. Acute uncomplicated cystitis is caused by bowel flora that colonizes periurethral tissues and ascends through the urethra, infecting the bladder. About 80% of cases of acute uncomplicated cystitis are caused by *Escherichia coli* and 10% by *Staphylococcus saprophyticus.*[2] Most of the remaining infections are caused by *Proteus mirabilis, Klebsiella pneumoniae, Enterobacter* species, and beta-hemolytic streptococi.[2]

Asymptomatic bacteriuria is a common occurrence among young, sexually active women. In one study, monthly cultures were performed for 6 months in asymptomatic women, and more than 20% of the women in the study had at least one positive culture finding.[3] However, only 8% of these positive cultures were followed by a symptomatic UTI. This finding supports the practice of treating bacteriuria only in symptomatic individuals. Only under special circumstances (e.g., pregnancy, preceding urologic procedures) is it appropriate to treat asymptomatic bacteriuria.

Epidemiology

The lifetime risk of UTI among women may be as high as 60%.[4] Up to 20% of these women will develop recurrent cystitis.[5] Risk factors for acute uncomplicated cystitis include sexual activity, the use of spermicide (especially with diaphragms), delayed micturition (especially after intercourse), recent antibiotic use (especially beta-lactams), and a prior history of UTI. Some women with recurrent UTI have been found to have epithelial glycoproteins and ABO serotype nonsecretion, which predispose them to infection. Certain strains of bacteria also have adherence factors that play a role in colonization and infection.[6]

History

Typical symptoms of cystitis are dysuria, frequency, urgency, suprapubic pain and, less often, gross hematuria. Symptoms of cystitis often follow sexual intercourse by a few days. Delayed micturition (as with travel) and dehydration may also precipitate symptoms. Menstrual history should be recorded, as this can affect urinalysis and treatment.

Pertinent negatives in the history should include the following:
- Vaginal discharge or irritation or pruritis (vaginitis)
- Back pain, fever, nausea, emesis (pyelonephritis)
- Headache, myalgia, photophobia (genital herpes)
- High-risk sexual exposure (urethritis)

Physical Examination

The physical examination in patients suspected of having cystitis is typically brief, focusing on temperature, abdominal examination, and palpation of the costovertebral angle. Although 15% to 20% of patients have mild suprapubic pain or tenderness,[7] the physical examination findings are generally unremarkable. If abdominal tenderness is diffuse or intense, other causes, such as pelvic inflammatory disease or nephrolithiasis, should be considered. Patients with vaginal discharge or significant abdominal tenderness may require a pelvic examination.

Urinalysis

In a dysuric woman with all the pertinent negatives on history and examination, pyuria is diagnostic of UTI. To minimize specimen contamination, urine should be collected using the midstream clean-catch technique. The most accurate method for assessing pyuria is placing unspun urine in a hemacytometer.[8] Ten or more leukocytes per milliliter is considered abnormal. However, most offices do not have a hemacytometer.

More practical methods of urinalysis are using a microscope or a dipstick test for leukocyte esterase. Although the sensitivity of leukocyte esterase for UTI is reported to be 72% to 97%, the true sensitivity is likely somewhat lower, since urethritis caused by chlamydia or gonorrhea may also produce pyuria.[9] Dipstick tests for nitrite may be only as sensitive as 30%. *S. saprophyticus* and *Enterococcus* do not produce nitrite at all.

If dipstick testing findings are negative, microscopy should be performed. Microscopy may also be needed if a patient is self-treating with pyridium, which stains urine and dipsticks with an orange pigment. For microscopy, urine is centrifuged for 2 minutes and examined under high power. White blood cell casts are indicative of upper urinary tract infection. Microscopic pyuria is defined as three or more white blood cells per high-power field (hpf).[10,11] However, some clinicians use a cutoff as low as two leukocytes,[12] whereas others raise the bar to 10 cells per high-power field in unspun urine.[8,13] Defining microscopic pyuria is difficult, since it depends on many factors: hydration status, centrifuge time and speed, resuspension volume, and the volume of urine placed on the slide.

Hematuria occurs in about 40% to 60% of cases of uncomplicated cystitis,[14] but this is unexpected in cases of urethritis and vaginitis. Hematuria is defined as three or more red blood cells in the urine per high-power field.[10] UTI with gross hematuria is termed *hemorrhagic cystitis.* Treatment is unaffected by gross blood, but reassurance is important for patients. In a hematuric patient without pyuria who has significant back, flank, or abdominal pain, it is important to consider renal calculi. False-positive hematuria may occur a few days before or after a menstrual period.

Urine Culture

Urine culture is unnecessary in uncomplicated cases of cystitis.[11–14] However, many clinicians opt to perform cultures in patients with no previous history of UTI. Traditionally, urine cultures were considered positive if there were greater than 10^3 colony-forming units (CFU) per milliliter. However, this cut-off was found to exclude 30%–50% of infections.[14] In symptomatic patients, a colony count of 10^2 CFU/ml is a more reliable predictor of UTI. Unfortunately, some laboratories do not report colony counts below 10^4 CFU/ml.

Differential Diagnosis

Other infectious causes of dysuria that may mimic acute uncomplicated cystitis include urethritis (*Chlamydia trachomatis, Neisseria gonorrhoeae,* or herpes simplex virus) and vaginitis (*Candida* species, bacterial vaginitis, or *Trichomonas vaginalis*). It is important to remember that up to 20% of women with *Chlamydia trachomatis* infection have urethritis only.[15] Such patients would have negative cervical tests for *Chlamydia* and would be unlikely to have vaginal discharge. If urine culture is negative or a patient does not respond to therapy, consider sending urine for chlamydia and gonorrhea nucleic acid testing. In such cases, a pelvic examination should also be performed.

Noninfectious causes of dysuria include interstitial cystitis, dehydration, atrophic vaginitis, sensitivity to topical preparations (e.g., sprays, soaps, scented toilet paper), and postcoital irritation.

Treatment

A single course of antibiotics has at least a 90% cure rate. A 3-day course of antibiotics seems to offer the best compromise between preventing relapse and minimizing side effects.[16] The incidence of side effects (especially gastrointestinal symptoms and yeast infections) increases dramatically after 7 days of therapy.

The traditional first-line treatment of UTI is a three-day course of trimethoprim-sulfamethoxazole (co-trimoxazole). Unfortunately, resistance to co-trimoxazole has increased to as high as 32% in the United States.[17] The Infectious Diseases Society of America has published guidelines for the treatment of UTI (Table 1).[16] If the co-trimaoxzole resistance in a given community is greater than 20%, another antibiotic should be used as the first-line agent.[16] Determination of local resistance can be difficult, since cultures are typically performed only in complicated or resistant cases.

In areas of high resistance to trimethoprim-sulfamethoxazole, fluoroquinolones (ciprofloxacin, norfloxacin, ofloxacin) are a good choice for empirical therapy.[16] It is unclear whether the newer fluoroquinolones achieve high enough urinary concentrations for adequate treatment. Single-dose therapy with other fluoroquinolones (fosfomycin, pefloxacin, rufloxacin) has been studied but not adequately enough to merit recommendation from the Infectious Diseases Society of America. Fosfomycin does have Food and Drug Administration approval for single-dose therapy in cases of acute cystitis, however.

TABLE 1. Empiric Treatment of Acute Uncomplicated Cystitis
1. Trimethoprim-sulfamethoxazole double-strength (Bactrim, Septra) twice daily for 3 days
2. Trimethoprim 100 mg twice daily for 3–7 days
3. Ofloxacin (Floxin) 200 mg twice daily for 3 days
4. Norfloxacin (Noroxin) 400 mg twice daily for 3 days
5. Ciprofloxacin (Cipro) 250 mg twice daily for 3 days
6. Nitrofurantoin (Macrodantin) 50–100 mg twice daily for 7 days (3-day regimen not as effective)
Adapted from Warren JW, Abrutyn E, Hebel JR, et al: Infectious Diseases Society of America practice guidelines for antimicrobial treatment of uncomplicated acute bacterial cystitis and acute pyelonephritis in women. Clin Infect Dis 29:745–758, 1999.

Nitrofurantoin is useful against *E. coli* and *Enterococcus* species. However, it is not effective against *S. saprophyticus* or *Proteus mirabilis.* Some strains of *Enterobacter, Klebsiella,* and gram-negative organisms are resistant to nitrofurantoin. Seven-day therapy is recommended when using nitrofurantoin.[16] Beta-lactam antibiotics can be useful in treating UTI caused by gram-positive organisms, but these are generally less useful in treating UTI.

Pyridium can be very helpful in treating the dysuria associated with UTI. It should only be used for the first 2 days of treatment or it may mask inadequate response to therapy. Patients should be cautioned that pyridium will give their urine and contact lenses an orange color.

Follow-Up

Patients whose symptoms worsen or fail to improve within 72 hours should be reevaluated. A urine culture should be performed at this point to test for antibiotic sensitivities. The alternative diagnoses discussed above should also be reconsidered. Women who respond to treatment do not need a follow-up urine culture for test of cure.

Prevention

A number of practices may help to prevent UTIs:
• Wiping from front to back after bowel movements
• Urinating after intercourse
• Avoiding serial anal-genital contact during sex
• Drinking cranberry juice
• Adequate fluid intake
• Avoiding wet clothing (e.g., bathing suits)

Recurrent Infection

A recurrent UTI occurs within 4 weeks after previous infection. Symptoms that occur sooner than this are likely to be relapses due to the original pathogen. In such cases, it is important to perform urine cultures and re-treat for at least 2 weeks.

Recurrent UTI is usually caused by factors that allow increased bacterial adherence to urinary epithelium. Investigation for anatomical or functional urinary tract abnormalities are generally of low yield. In less than 1% of cases, a surgically correctable lesion is found.[18]

Patients with recurrent UTI can be instructed on patient-initiated therapy. At the onset of typical UTI symptoms, patients simply begin a 3-day course of antibiotics. Patients with more than two episodes of cystitis per year can be offered antibiotic prophylaxis.[19] If the infections are temporally related to intercourse, a single dose of antibiotics should be taken within 2 hours after intercourse. If the infections are unrelated to intercourse, patients can be given continuous daily prophylaxis (Figure 1). Prophylaxis is 95% effective in reducing recurrences without causing an increase in bacterial resisitance.[14] Unfortunately, recurrences tend to happen when prophylaxis is stopped.

Figure 1.   Treatment of recurrent uncomplicated cystitis. (Adapted from Stamm WE, Hooton TM: Current concepts: Management of urinary tract infections in adults. N Engl J Med 329:1328–1334, 1993; Hynes NA: Urinary tract infection, recurrent [women]. In the Johns Hopkins University, Division of Infectious Diseases, Antibiotic Guide. Accessed Sept 17, 2002 at www. hopkins_abxguide.org.

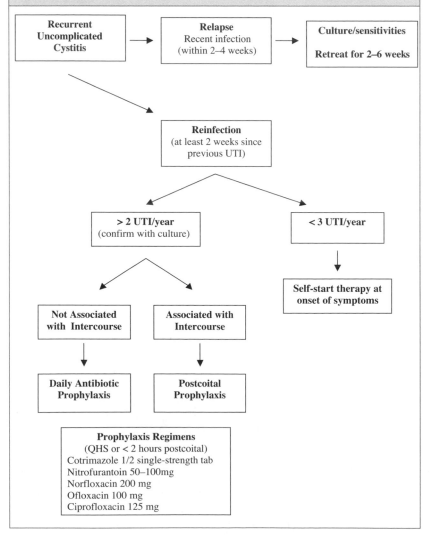

Acute Pyelonephritis

Pyelonephritis is an inflammation of the kidney that is almost always caused by urinary tract infection ascending from the bladder. As with uncomplicated cystitis, pyelonephritis can be classified as uncomplicated if it occurs in a young, healthy nonpregnant woman. Most cases of pyelonephritis occur in women with normal urinary tracts. The causative organisms in pyelonephritis are similar to those in cystitis except that *S. saprophyticus* is less common.

The distinction between cystitis and pyelonephritis is often indiscernible in the clinical setting. Investigational radiologic studies have shown that subclinical upper urinary tract infections occur in about one third of patients who otherwise seem to have uncomplicated cystitis.[20]

Symptoms

It is important to remember that pyelonephritis can occur without symptoms of lower urinary tract infection. This may be a more common presentation in initial UTI, since patients may ignore mild dysuria.

Typical symptoms of pyelonephritis include the following:

- Unilateral back/flank/abdominal pain
- Fever
- Nausea
- Emesis
- Lower urinary tract symptoms (may not be present)

Urinalysis

Urinalysis in cases of pyelonephritis is similar to that in cystitis: pyuria, hematuria, bacteriuria, and nitrite. In cases of pyelonephritis, white blood cell casts may also be found.

Culture

Unlike for cystitis, urine culture with antibiotic susceptibility testing should *always* be performed in cases of pyelonephritis.[16] Although complications are not common, they are more likely to occur if treatment is inadequate. Complications include renal scarring and, rarely, chronic renal failure. Typically, colony counts are higher (>100,000 CFU/ml) than those in cystitis. However, up to 20% of cases have counts less than 10,000.

Blood Testing

Most patients with pyelonephritis do not require blood testing, but in toxic-appearing patients or those who are hospitalized, complete blood cell count and two sets of blood cultures should be performed. Blood culture findings are positive in 12% to 20% of pyelonephritis cases.[8,19] Bacteremia in pyelonephritis does not alter treatment or outcome, however.[8]

Treatment

Outpatient Therapy. Most pyelonephritis patients can be treated as outpatients. Compliant women with pyelonephritis who have only slight elevations in temperature and white blood cell count and who have no nausea or vomiting can be treated as outpatients with 7 to 14 days of oral antibiotics. Antibiotic treatment should be aimed at the same pathogens that cause acute cystitis (e.g., *E. coli, S. saprophyticus*). Fluoroquinolones are the drugs of choice for empirical therapy.[16] Co-trimoxazole should be used only if the causative organism is known to be susceptible. If a gram-positive organism is causative, amoxicillin or amoxicillin-clavulanate can be used.[16] Patients who do not improve with 48 to 72 hours of appropriate therapy should be investigated for obstruction or renal abscess with either renal ultrasonography or abdominal computed tomography (CT).

To avoid hospitalizations, some clinicians will observe patients for up to 24 hours on intravenous therapy to assess response to treatment. If the response is rapid, admission can be avoided. Another option in reliable patients is to give once-daily intravenous or intramuscular dosing (e.g., ceftriaxone, levofloxacin) in the outpatient setting. Other clinicians simply administer a single dose of parenteral antibiotics before starting oral antibiotics. All of these options are reasonable.

Inpatient Therapy. Hospital admission for intravenous antibiotics and fluids is required in patients who appear toxic or cannot ingest medications or adequate fluids. Several antibiotic regimens can be used in the inpatient setting. These include fluoroquinolones, an aminoglycoside (with or without ampicillin), or a broad-spectrum cephalosporin (with or without an aminoglycoside).[16] Once antibiotics and hydration are started, most patients improve within 72 hours. Once a patient's condition has improved, treatment can be switched to oral antibiotics tailored to the pathogen's antibiotic susceptibility.

As with outpatient therapy, renal ultrasonography or abdominal CT should be performed if a patient does not improve within 72 hours. Rarely, patients with renal parenchymal involvement will continue to mount low-grade fevers after several days of appropriate therapy. If these patients are otherwise improving (e.g., decreased pain, advancement of diet), it is reasonable to discharge them on oral antibiotics and follow them closely as outpatients.

Follow-Up

Once symptoms have completely resolved, routine follow-up is not necessary after an isolated case of pyelonephritis. However, patients with several cases or resistant cases of pyelonephritis warrant a urologic work-up.

Urinary Tract Infections in Men

From adolescence through middle age, UTI is much more common in women. However, the incidence of UTI among elderly men and women is almost equal. The main reason for this change in epidemiology is benign prostatic hypertrophy. As with women, sexual activity (especially anal sex) is a risk factor for men. Other risk factors include being uncircumcised and having sex with men.

The male urinary tract is less prone to UTI for a number of reasons: the urethral meatus is farther removed from the perineum, the urethra is longer, and prostatic secretions possess antibacterial activity. The pathogens causing infection in men differ slightly from those in women. Gram-negative rods cause about 75% of infections in men, but only half of these are caused by E. coli.[21] Gram-positive bacteria cause about 20% of infections in men, but S. saprophyticus is rarely involved.[21]

Symptoms

In addition to the irritative symptoms that women with UTI suffer, men may also report obstructive symptoms (weak stream, hesitance, dribbling, nocturia) related to the prostate gland. Obstructive symptoms may be directly related to secondary infection of the prostate or may reflect underlying prostate pathology. Predominance of either irritative or obstructive symptoms does not aid in predicting bacteriuria.[22] Patients reporting irritative or obstructive symptoms should be assessed for UTI, prostatitis, and benign prostatic hypertrophy.

Physical Examination

As with women, examination of men with a potential UTI should include temperature measurement, abdominal examination, and palpation of the costovertebral angles. In men, however, the genitals should always be examined as well.

The examination should include assessment for the following:
- Penile lesions
- Inflammation of the glans (retract foreskin if uncircumcised)
- Urethral discharge
- Meatal erythema
- Tender/swollen testicle
- Tender/swollen epididymis
- Tender/swollen prostate
- Inguinal adenopathy

Laboratory Tests

In men, urine cultures should always be performed. Midstream urine collection is unnecessary in men. Even in uncircumcised men, the likelihood of contamination is low.[22] Culture is considered positive with a CFU exceeding 10^3/ml of one organism.[23]

Based on history and physical examination findings, acute uncomplicated cystitis is difficult to differentiate from prostatitis. Three-glass or four-glass testing can help to localize the infection.[21] First-void (urethral), midstream (bladder), and end-stream (bladder) urine samples are collected and cultured. A fourth sample is obtained by expressing secretions through prostatic massage. Infection is localized to the prostate if the prostatic samples (end-void or prostatic secretions) yield a 10-fold greater colony count than the first-void sample. Most clinicians do not routinely perform these tests because they are cumbersome, expensive, and not well standardized. Some clinicians opt to perform simple urinalysis on three- or four-glass specimens. In men whose culture findings are negative, testing for gonorrhea and chlamydia should be performed. Other possible pathogens include *Ureaplasma, Trichomonas,* and herpes simplex virus.

Treatment

Antibiotic choice in men is similar to that in women. However, beta-lactams and nitrofurantoin tend to be less effective, since they do not achieve high concentrations within the prostate gland.[8] Fluoroquinolones are generally favored, and men are typically treated for 7 to 14 days. Recurrent infection likely represents residual prostatic infection, in which case retreatment for 4 to 6 weeks is prudent.

Follow-Up

About one third of young men with one UTI have demonstrable (on renal ultrasonogram, intravenous pyelogram, or voiding cystourethrogram) urinary tract defects.[23] However, these numbers may not differ much from women's and usually do not affect treatment. Isolated infections are treated with 7 to 10 days of antibiotics, and frequent infections (more than two per year) are treated with prophylaxis. Most experts do not recommend urologic evaluation for men with a single UTI.[8,23]

Prostatitis

Definition

About half of all men will develop symptoms of prostatitis at some point in their lives.[21] In 1995, the National Institutes of Health (NIH) created a classification system for prostatitis[24]:

a. Acute bacterial prostatitis
b. Chronic bacterial prostatitis
c. Chronic nonbacterial prostatitis/chronic pelvic pain syndrome
    i. Inflammatory prostatitis (leukocytes in expressed prostatic secretions or voided bladder urine-3)
    ii. Noninflammatory prostatitis (no leukocytes)
d. Asymptomatic inflammatory prostatitis

Infectious causes of prostatitis include those organisms that cause cystitis (e.g., *E. coli*) and those that cause sexually transmitted infection (e.g., *C. trachomatis, N. gonorrhoeae*).

Symptoms

The symptoms of prostatitis can be classified into two groups:
* Irritative
  * Dysuria
  * Frequency
  * Urgency
* Obstructive
  * Hesitance
  * Dribbling
  * Weak stream
  * Nocturia

Acute Prostatitis

Acute prostatitis, an uncommon presentation, is a severe systemic illness. Aside from the typical UTI and prostatitis symptoms, patients may also present with urinary retention, fever, and rigors.

On examination, patients may appear toxic. Examiners should forgo prostatic massage, and prostate examination should be gentle to avoid inducing bacteremia. The prostate is usually exquisitely tender and swollen and may be warm to the touch.

Urine testing for pyuria and bacterial culture is generally positive. Acute prostatitis is caused by the same organisms that cause UTI (see earlier). If a patient can tolerate oral medications, a fluoroquinolone, co-trimoxazole, or trimethoprim is used for 28 days. Those patients requiring hospitalization should be started on a broad-spectrum cephalosporin plus gentamicin.[24] Treatment should also include bed rest, pain control, stool softeners, and hydration.

For cases of acute urinary retention, catheterization should be suprapubic to avoid prostate damage.[24] If response to therapy is poor, transrectal ultrasonography or abdominal CT should be used to rule out a prostatic abscess. Once fully recovered, patients should undergo urologic evaluation.

Chronic Bacterial Prostatitis

This is a subacute infection with milder symptoms and a more insidious onset than acute prostatitis. The NIH has developed a chronic prostatitis symptom index to measure the symptoms and their impact on daily life.[26] Although produced for research purposes, the scale has been found to be useful in localizing urinary symptoms to the prostate gland. A score of more than 4 on the pain questions (the first four questions), has been found to be indicative of prostatitis.[27] The remainder of the questions can be used to assess the severity of symptoms and gauge response to treatment.

Urine cultures should be performed to rule out UTI. If sexual history warrants, testing for gonorrhea and chlamydia should be performed. The physical examination findings in cases of chronic bacterial prostatitis are generally unremarkable except for the prostate gland, which may be boggy and slightly tender.

First-line treatment of chronic bacterial prostatitis is 4 to 12 weeks[23] of therapy with a fluorquinolone.[25] Alternatives include minocycline, doxycycline, trimethoprim, and co-trimoxazole.

Chronic Nonbacterial Prostatitis

More than 90% of cases of prostatitis are chronic nonbacterial cases.[28] Unfortunately, the cause and appropriate treatment remain elusive. In some cases, occult infection may be the cause. When nucleic acid testing is performed on prostate biopsy specimens, evidence of infection is found in up to 77% cases.[29,30] These studies were not well controlled, and response to antibiotic treatment was found to be poor. Other possible causes include atypical infections (*Chlamydia, Trichomonas, Mycoplasma, Ureaplasma*), reflux secondary to urethral spasm, excessive ejaculation, infrequent ejaculation, prostate trauma (as with receptive anal intercourse), interstitial cystitis, allergy, and stress.

Symptoms and signs in patients with chronic nonbacterial prostatitis are the same as those for bacterial causes. Urine and prostatic fluid cultures are negative in nonbacterial cases. The NIH chronic prostatitis symptom scale can also be applied to nonbacterial cases.

Treatment of chronic nonbacterial prostatitis is generally disappointing, since the response rate is so poor. Many clinicians believe that a 1-month trial of antibiotics to cover for occult infection is reasonable.[23] Other treatments include sitz-baths, anti-inflammatory agents, Quercetin (a bioflavinoid), stress reduction, alpha-blockers, allopurinol, avoiding caffeine, and transurethral microwave thermatherapy. The number and variety of treatments reflect the confusion surrounding this illness. More research is needed to improve the quality of life in men suffering from this disease.

Complicated Urinary Tract Infection

The distinguishing feature of complicated infections is that they are resistant to treatment. Longer treatment regimens are indicated and close follow-up is prudent. Treatment should be prolonged for 7 to 14 days in most cases.

Factors that complicate a UTI include the following[31]:

- Pregnancy
- Male gender
- Advanced age
- Pediatric age group
- Symptoms for more than 7 days
- Indwelling urinary catheter
- Diabetes mellitus
- Relapsing infection
- Immunosuppression
- Recent hospitalization (within 2 weeks)
- Recent nephrolithiasis
- Urinary tract stents
- Unusual pathogens (yeasts, *Myoplasma, Pseudomonas*)

Classifying a UTI as complicated can be troublesome. There are no specific guidelines for dealing with each complication. But with prolonged treatment of up to 14 days, cure can be achieved in 80% to 90% of cases.[31]

UTI in Diabetes Mellitus

Patients with diabetes mellitus are more likely to have anatomic abnormalities of the urinary tract and unusual organisms. Pathogens causing UTI in this population include *Pseudomonas* and *Candida*. Some practitioners recommend that diabetes mellitus patients with UTI should have urine cultures performed before and after therapy.[32] Broad-spectrum antibiotics (e.g., fluoroquinolones) are a reasonable choice for empiric therapy, and treatment should last at least 7 days.

UTI in Pregnancy

A urine culture is routinely performed to screen asymptomatic patients during pregnancy, and asymptomatic bacteriuria is present in up to 10% of pregnant women.[33] Urine culture should be performed at the first prenatal visit or between 12 and 16 weeks of gestation, as well as once during the third trimester.[33] Treating these infections has been shown to decrease the incidence of preterm birth and low birth weight infants. Pregnant women with UTI should be treated for 14 days. Fluoroquinolones should not be used in pregnant patients. Antibiotics that are generally considered to be safe in pregnancy (class B) include cephalexin, erythromycin, nitrofurantoin, amoxicillin-clavulonate, and fosfomycin.

References

1. Foxman B: Epidemiology of urinary tract infections: Incidence, morbidity, and economic costs. Am J Med 113:5S–13S, 2002.
2. Kurowski K: The woman with dysuria. Am Fam Phys 57:2155–2164, 1998.
3. Hooton TM, Scholes D, Stapleton AE, et al: A prospective study of asymptomatic bacteriuria in sexually active young women. N Engl J Med 343:992–997, 2000.
4. Foxman B, Barlow R, D'Arcy H, et al: Urinary tract infection: Self-reported incidence and associated costs. Ann Epidemiol 10:509–515, 2000.
5. Orenstein R, Wong ES: Urinary tract infections in adults. Am Fam Phys 59:1225–1234, 1237, 1999.
6. Johnson JR: Virulence factors in E. coli urinary tract infection. Clin Microbiol Rev 4:80–128, 1991.
7. Wigton RS, Hoellerich VL, Ornato JP, et al: Use of clinical findings in the diagnosis of urinary tract infections in women. Arch Intern Med 145:2222–2227, 1985.
8. Hooton TM, Stamm WE: Diagnosis and treatment of uncomplicated urinary tract infection. Infect Dis Clin North Am 11:551–581, 1997.
9. Pels RJ, Bor DH, Woolhandler S, et al: Dipstick urinalysis screening of asymptomatic adults for urinary tract disorders. JAMA 262:1221–1224, 1989.
10. Bakerman S, Bakerman P, Strausbauch P: Bakerman's ABC's of Interpretive Laboratory Data, 2nd ed. Myrtle Beach, SC: Interpretive Laboratory Data, 1994:516–519.
11. Bremner JD, Sadovsky R: Evaluation of dysuria in adults. Am Fam Phys 65:1589–1596, 2002.
12. Komaroff AL: Urinalysis and urine culture in women with dysuria. Ann Intern Med 104:212–218, 1986.
13. Bent S, Saint S: The optimal use of diagnostic testing in women with acute uncomplicated cystitis. Am J Med 113:20S–28S, 2002.
14. Schaeffer A: Urinary tract infections. In: Campbell's Urology, 8th ed. Philadelphia: WB Saunders, 2002:515–592.
15. Brokenshire MK, Say PJ, Van Vonno AH, Wong C: Evaluation of microparticle enzyme immunoassay Abbott IMx Select Chlamydia and the importance of urethral site sampling to detect Chlamydia trachomatis in women. Genitourinary Med 73:498–502, 1997.
16. Warren JW, Abrutyn E, Hebel JR, et al: Infectious Diseases Society of America practice guidelines for antimicrobial treatment of uncomplicated acute bacterial cystitis and acute pyelonephritis in women. Clin Infect Dis 29:745–758, 1999.
17. Talan DA, Stamm WE, Hooton TM, et al: Comparison of ciprofloxacin (7 days) and trimethoprim-sulfamethoxazole (14 days) for acute uncomplicated pyelonephritis in women. JAMA 283:1583–1590, 2000.
18. Fowler JE: Excretory urography, cystography, and cystoscopy in the evaluation of women with urinary tract infection: A prospective study. N Engl J Med 304:462–465,

1981.
19. Stamm WE, Hooton TM: Current concepts: Management of urinary tract infections in adults. N Engl J Med 329:1328–1334, 1993.
20. Ronald AR, Boutros P, Mourtada H: Bacteriuria localization and response to single-dose therapy in women. JAMA 235:1854–1856, 1976.
21. Lipsky BA: Urinary tract infections in men. Ann Intern Med 110:138–150, 1989.
22. Lipsky BA, Ireton RC, Fihn SD, et al: Diagnosis of bacteriuria in men: Specimen collection and culture interpretation. J Infect Dis 155:847–854, 1987.
23. Lipsky BA: Prostatitis and urinary tract infections in men: What's new; what's true. Am J Med 106:327–334, 1999.
24. National Institutes of Health Summary Statement: National Institutes of Health/National Institute of Diabetes and Digestive and Kidney Diseases workshop on chronic prostatitis. Executive summary, Bethesda, Maryland, December 1995. Accessed Oct 2002 at http:www.niddk.nih.gov/health/urology/pubs/cpwork/cpwork.htm.
25. Association of Genitourinary Medicine and the Medical Society for the Study of Venereal Diseases: National guidelines for the management of prostatitis. Clinical Effectiveness Group. Sexually Transmitted Infections 75:S46–50, 1999.
26. Litwin MS, Naughton-Collins M, Fowler FJ, et al: The National Institutes of Health chronic prostatitis symptom index: Development and validation of a new outcome measure. J Urol 162:369–375, 1999.
27. Nickel JC, Downey J, Hunter D, Clark J: Prevalence of prostatitis-like symptoms in a population based study using the National Institutes of Health chronic prostatitis symptom index. J Urol 165:842–845, 2001.
28. McNaughton Collins M, MacDonald R, Wilt IJ: Diagnosis and treatment of chronic abacterial prostatitis: A systematic review. Ann Intern Med 133:367–381, 2000.
29. Krieger JN, Riley DE, Vesella RL, et al: Bacterial DNA sequencing in prostate tissue from patients with prostate cancer and chronic prostatitis. J Urol 164:1221–1228, 2000.
30. Krieger JN, Riley DE, Roberts MC, et al: Prokaryotic DNA sequence in patients with chronic idiopathic prostatitis. J Clin Microbiol 34:3120–3128, 1996.
31. Ronald AR, Harding GKM: Complicated urinary tract infections. Infect Dis Clin North Am 1:583–592, 1997.
32. Stapleton A: Urinary tract infections in patients with diabetes. Am J Med 113:80S–84S, 2002.
33. Delzell JE, Letevre ML: Urinary tract infections during pregnancy. Am Fam Phys 61:713–721, 2000.

Sexually Transmitted Diseases

chapter

22

Barry E. Kenneally, M.D.

Sexually transmitted infections (STIs) are always a "hot topic" in primary care, since practitioners deal with a broad range of STIs. Diagnosing and treating these infections can be challenging, because organisms, treatments, and diagnostic technologies constantly evolve. However, these cases offer an opportunity to counsel patients on safer sex practices and other risk behaviors. The following pages are a review of common STIs seen in primary care. Special attention is given to the new guidelines published by the Centers for Disease Control and Prevention (CDC) in May 2002.[1]

Pelvic Inflammatory Disease

Pelvic inflammatory disease (PID) is an inflammatory disorder of the female upper genital tract that can include endometritis, salpingitis, tubo-ovarian abscess, and pelvic peritonitis. Sexually transmitted organisms such as *Neisseria gonorrhoeae, Chlamydia trachomatis, Mycoplasma hominis,* and *Ureaplasma urealyticum* cause many cases of PID. However, organisms that comprise the normal vaginal flora (*Gardnerella vaginalis, Haemophilus influenzae, Streptococcus agalactiae,* enteric gram-negative rods) have also been implicated.

Pelvic inflammatory disease has a number of severe long-term sequelae. Of women who develop PID, 20% develop infertility, 18% suffer from chronic pelvic pain, and 9% will have an ectopic pregnancy.[2] Because of these devastating sequelae, the CDC has cautioned clinicians to maintain a low threshold for its diagnosis and treatment, and this should be especially true among sexually active young women. Preventing these sequelae is the reason that *C. trachomatis* screening in asymptomatic women has been implemented, as *C. trachomatis* causes about 40% of PID cases.[1]

Risk Factors

A number of risk factors for PID have been identified and should be recognized by practitioners:
- Age less than 35 years
- Nonbarrier contraception
- New, multiple, or symptomatic sexual partners
- History of PID

Clinical Findings

Bilateral lower abdominal pain is the most typical symptom in PID. The pain may be mild and is sometimes present only during intercourse or menses. Other symptoms include vaginal discharge, fever, and dysuria. On examination, patients with PID may appear well or toxic. If abdominal tenderness is present, it is typically diffuse. Fever and vaginal discharge are important signs to look for.

Diagnosis

The diagnosis of PID can often be challenging, since a wide variety of symptoms, which may be mild, are often seen. Although only 50% sensitive and specific, the diagnosis is usually made clinically.[3]

In women at risk for PID who have no apparent alternative diagnosis, the CDC has suggested several findings on physical examination that are suggestive of PID[1]:
- Uterine tenderness
- Adnexal tenderness
- Cervical motion tenderness

Use of these criteria makes it very unlikely that a case of PID will go undetected.[3]

Additional criteria that support the diagnosis of PID are the following:
- Temperature greater than 101°F
- Abnormal mucopurulent cervical or vaginal discharge (Most women with PID will have visible mucopurulent discharge or vaginal secretions with white blood cells. If neither of these finding is present, serious consideration should be given to an alternate diagnosis.[1])
- White blood cells in vaginal secretions
- Elevated erythrocyte sedimentation rate
- Elevated C-reactive protein
- Positive tests for *N. gonorrhoeae* or *C. trachomatis* (However, negative endocervical *N. gonorrhoeae* or *C. trachomatis* tests do not rule out infection of the upper genital tract.)

Several other tests may be helpful in supporting a diagnosis of PID, and these include laparoscopy, endometrial biopsy, transvaginal ultrasonography, and magnetic resonance imaging. Laparoscopy is very useful, but it is not always readily available, and it is difficult to justify in mild cases. Imaging studies such as ultrasonography or magnetic resonance imaging may be used to look for distinct abnormalities: fallopian tubes that are thickened or fluid-filled; free pelvic fluid; or a tubo-ovarian complex. Power Doppler ultrasonography to detect fallopian tube hyperemia is a newer technology that may prove useful.[3]

Treatment

Early treatment is imperative to prevent the long-term sequelae of PID. Most patients can be treated on an outpatient basis, and only 10% to 25% of patients with PID are now hospitalized for treatment.[4]

Factors that might warrant hospitalization include the following:
- Pregnancy
- Severe illness with vomiting or high fever
- Tubo-ovarian abscess
- Intolerance to oral antibiotic regimen
- Poor response to oral antibiotics
- Surgical abdomen not excluded

Empiric treatment needs to cover a wide range of bacteria, including N. gonorrhoeae, C. trachomatis, anaerobes, gram-negative facultative bacteria, and streptococci. There are no efficacy data that compare parenteral and oral regimens, but the efficacy of each has been demonstrated in many clinical trials. If treatment is initiated with parenteral drugs, the transition to oral medications can be made within 24 hours of clinical improvement. The total duration of antibiotic treatment should be 14 days.

Parenteral Regimens. The decision to use parenteral therapy can be guided by the criteria for hospitalization. The CDC recommends two parenteral regimens (Table 1): doxycycline plus cefotetan (Cefotan) or cefoxitan (Mefoxin); and clindamycin (Cleocin) plus gentamicin.[1] If possible, doxycycline should be administered orally because of the pain associated with intravenous infusion. Alternative parenteral regimens are also given in Table 1.

Once a clinical improvement occurs, patients can be switched to an oral regimen of doxycycline (100 mg every 12 hours) or clindamycin (450 mg every 6 hours) for a total of 14 days of therapy.[1] Clindamycin for anaerobic coverage may be more appropriate if a tubo-ovarian abscess is present.

There are limited data to support the use of other parenteral regimens, but the three alternative regimens listed by the CDC are (1) ofloxacin (Floxin) with or without metronidazole (Flagyl); (2) levofloxacin (Levaquin) with or without metronidazole; and (3) ampicillin/sulbactam (Unasyn) plus doxycycline.[1] Although some clinicians treat PID with

TABLE 1. Parenteral Treatment of Pelvic Inflammatory Disease.

Recommended by CDC	Alternative
Regimen A Cefotetan (Cefotan) 2 g IV every 12 hours *or* Cefoxitin (Mefoxin) 2 g IV every 6 hours *plus* Doxycycline 100 mg IV or PO every 12 hours (oral doxycycline is preferred, since IV doxycycline can be very painful) **Regimen B** Clindamycin 900 mg IV every 8 hours *plus* Gentamicin 2 mg/kg IM or IV loading dose followed by 1.5 mg/kg IV every 8 hours (once-daily gentamicin can also be used)	**Regimen A** Ofloxacin (Floxin) 400 mg IV every 12 hours *with or without* Metronidazole (Flagyl) 500 mg IV every 8 hours **Regimen B** Levofloxacin (Floxin) 500 mg IV once daily *with or without* Metronidazole (Flagyl) 500 mg IV every 8 hours **Regimen C** Ampicillin/sulbactam (Unasyn) 3 g IV every 6 hours *plus* Doxycycline 100 mg PO or IV every 12 hours

Adapted from Centers for Disease Control and Prevention: Sexually transmitted disease treatment guidelines 2002. MMWR Morbid Mortal Wkly Rep 51(RR-6):1–78, 2002.

fluoroquinolones alone, the addition of metronidazole offers better coverage of anaerobes.

Oral Regimens. Two CDC-recommended oral regimens for PID are ofloxacin with or without metronidazole and levofloxacin with or without metronidazole (Table 2). Each regimen is administered for 14 days. As with parenteral regimens, the addition of metronidazole offers better coverage of anaerobes.

Combined Oral and Parenteral Regimens. Another set of CDC-recommended regimens combine single-dose intramuscular medications with oral medications (Table 3).

TABLE 2. Oral Antibiotic Regimens for Pelvic Inflammatory Disease

Ofloxacin (Floxin) 400 mg orally twice a day for 14 days
or
Levofloxacin (Levaquin) 500 mg orally once daily for 14 days
with or without
Metronidazole (Flagyl) 500 mg orally twice daily for 14 days

Adapted from Centers for Disease Control and Prevention. Sexually transmitted disease treatment guidelines 2002. MMWR Morbid Mortal Wkly Rep 51(RR-6):1–78, 2002.

TABLE 3. Combined Parenteral and Oral Regimens for Pelvic Inflammatory Disease
Ceftriaxone (Rocephin) in a single intramuscular dose of 250 mg
or
Cefoxitin (Mefoxin) in a single intramuscular dose of 2 g (with Probenecid 1 g orally)
or
Another parenteral third-generation cephalosporin (e.g. ceftizoxime [Cefizox], cefotaxime [Claforan])
plus
Doxycycline 100 mg PO twice daily for 14 days
with or without
Metronidazole (Flagyl) 500 mg PO twice daily for 14 days
Adapted from Centers for Disease Control and Prevention. Sexually transmitted disease treatment guidelines 2002. MMWR Morbid Mortal Wkly Rep 51(RR-6):1–78, 2002.

Follow-Up

Patients receiving outpatient therapy should be seen within 3 days for re-evaluation. If there has been no substantial improvement, hospitalization for intravenous antibiotics and further evaluation is warranted. If *N. gonorrhoeae* or *C. trachomatis* is detected, many clinicians recommend testing for cure 4 to 6 weeks after therapy is completed. Recent (60 days) sexual partners should also be evaluated. During follow-up evaluations, consideration should he given to testing for other sexually transmitted infections such as human immunodeficiency virus, human papillomavirus, syphilis, and hepatitis B virus.

Urethritis

Urethritis is an inflammation of the urethra characterized by mucopurulent or purulent urethral discharge, dysuria, or urethral pruritis. It is usually caused by infection, and patients are asymptomatic in about 50% of cases.[1] The organisms causing urethritis in men typically cause cervicitis in women. However, over 20% of infected women may have urethral infection only.[5]

Urethritis is usually caused by sexually transmitted organisms. Gonococcal urethritis is caused by *N. gonorrhoeae,* which is isolated in 20% of men with urethritis.[6] In contrast, nongonococcal urethritis may be caused by *C. trachomatis, U. urealyticum, Mycoplasma genitalium, M. hominis, Trichomonas vaginalis,* and herpes simplex virus. *C. trachomatis* is isolated in 30% to 50% of nongonococcal urethritis cases.[7]

Clinical Findings

Patients with urethritis may complain of a mucopurulent or purulent urethral discharge, dysuria, or urethral pruritis. Male patients with urethritis may present with prostatitis symptoms such as weak urinary stream, perineal pain, and ejaculatory pain. A sexual history of recent contacts is also important. Nongonococcal urethritis tends to have a more insidious onset and milder symptoms. In cases of gonococcal infection, 3% of patients will develop generalized symptoms such as fever, rash, and polyarthritis.[8]

Men with symptoms of urethritis should have a thorough genital examination. The penis should be assessed for lesions suggestive of warts or herpes. Erythema of the distal urethra may be noted. If there is no spontaneous urethral discharge, the glans penis should be gently squeezed to express fluid. Any fluid should be collected for microscopic examination. Inguinal lymphadenopathy may be present. If there are symptoms suggestive of prostate involvement, a rectal examination should be performed. This is important because prostate involvement may necessitate prolonged antibiotic therapy.

Fever, a pustular or papular rash, and tenosynovitis are signs of gonococcemia. Reiter's syndrome is an autoimmune response that is often seen in cases of urethritis, especially with *C. trachomatis* infection. Reiter's syndrome manifests as synovitis, nonarticular bone pain (especially the heel), iritis, conjunctivitis, and ulcerations of the oral or genital mucosae.

Diagnosis

Urethritis can be diagnosed if any of the following criteria are present[1]:
- Visible mucopurulent or purulent urethral discharge
- Gram stain of urethral secretions showing more than four leukocytes per oil immersion field
- Positive leukocyte esterase test on first-void urine
- First-void urine with more than nine leukocytes per high-power field

The CDC considers Gram stain to be the best rapid test for diagnosing urethritis. Demonstration of gram-negative intracellular diplococci has 99.6% correlation with Gen-Probe for *N. gonorrhoeaea*.[9] However, many clinicians do not have office-based Gram stain capabilities. If none of the above criteria are met, treatment can be deferred pending the results of specific testing for *N. gonorrhoeae* and *C. trachomatis*. But many clinicians will initiate empiric treatment at this point, especially if patient follow-up is questionable. Empiric treatment will cover some of those organisms that are not routinely cultured, such as *M. hominis, M. genitalium,* and *U. urealyticum.*

Nucleic acid amplification tests, which target and amplify sequences of DNA or RNA that are specific to *N. gonorrhoeae* or *C. trachomatis,* are easier, cheaper, and more sensitive than traditional culture methods.[10] Amplification techniques include ligase chain reaction, polymerase chain reaction, and transcription-mediated amplification. Rapid 30-minute nucleic acid tests for office use are available but are not as sensitive as laboratory-based tests.[10] Testing first-void urine specimens may be slightly less sensitive than using urethral swab samples.[10] However, many clinicians (and patients) prefer urine sampling for its ease of use. First-void urine sampling involves collecting the first 10 to 20 mL of a void. Patients should not have urinated for 30 to 60 minutes before the sample is collected.

Treatment

Treatment of Gonococcal Urethritis. Because of resistance, the CDC does not recommend the use of fluoroquinolones for infections acquired in Asia or the Pacific (including Hawaii).[1] In addition, the CDC has stated that it is "probably inadvisable" to use fluoroquinolones for infections acquired in California.[1] Antibiotics for the treatment of gonococcal infection include cefixime (Suprax), ceftriaxone (Rocephin), ciprofloxacin (Cipro), levofloxacin (Levaquin), and ofloxacin (Floxin) (Table 4).[1] Alternative antibiotics for *N. gonorrhoeae* infection include spectinomycin, ceftizoxime, cefoxitin (with probenecid), cefotaxime, gatifloxacin, norfloxacin, and lomefloxacin.[1] Since coinfection with *C. trachomatis* occurs in 10% to 30% of gonococcal urethritis cases, treatment for both infections should be provided.[7] A single 2 g dose of azithromycin treats both gonococcal and chlamydial infection, but this is not recommended by the CDC, presumably because of the significant gastrointestinal side effects. Instead, the CDC recommends combining the regimens for gonococcal and nongonoccal urethrits.

Treatment of Nongonococcal Urethritis. The first-line regimens for the treatment of nongonococcal urethritis are either azithromycin (Zithromax) in a single 1 g oral dose or doxycycline 100 mg orally twice daily for 7 days (Table 5).[1] Clearly, azithromycin is a better choice if

---

TABLE 4. Treatment of Uncomplicated Gonococcal Infections of the Urethra, Cervix, and Rectum*
Cefixime (Suprax) in a single 400-mg oral dose
Ceftriaxone (Rocephin) in a single 125-mg IM dose
Ciprofloxacin (Cipro) in a single 500-mg oral dose[†]
Ofloxacin (Floxin) in a single 400-mg oral dose[†]
Levofloxacin (Levaquin) in a single 250-mg oral dose[†]

*If *Chlamydia* infection is not ruled out, treat empirically with azithromycin or doxycycline.
[†]Quinolones are not recommended for infections acquired in Asia, the Pacific (including Hawaii), and perhaps California.
Adapted from Centers for Disease Control and Prevention. Sexually transmitted disease treatment guidelines 2002. MMWR Morbid Mortal Wkly Rep 51(RR-6):1–78, 2002.

TABLE 5. Treatment of Nongonococcal Urethritis	
Recommended Regimens	**Alternative Regimens**
Azithromycin (Zithromax) in a single oral 1 g dose	Erythromycin base 500 mg PO four times a day for 7 days
Doxycycline 100 mg orally twice daily for 7 days	Erythromycin ethylsuccinate 800 mg PO four times daily for 7 days
	Ofloxacin (Floxin) 300 mg PO twice daily for 7 days
	Levofloxacin 500 mg PO once daily for 7 days

Adapted from Centers for Disease Control and Prevention. Sexually transmitted disease treatment guidelines 2002. MMWR Morbid Mortal Wkly Rep 51(RR-6):1–78, 2002.

compliance is an issue, and it even offers the opportunity for directly observed therapy. Alternative treatments for nongonococcal urethritis are 7-day regimens of erythromycin, ofloxacin (Floxin), or levofloxacin (Levaquin).[1] Patients who have persistent symptoms (without treatment) and negative findings on tests for *N. gonorrhoeae* and *C. trachomatis* are generally treated for nongonococcal urethritis.

Follow-Up

If testing reveals infection with either *C. trachomatis* or *N. gonorrhoeae,* partner notification is imperative. If symptoms resolve with treatment, there is no need for test-of-cure. When a patient has confirmed infection with *N. gonorrhoeae,* clinicians should consider testing for human immunodeficiency virus and syphilis as well.

Recurrent or Persistent Urethritis

Patients with recurrent or persistent symptoms should be reevaluated for objective signs of urethritis. If re-exposure or poor compliance is suspected, retreatment with the original regimen is reasonable (Table 6). Dual treatment for gonococcal and nongonococcal infection should also be considered if it was not already used. Retesting for *C. trachomatis* and *N. gonorrhoeae* should be done with caution, since nucleic acid amplification tests will remain positive up to 3 weeks after effective treatment.[10] If persistent gonococcal infection is suspected, a culture should be performed instead of nucleic acid amplification so that antibiotic susceptibility can be assessed.

If a compliant patient without re-exposure has persistent objective signs of infection, clinicians should test for *Trichomonas vaginalis* with cultures of first-void urine and intraurethral swab specimens.[1] In such cases, presumptive treatment with metronidazole and erythromycin will eradicate both *T. vaginalis* and tetracycline-resistant *U. urealyticum.*[1]

TABLE 6. Treatment of Recurrent or Persistent Urethritis
Metronidazole in a single oral 2 g dose *plus* Erythromycin base 500 mg PO four times daily for 7 days *or* Erythromycin ethylsuccinate 800 mg PO four times daily for 7 days
Adapted from Centers for Disease Control and Prevention. Sexually transmitted disease treatment guidelines 2002. MMWR Morbid Mortal Wkly Rep 51(RR-6):1–78, 2002.

Cervicitis

Cervicitis is characterized by purulent or mucopurulent discharge from the cervix. *N. gonorrhoeae* and *C. trachomatis* most commonly cause cervicitis, but in most cases, neither is isolated. Another cause of cervicitis is inflammation in the zone of ectopy, and this should especially be suspected in chronic cases that are resistant to antibiotics.

The CDC recommends antibiotic treatment for cervicitis only if *N. gonorrhoeae* or *C. trachomatis* is isolated.[1] However, empiric treatment can be considered in patient populations with a high incidence of infection or in patients who may not return for test results. Treatment regimens are the same as those for urethritis. Test-of-cure is not necessary. Partners should be appropriately notified, and sexual abstinence is recommended until 7 days after completion of therapy.

Epididymitis

The epididymis is a convoluted duct on the posterior and superior surfaces of the testes that serves as a reservoir for spermatozoa. Epididymitis is an inflammation of this structure characterized by pain and swelling. Epididymitis can be caused by sterile urinary reflux or by ascending infection. In men younger than 35 years of age, *C. trachomatis* and *N. gonorrhoeae* are responsible for most cases.[1] Older men and children are more likely to have infection with the coliform bacteria that cause urinary tract infections. Coliform bacteria may also be the most common pathogen among men who have unprotected anal sex.[7]

Men complaining of a painful epididymis should be questioned about symptoms of urethritis, cystitis, and prostatitis. Occasionally, generalized symptoms such as fever and chills may be noted. In epididymitis, swelling and tenderness is typically limited to the epididymis. A very important diagnostic consideration is testicular torsion, which can lead to infarction and loss of the testicle if undiagnosed. Swelling can be limited to the epididymis in early torsion.[7] Prompt ultrasonography is imperative if the diagnosis is in doubt. Color duplex Doppler ultrasonography is very sensitive and specific for both epididymitis and testicular torsion. Gram stain of urethral discharge and first-void urine for leukocytes can be helpful. Urine culture as well as testing for *C. trachomatis* and *N. gonorrhoeae* should also be performed. But antibiotics should be started empirically before the results of these tests are back. Depending on the clinical scenario, treatment is aimed at either coliform bacteria or sexually transmitted organisms (Table 7). Patients who do not improve within 3 days should be reevaluated. Patients with generalized symptoms sometimes require hospitalization.

Vaginitis

In the primary care setting, vaginitis is the most common gynecologic diagnosis.[11] Vaginitis is an inflammatory condition of the vagina characterized by vaginal discomfort, pruritis, and discharge. Infection causes 90% of cases and the offending organisms include bacteria, fungi, and parasites, and most of these infections are not sexually transmitted. Bacterial vaginosis (40–50% of cases) is the most common cause of vaginitis, followed by vulvovaginal candidiasis (20–25% of cases) and trichomoniasis (15–20% of cases).[12] Bacterial vaginosis is typically caused by an overgrowth of *Gardnerella vaginalis,* although other bacteria, especially anaerobes, may play a role. *G. vaginalis* is sometimes sexually transmitted.[13] Up to 50% of women colonized with *G. vaginalis* are asymptomatic. *Candida albicans* causes 80% to 90% of vaginal yeast infections.[13] Another cause of vaginitis is *Trichomonas vaginalis,* a parasite that is almost always sexually transmitted. Noninfectious causes of vaginitis include atrophic vaginitis, allergy, chemical irritation, desquamative inflammatory vaginitis, lichen planus, and collagen vascular disease.

TABLE 7.   Treatment of Epididymitis
For sexually transmitted infection:
Ceftriaxone (Rocephin) 250 mg IM in a single dose
plus
Doxycycline 100 mg PO twice a day for 10 days
For enteric organisms, cephalosporin or tetracycline allergy, or patients > 35 years:
Ofloxacin (Floxin) 300 mg PO twice daily for 10 days
or
Levofloxacin (Levaquin) 500 mg PO once daily for 10 days
Adapted from Centers for Disease Control and Prevention. Sexually transmitted disease treatment guidelines 2002. MMWR Morbid Mortal Wkly Rep 51(RR-6):1–78, 2002.

Clinical Findings

The symptoms of vaginitis are nonspecific and include vaginal discharge and pain or pruritis that may be exacerbated by urination. The dysuria of vaginitis is described as external, occurring when urine touches the vulva. The dysuria of cystitis is usually described as a more internal pain that begins before urine leaves the urethra. About 25% of women with *T. vaginalis* and 50% with *G. vaginalis* are asymptomatic.[13] The history in women with vaginitis should also include questions regarding menstrual history, sexual history, abdominal or pelvic pain, and fever.

Although not diagnostic, the physical examination is important in localizing the site of involvement to the vagina, vulva, or cervix. In cases of candidal infection, the vulva and vagina are erythematous and edematous, with fissures and a thick, white, adherent discharge. In cases of trichomoniasis, the vulva and vagina are also erythematous and edematous, but the discharge tends to be frothy and purulent. Up to 25% of women with trichomoniasis will also have "strawberry cervix."[11] In cases of bacterial vaginosis, the vulvar and vaginal tissues appear normal but have a gray, adherent, malodorous discharge.

Diagnosis

Wet Mount. A wet-mount preparation is performed by combining vaginal discharge and one or two drops of normal saline on a microscope slide. Several microscope fields should be examined for motile trichomonads and for the clue cells of bacterial vaginosis. The sensitivity of these tests is about 60% for trichomoniasis and bacterial vaginosis, but the specificity is 98%.[11] Other possible findings on the wet-mount examination include fungal hyphae (candidiasis), numerous white blood cells (trichomoniasis), and parabasal cells (atrophic vaginitis).

Potassium Hydroxide (KOH) Preparation. To perform a "KOH prep," a sample of vaginal discharge is combined with one or two drops of 10% to 20% potassium hydroxide (KOH) on a microscope slide. The whiff test is performed at this point by smelling for a fishy amine odor, which occurs in bacterial vaginosis. Once the slide has been dried by flame or air, it is examined under low power for candidal hyphae, spores, and mycelia. Scanning for these fungal elements is about 60% sensitive for candidiasis.[12]

Litmus Testing. The pH level of vaginal secretions is measured by placing litmus paper in pooled secretions or against the vaginal wall. Normal vaginal pH is 3.8 to 4.2, whereas in bacterial vaginosis, the pH is above 4.5 in about 90% of cases.[13] The vaginal pH can also be elevated in trichomoniasis and atrophic vaginitis, but to a lesser degree.

Culture. Cultures are not typically done to diagnose vaginitis but can be helpful in cases in which the diagnosis is in question or when treatment has failed. Cultures for *T. vaginalis* on Diamond's medium and DNA probes have sensitivities of 90% and 95% respectively.[12]

Cultures can also be useful in cases of candidiasis but many women without vulvovaginal candidiasis are colonized with *Candida*. Many clinicians will treat presumptively for yeast if vaginal pH is normal and nondiagnostic organisms are found on microscopy.

Cultures for *G. vaginalis* are not helpful for diagnosis, since they are positive in 50% of women without symptoms.[13] Diagnostic cards (Femcard) have recently been introduced that can detect elevated pH and amines in vaginal fluid. These cards have a sensitivity of 87% and a specificity of 92%.[14]

In general, Amsel's criteria can be useful, and the presence of three of these criteria is 90% sensitive for bacterial vaginosis[15]:
- Thin, homogeneous discharge
- Positive whiff test
- Clue cells
- Vaginal pH greater than 4.5

Treatment

Bacterial Vaginosis. Oral or vaginal metronidazole (Flagyl) and vaginal clindamycin (Cleocin) are the recommended regimens for treating bacterial vaginosis (Table 8).[1] Single-dose metronidazole and clindamycin are less effective than the above regimens but can be used if compliance is a problem.

Candidiasis. Many topical and systemic therapies are now available for yeast infections. The efficacy of oral and topical therapies is equivalent, although side effects are more common with systemic therapy (Table 9). Treatment with topical azoles results in cure in 80% to 90% of patients.[1] The efficiency of oral regimens, especially single-dose flu-

| TABLE 8. Treatment of Bacterial Vaginosis ||
Recommended Regimens	Alternative Regimens
Metronidazole (Flagyl) 500 mg PO twice daily for 7 days	Metronidazole 2 g PO in a single dose
Metronidazole 0.75% gel 5 g intravaginally once daily for 5 days	Clindamycin 300 mg PO twice daily for 7 days
Clindamycin (Cleocin) 2% cream 5 g intravaginally once daily for 7 days	Clindamycin ovules 100 g intravaginally once daily for 3 days
Adapted from Centers for Disease Control and Prevention. Sexually transmitted disease treatment guidelines 2002. MMWR Morbid Mortal Wkly Rep 51(RR-6):1–78, 2002.	

TABLE 9. Treatment Options for Vulvovaginal Candidiasis

Butoconazole 2% cream 5 g intravaginally daily for 3 days*
Butoconazole 2% cream 5 g (Butoconazole-1 sustained release), a single intravaginal application
Clotrimazole (Mycelex, Lotrimin) 1% cream 5 g intravaginally daily for 7–14 days*
Clotrimazole 100 mg vaginal tablet daily for 7 days
Clotrimazole 100 mg vaginal tablet, 2 tablets daily for 3 days
Clotrimazole 500 mg vaginal tablet in a single dose
Miconazole (Monistat) 2% cream 5 g intravaginally once daily for 7 days*
Miconazole 100 mg vaginal suppository once daily for 7 days*
Miconazole 200 mg vaginal suppository once daily for 3 days*
Nystatin (Mycostatin) 100,000-unit vaginal tablet once daily for 14 days
Tioconazole 6.5% ointment 5 g intravaginally in a single dose*
Terconazole 0.4% cream 5 g intravaginally once daily for 7 days
Terconazole 0.8% cream 5 g intravaginally once daily for 3 days
Terconazole 80 mg vaginal suppository once daily for 3 days
Fluconazole (Diflucan) 150 mg orally as a single dose

*Over-the-counter preparations
Adapted from Centers for Disease Control and Prevention. Sexually transmitted disease treatment guidelines 2002. MMWR Morbid Mortal Wkly Rep 51(RR-6):1–78, 2002.

conazole, has made them very popular among patients. Unless an infection is complicated, it is reasonable to treat according to patient preference.[14]

In complicated cases (e.g., recurrence, diabetes), treatment should be with a topical agent for 14 days. In most cases, sexual partners need not be treated. However, *Candida* can be transmitted sexually, and partner treatment should be considered in recurrent or resistant cases.

Trichomoniais. Systemic therapy with metronidazole (Flagyl) is the treatment of choice in cases of trichomoniasis, and the 2 g single-dose oral regimen is very effective.[1] An alternative is 500 mg orally twice daily for 7 days. Topical preparations of metronidazole do not penetrate the urethra or periurethral glands, which can serve as reservoirs for infection and relapse. Sexual partners should be treated simultaneously. Male partners of women with trichomoniasis have detectable infection about one third of the time.[1]

Genital Ulcer Disease

Most genital ulcers in the United States are caused by sexually transmitted infection with herpes simplex virus (HSV), *Treponema pallidum* (syphilis), and *Haemophilus ducreyi* (chancroid). Less common noninfectious causes include Behçet's syndrome, trauma, squamous cell carcinoma, and fixed drug eruption. Even after a full evaluation, at least

25% of patients have no laboratory-confirmed diagnosis, and clinicians must often treat presumptively and for more than one condition.[1]

Herpes Simplex Virus

At least 50 million Americans have genital herpes simplex infection.[1] These infections can be caused by two serotypes: HSV-1 and HSV-2. Although HSV-1 more commonly infects the oral mucosa, it also causes up to 30% of genital infections.[1] Almost all HSV-2 infection is sexually acquired.[1]

Clinical Findings. In one large study following HSV seronegative patients, approximately 70% of patients developed symptoms when they became infected with HSV-1, whereas about 40% of patients infected with HSV-2 developed symptoms.[16] Clinicians should suspect HSV whenever an ulcerating genital lesion is noted. Most patients with symptomatic primary infections will have painful genital lesions, itching, and inguinal adenopathy. The classic presentation of genital HSV is a cluster of vesicles on an erythematous base. But these classic lesions are present in only 60% to 70% of symptomatic cases.[18] About one half of patients will have fever, and one third will report photophobia and headache.[17]

Diagnosis. Clinical diagnosis should not be relied upon because it is insensitive and nonspecific for serotype. Serotyping is important to properly counsel patients, since HSV-2 is much more likely than HSV-1 to recur. Tests that can distinguish serotypes include viral culture, direct fluorescent antibody tests, and serum antibody titers. Tzanck smears and some HSV antigen tests do not distinguish between serotypes of HSV. Viral culture becomes less sensitive as lesions heal, so false-negative results are common. Type-specific serologic testing should be considered in such cases. Antibodies to HSV develop within the several weeks of infection and persist indefinitely. Polymerase chain reaction may replace culture as the test of choice for herpes.[19]

Treatment. Treatment with antiviral medications can minimize symptoms and shorten the course of both primary and recurrent episodes of herpes. Three drugs—acyclovir, famciclovir, and valacyclovir—have all been found to be effective therapy for HSV. The recommended regimens are different for primary and recurrent episodes (Table 10).

Recurrence. About 90% of patients with HSV-2 infection will have at least one recurrence within 1 year.[20] The median number of recurrences is four, and more than one third of patients will have more than six episodes per year.[20] Frequent recurrence is more likely if the primary infection was severe. The recurrence rate is much lower in patients with HSV-1 infection. Infrequent recurrences can be treated by patient-initiated therapy. Patients should be given a supply of medication and instructed

TABLE 10. Recommended Therapy for Genital Herpes Infection	
Primary Infection	**Secondary Infection**
Acyclovir (Zovirax) 400 mg PO three times a day for 7–10 days	Acyclovir (Zovirax) 400 mg PO three times a day for 5 days
Acyclovir 200 mg five times a day for 7–10 days	Acyclovir 200 mg PO five times a day for 5 days
Famciclovir (Famvir) 250 mg three times daily for 7–10 days	Acyclovir 800 mg PO twice a day for 5 days
Valacyclovir (Valtrex) 1 g PO twice a day for 7–10 days	Famciclovir (Famvir) 125 mg PO twice a day for 5 days
(All regimens can be extended if healing is not complete after 10 days)	Valacyclovir (Valtrex) 500 mg PO twice a day for 3–5 days
	Valacyclovir 1 g PO once a day for 5 days

Adapted from Centers for Disease Control and Prevention. Sexually transmitted disease treatment guidelines 2002. MMWR Morbid Mortal Wkly Rep 51(RR-6):1–78, 2002.

to start the medication within 1 day of lesion onset (Table 10). Often, patients will notice a tingling or burning sensation 1 to 2 days before lesions appear.

Frequent recurrences (more than five per year) can be treated using suppressive therapy. Suppression requires daily antiviral medication (Table 11), but this can reduce recurrences by 70% to 80%.[1] Patients taking suppressive therapy report an improved quality of life. Suppressive therapy lowers, but does not eliminate, viral shedding. It is unknown whether suppression affects HSV transmission.

Counseling. The psychological effect of herpes is often more substantial than the infection itself. Herpes is a lifelong, recurrent infection, and patients need time and guidance to deal with it properly. It is often helpful to counsel couples together. Abstinence or condom use during recurrences can help prevent transmission to partners. But patients should know that viral shedding and transmission also occur during asymptomatic phases. Pregnant women in their third trimester should avoid sexual contact with men who have a history of herpes.

TABLE 11. Suppressive Therapy for Recurrent Genital Herpes
Acyclovir (Zovirax) 400 mg PO twice a day
Famciclovir (Famvir) 250 mg PO twice a day
Valacyclovir (Valtrex) 500 mg PO once a day
Valacyclovir 1 g PO once a day (more effective than 500 mg dose if > 9 episodes per year)

Adapted from Centers for Disease Control and Prevention. Sexually transmitted disease treatment guidelines 2002. MMWR Morbid Mortal Wkly Rep 51(RR-6):1–78, 2002.

Syphilis

The rate of syphilis declined a dramatic 89% between 1990 and 2000.[21] But in 2001, for the first year since 1990, there was a slight increase in the rate of primary and secondary syphilis.[22] It is hoped that this does not represent a new trend. Syphilis is caused by infection with the spirochete *T. pallidum*. The organism is transmitted through the skin or mucous membranes and causes systemic infection if left untreated.

Clinical Findings. Primary syphilis occurs 2 to 4 weeks after sexual exposure, manifesting as a painless genital sore or chancre. Chancres can occur anywhere on the genitals as well as the mouth and lips. Once the chancre heals, syphilis enters a latent stage. Latent infection is divided into early (contracted within 1 year) and late latent infection. This is an important distinction, since late infection may require a longer duration of therapy.

Weeks to months later, 25% of untreated patients will develop secondary syphilis.[23] The classic sign of secondary syphilis is a rash of 5 to 20 mm red or red-brown papules that affects the entire body. Involvement of the palms and soles is characteristic. Other symptoms of secondary syphilis include lymphadenopathy, fever, sore throat, headache, malaise, weight loss, and a patchy alopecia. Secondary syphilis resolves spontaneously, but without treatment, patients may suffer recurrent episodes for years. Tertiary syphilis is characterized by visceral and cardiac involvement. Occasionally gummas, erosions or granulomatous lesions, may appear on the skin or in visceral organs.

In neurosyphilis, *T. pallidum* infects the central nervous system. Neurologic involvement can manifest as meningitis, general paresis, meningovascular strokes, tabes dorsalis, and a host of other neurologic symptoms.

Diagnosis. All patients with syphilis should be tested for HIV infection.[1] The variety of presentations can make syphilis a difficult diagnosis to make. Laboratory testing is imperative. In primary syphilis, the presence of a chancre allows for easier diagnosis and laboratory testing. The definitive tests for early syphilis are darkfield examination and direct fluorescent antibody tests of lesion exudates or tissue.[1] If there are no skin lesions, serology must be used. Because many diseases can cause positive syphilis tests, two types of serologic tests, treponemal and nontreponemal, should be used to diagnose syphilis:

- Treponemal serologic tests
  - Fluorescent treponemal antibody absorbed (FTA-ABS)
  - *T. pallidum* particle agglutination
- Nontreponemal serologic tests
  - Veneral Disease Research Laboratory (VDRL)
  - Rapid plasma reagin (RPR)

Nontreponemal tests change with disease activity and should be reported numerically. A fourfold change in titer (e.g., two dilutions) is necessary to demonstrate a clinically significant difference. The RPR and VDRL tests cannot be compared directly because RPR titers tend to run higher. Although these test results usually become negative after treatment, occasionally they will remain positive for life (serofast reaction). Treponemal serologies tend to remain positive for life, regardless of treatment. These treponemal tests do not correlate with disease activity.

Neurosyphilis is a challenging diagnosis. VDRL can be performed on cerebrospinal fluid. The test is highly specific but insensitive. A positive VDRL result on cerebrospinal fluid is diagnostic of neurosyphilis.[1] If the VDRL is negative, FTA-ABS can be performed on the sample. The FTA-ABS is less specific but is highly sensitive. Some experts believe that a negative FTA-ABS finding on cerebrospinal fluid excludes neurosyphilis.[1] Patients with uveitis should be considered to have neurosyphilis and have cerebrospinal fluid examination.

Treatment. Although there are different antibiotic regimens for each stage of syphilis, penicillin is the mainstay of treatment for each (Table 12). Patients should be followed for resolution or absence of symptoms. Nontreponemal serologies should be rechecked at 6 and 12 months following therapy. If symptoms or titers remain unchanged, a cerebrospinal fluid analysis should be performed. Treatment of partners to prevent reinfection is also very important in resistant cases. In patients with neurosyphilis, reevaluation of cerebrospinal fluid should also be performed.

Chancroid

Chancroid is caused by infection with a gram-negative rod, *Haemophilus ducreyi*. In the United Sates, *H. ducreyi* infection tends to occur in discrete outbreaks, and it is often acquired from asymptomatic carriers. About 10% of people with chancroid in the United States are coinfected with *T. pallidum* or HSV, and it is also associated with human immunodeficiency virus infection.[1]

Clinical Findings. The incubation period for chancroid is only a few days, and the genital ulcers that form tend to be deep and painful. Autoinoculation gives rise to more lesions on the genitals and surrounding

TABLE 12. Treatment of Syphilis
Primary, Secondary, or Early Latent Syphilis Benzathine penicillin G 2.4 million units IM in a single dose **Late Latent and Tertiary Syphilis** Benzathine penicillin G 2.4 million units IM weekly for three doses **Neurosyphilis** Aqueous crystalline penicillin G 18–24 million units per day for 10–14 days
Adapted from Centers for Disease Control and Prevention. Sexually transmitted disease treatment guidelines 2002. MMWR Morbid Mortal Wkly Rep 51(RR-6):1–78, 2002.

TABLE 13. Treatment of Chancroid

Azithromycin (Zithromax) 1 g PO in a single dose
Ceftriaxone (Rocephin) 250 mg IM in a single dose
Ciprofloxacin (Cipro) 500 mg PO twice daily for 3 days
Eythromycin base 500 mg PO three times a day for 7 days

Adapted from Centers for Disease Control and Prevention. Sexually transmitted disease treatment guidelines 2002. MMWR Morbid Mortal Wkly Rep 51(RR-6):1–78, 2002.

---

skin. Generalized symptoms such as fever are sometimes present, and tender inguinal adenopathy occurs in 50% of cases. Suppuration of these nodes is almost diagnostic of chancroid.

Diagnosis. *H. ducreyi* cannot be cultured on routine medium, and its nutritional requirements seem to be geographically defined.[24] Culture is 80% sensitive at best.[1] Polymerase chain reaction is a promising alternative, but there are no tests yet available that are approved by the Food and Drug Administration.

A probable diagnosis of chancroid can be made if all of the following criteria are met[1]:

- One or more painful genital ulcers
- Negative testing for *T. pallidum* by darkfield examination or a serologic test for syphilis performed at least 7 days after onset of ulcer
- Clinical presentation and ulcer appearance are typical of chancroid
- Negative test for HSV performed on the ulcer exudates

Treatment. Chancroid can be treated with short courses of azithromycin (Zithromax), ceftriaxone (Rocephin), ciprofloxacin (Cipro), or erythromycin (Table 13). Intermediate resistance to ciprofloxacin and erythromycin have been reported. Patients should be reevaluated within 1 week of diagnosis. Recent (10 days) sexual partners should be evaluated and treated. HIV and syphilis testing should be repeated at 3 months.

References

1. Centers for Disease Control and Prevention: Sexually transmitted disease treatment guidelines 2002. MMWR Morbid Mortal Wkly Rep 51(RR-6):1–78, 2002.
2. Westrom L, Joesoef R, Reynolds G, et al: Pelvic inflammatory disease and infertility: A cohort of 1,844 women with laparoscopically verified disease and 657 control women with normal laparoscopy results. Sexually Transmitted Diseases 19:185–192, 1992.
3. Ross JDC: An update on pelvic inflammatory disease. Sexually Transmitted Infection 78:18–19, 2001.
4. Livengood CH: Treatment and sequelae of pelvic inflammatory disease in adults. In UpToDate. Accessed Sept. 18, 2002 at www.uptodate.com.
5. Brokenshire MK, Say PJ, Van Vonno AH, Wong C: Evaluation of microparticle en-

zyme immunoassay Abbott IMx Select Chlamydia and the importance of urethral site sampling to detect *Chlamydia trachomatis* in women. Genitourinary Med 73:498–502, 1997.

6. Pfeffer DM: Sexually transmitted diseases. In Stein BS, ed: Clinical urologic practice. New York: WW Norton & Co., 1995:355–394.

7. Berger RE, Lee JC: Sexually transmitted diseases: The classic diseases. In Walsh PC, Retik AB, Vaughn ED Jr, Wein AJ, eds: Campbell's Urology, 8th ed. St. Louis: WB Saunders, 2002:671–691.

8. Goodson JD: Approach to the male patient with urethritis. In Goroll AH, Mulley AG, ed: Primary Care Medicine Office Evaluation and Management of the Adult Patient, 4th ed. Philadelphia: Lippincott Williams & Wilkins, 2000:787–790.

9. Juchau SV, Nackman R, Ruppart D: Comparison of Gram stain with DNA probe for detection of *Neisseria gonorrhoeae* in the urethras of symptomatic males. J Clin Microbiol 33:3068–3069, 1995.

10. Centers for Disease Control and Prevention: Screening test to detect *Chlamydia trachomatis* and *Neisseria gonorrhoeae* infections—2002. MMWR Morbid Mortal Wkly Rep 51(RR-15):1–40, 2002.

11. Egan ME, Lipsky MS: Diagnosis of vaginitis. Am Fam Phys 62:1095–1104, 2000.

12. Sobel JD: Current concepts: Vaginitis. N Engl J Med 337:1896–1903, 1997.

13. Rein MF: Vulvovaginitis and cervicitis. In Mandell GL, Bennett JE, Dolin R, eds: Mandell, Douglas, and Bennett's Principles and Practice of Infectious Diseases, 5th ed. Philadelphia: Churchill Livingstone, 2000:1219–1233.

14. Sobel JD: Overview of vaginitis. In UpToDate. Accessed Oct. 6, 2002 at www. uptodate.com.

15. Amsel R, Totten PA, Spiegel CA, et al: Nonspecific vaginitis: Diagnostic criteria and microbial and epidemiologic associations. Am J Med 74:14–22, 1983.

16. Langenberg AGM, Corey L, Ashley RL, et al: A prospective study of new infections with herpes virus type one and type 2. N Engl J Med 341:1432–1438, 1999.

17. Benedetti J, Corey L, Ashley R: Recurrence rates in genital herpes after symptomatic first-episode infection. Ann Intern Med 121:847–854, 1994.

18. Wald A: New therapies and prevention strategies for genital herpes. Clin Infect Dis 28(S1):S4–13, 1999.

19. Albrecht MA: Clinical manifestations and diagnosis of genital herpes simplex virus infection. In UpToDate. Accessed Sept. 23, 2002 at www.uptodate.com.

20. Benedetti J, Corey L, Ashley R: Recurrence rates in genital herpes after symptomatic first-episode infection. Ann Intern Med 121:847–854, 1994.

21. Centers for Disease Control and Prevention: Sexually transmitted disease surveillance—2000. Atlanta, GA: US Department of Health and Human Services, Public Health Service, CDC, 2001.

22. Primary and secondary syphilis–United States, 2000–2001. MMWR Morbid Mortal Wkly Rep 51(43):171–973, 2002.

23. Hicks CD, Sparling PF: Early syphilis. In UpToDate. Accessed Oct. 5, 2002 at www.uptodate.com.

24. Habif TP: Clinical Dermatology: A Color Guide to Diagnosis and Therapy, 3rd ed. St. Louis: Mosby, 1996.

Fever of Unknown Origin

Valerianna Amorosa, M.D.

chapter

23

In a day in which one sees much of medical practice moving toward protocols and algorithms for diagnosing and treating disease, what make fever of unknown origin (FUO) a "hot topic" is that it does not submit easily to diagnostic and therapeutic protocols. We are challenged to put into practice both the art and the science of clinical medicine—that is, to assess our patient with absolute thoroughness, to be familiar with the most cutting-edge approaches to diagnoses, and to judge what is an appropriate course of action in each unique situation. Thanks to advances in radiology, microbiology, serology, and molecular diagnostics, many diseases that were once found only after exhaustive study are now discovered earlier in a fever evaluation.

Fever of unknown origin is defined as an illness of greater than 3 weeks' duration with fevers exceeding 38.1°C (101°F) on repeated occasions without a diagnosis after 1 week of testing in the hospital.[1] This definition has evolved to allow testing to occur in an outpatient environment.[2,3] Frequently, an FUO is an atypical presentation of a more common illness, and the clinical experience of a specialist who has seen many presentations of disease can be insightful. Thus, during the evaluation of an FUO, it is reasonable to involve the help of consultants in infectious diseases, hematology and oncology, and rheumatology.

This chapter focuses on the overall approach to the diagnosis of an FUO. Emphasis is placed on the initial history, physical examination, and diagnostic studies that should be completed and confirmed during the evaluation. In addition, the common causes of FUO are reviewed.

Approach to the Diagnosis

Fever Patterns

The fever and its pattern may be helpful in the diagnostic work-up. A fever above 38.1°C must be observed on at least three occasions over 3 weeks. In elderly patients, because of a blunted febrile response, it is sug-

251

gested that the temperature criterion should be any increase of 1.3°C from the baseline temperature or a persistent rectal temperature greater than 37.5°C.[4]

The fever pattern may occasionally point to the diagnosis, and a number of fever patterns have been described. Cyclical fevers due to malaria can occur at 48-hour intervals (*tertian fevers*) in the case of *Plasmodium vivax* or *Plasmodium ovale* infection and at 72-hour intervals (*quartan fevers*) in the case of *Plasmodium malariae* infection.[2] The Pel-Ebstein fever pattern of Hodgkin's disease is characterized by 3 to 10 days of fever followed by 3 to 10 afebrile days.[5] The relapsing fever pattern due to *Borrelia* species is characterized by 2 to 3 days of fever followed by a 7- to 9-day afebrile interval before symptoms recur.[2]

The duration of the fever may also be helpful. Although a prolonged fever (occurring over months to years) without other concomitant symptoms is less suggestive of infection or malignancy, chronic "smoldering" osteomyelitis, an occult abscess, parasitic infections, or Whipple's disease can have indolent courses and should be considered. Still's disease, Crohn's disease, hereditary fever syndromes, and Behçet's disease may also have long recurrent courses of fever interspersed with afebrile periods.[7]

History

Once a patient has been diagnosed with an FUO, attention should be paid to every aspect of the medical history. A thorough medical history, even in a patient one has known for years, may catch potentially unknown historical features. Within the medical history, the clinician is searching for diagnostic clues. In particular, the medical history should address the following:

- **Fever**—The febrile illness, including its onset, course, and response to therapeutic trials.
- **Exposure history**—All exposures should also be obtained, including information about sick contacts, sexual activity, lifetime tuberculosis contacts, occupational and recreational activities, and exposure to animals.
- **Prodromes**—Recent prodromal symptoms, such as a sore throat, myalgias, or arthralgias, may be useful.
- **Diet**—Dietary history, including specifics about the origin of meat, dairy products, and vegetables consumed may provide important historical clues.
- **Travel history**—A complete lifetime travel history, including itineraries within and outside the home country, should be ascertained.[2]
- **Military service**—This should be determined because it may point to a number of exposures.

- **Past medical history**—Prior illnesses, infections, malignancies, surgeries, invasive procedures, implantation of prosthetic devices, and blood transfusions should also be ascertained.
- **Medication history**—A detailed history of medications, including any herbal supplements, is important in determining potential clues for drug fever. Exposure to any immunosuppressive drugs can broaden the likely differential diagnosis.
- **Illicit drugs**—Illicit inhaled and intravenous drug use during the patient's lifetime should be identified.
- **Family history**—An exhaustive family history should include any family members with prior tuberculosis or other infections, collagen vascular diseases, malignancies, or febrile syndromes. Ethnic origin should also be noted.
- **Review of systems**—A complete review of systems is often helpful in obtaining potential diagnostic clues to guide further investigation. Repeatedly revising the review of systems may be helpful in finding clues not previously appreciated on prior interviews. Positive findings might lead to clues of local disease or a constellation of findings suggestive of certain systemic illnesses. Uncommon symptoms may be discovered.

Physical Examination

As with the history, the physical examination should be done repeatedly and systematically. Diagnostic clues can be noticed for the first time, can be transiently present, or can evolve over time. One should view the whole body, removing all clothing, prosthetic limbs, dentures, and bandages. Tooth pain (possible abscess), temporal artery pain or nodularity (suggesting giant cell arteritis), skin rashes or pigmentations, oral or genital ulcerations, pain along any veins (suggestive of septic thrombophlebitis), lymphadenopathy, new cardiac murmurs (possible endocarditis), pelvic pain or abnormalities in women, and testicular pain or genital abnormalities in men can all give clues to various causes of FUO.[6,9] Given the variety of diagnostic clues that may be gleaned from ophthalmologic examination, it is also not unreasonable to have a thorough fundoscopic evaluation performed by an ophthalmologist. Table 1 lists a number of key physical findings and their associated diseases.

Laboratory Diagnosis

As with the medical history and physical examination, basic laboratory studies should be performed before progressing to advanced diagnostic testing. Very often, clues from the history and physical examination can guide laboratory testing. Various authors have provided opinions on the initial group of tests that should be performed. These in-

TABLE 1. Selected Physical Examination Clues to the Diagnosis of Fever of Unknown Origin

Physical Findings	Suggested Diagnoses
Neurologic Examination	
Subtle neurologic, behavioral symptoms, mononeuritis, peripheral neuropathy, cerebellar signs	Chronic meningitis, Whipple's disease, vasculitis, paraneoplastic disease, intracranial process, chronic meningitis
Eye Examination	
Pettechiae, lymphoid hyperplasia	Endocarditis, lymphoma
Scleritis	Rheumatologic disease
Uveitis	Tuberculosis, disseminated fungal infection, syphilis, other granulomatous diseases, seronegative spondylarthropathies, rheumatoid arthritis
Retinal Examination	
Roth spots (white-centered hemorrhagic lesions)	Infective endocarditis
Yellow-white choroidal lesions	Tuberculosis and disseminated fungal infection
Active retinitis	Disseminated toxoplasmosis, cytomegalovirus in immunocompromised host
Intraretinal hemorrhages, Roth spots, leukemic infiltrates	Leukemia
Choroidal metastases	Metastatic breast or lung cancer
Cotton wool exudates, intraretinal hemorrhage	Vasculitis
Perivascular sheathing, choroidal nodules	Sarcoidosis
Skin and Mucosal Surfaces	
Osler's nodes, Janeway lesions, splinter hemorrhages, palatal petechiae	Endocarditis
Rose spots—2–3 mm on trunk, blanching pink papules then faded brown after few days	Salmonellosis
Diffuse cutaneous hyperpigmentation	Whipple's disease, Addison's disease
Macules, papules, and nodules on trunk, extremities	Chronic meningococcemia, secondary syphillis
Painful red macules or petechiae evolving to pustules on distal extremities	Gonoccoccal disease
Papules progressing to verrucous, crusted growths	Blastomycosis
Warty nodules and subcutaneous abscesses	Coccidioidomycocosis
Erythematous papules, pustules, sub-cutaneous nodules and cellulitis	Cryptococcosis
Moveable firm and painless nodules, typically in clusters—particular attention to umbilicus, scalp	Intra-abdominal primary tumor; lung, kidney, and breast primary; scalp metastases
Oral ulcerations	Histoplasmosis, lupus, Behçet's disease

(continued)

TABLE 1. Selected Physical Examination Clues to the Diagnosis of Fever of Unknown Origin (*Continued*)	
Physical Findings	**Suggested Diagnoses**
Skin and Mucosal Surfaces (*continued*)	
Purplish papules, nodules and plaques, ecchymoses	Leukemia cutis
Erythematous painful plaques with bumps, pustules, vesicles on their surface	Sweet's syndrome
Palpable purpura of the lower exremities and areas of dependency (e.g., buttocks), urticaria, ulcers, infarcts, nodules, livido reticularis	Cutaneous vasculitis related to multiple potential pathologies
Cardiac Examination	
Heart failure, murmurs, plops	Endocarditis, atrial myxoma
Abdominal Examination	
Liver size, texture, splenomegaly, nodules, scars	Malignancy, disseminated infectious disease, prior surgeries
Genital Examination	
Masses, adnexal, testicular tenderness	Malignancy, granulomatous and other infectious disease Testicular tenderness associated with polyarteritis nodosa
Rectal Examination	
Perirectal or prostatic tenderness or fluctuance	Prostatitis, prostatic or perirectal abscess
Venous Examination	
Swelling, asymetrical edema, pain	Venous thrombosis or thrombophlebitis

Adapted from Hirschmann JV: Fever of unknown origin in adults. Clin Infect Dis 24:291–302, 1997.

vestigators have attempted to determine the diagnostic utility of various laboratory studies in the work-up of an FUO.[6,10] Generally accepted first-line tests that may be helpful in reaching the diagnosis of an FUO are presented in Table 2.

A complete blood cell count and a peripheral smear should be performed, since these may provide valuable clues. Atypical lymphocytes suggestive of a viral infection can be identified. A monocytosis may be suggestive of mycobacterial or fungal infection, and eosinophilia may prompt consideration of a parasitic or allergic disease. Rarely, one might observe parasites directly on a peripheral smear. Malaria and *Babesia* parasites are the most common organisms seen on a peripheral smear. Abnormal hematopoietic cells or their precursors can suggest a hematologic malignancy. Anemia may prompt consideration of myelophthisis or hemolysis. The presence of schistocytes, or torn red blood cells, could suggest microangiopathic or autoimmune hemolysis. Thrombocytopenia can also be noted on peripheral smear.

TABLE 2. Commonly Performed Tests that May Aid in Diagnosis of Fever of Unknown Origin*
Complete blood cell count
Routine chemistries, renal function, uric acid, creatine phosphokinase
Liver enzymes, bilirubin, lactose dehydrogenase
Coagulation panel
Urinalysis with microscopic examination
Erythrocyte sedimentation rate, C-reactive protein, ferritin
Antinuclear antibodies
Rheumatoid factor
Rapid plasma reagent
Three anaerobic and aerobic sets of routine blood cultures off antibiotics
Specific isolator blood cultures for mycobacteria, other fastidious organisms
Human immunodeficiency virus antibodies or virus detection assay
Cytomegalovirus serologies or direct viral detection
Heterophile antibodies in younger age group
Angiotensin converting enzyme level
Feces for occult blood
Urine culture, sputum culture, feces culture when indicated
Chest radiograph
Abdominal computed tomography or ultrasonography
Purified protein derivative
Mammogram in women

*Taken from Mackowiak and Durack,[2] Arrow and Flaherty,[6] Hirschman,[9] and DeKleijn et al.[10]

Serum chemistries should also be performed to assess for abnormalities. Liver function test abnormalities are vague diagnostic clues in FUO but can nonetheless be helpful. Abnormalities can prompt earlier assessment of hepatobiliary system.[10] A urinalysis can specifically be useful in determining the presence of genitourinary disease. The erythrocyte sedimentation rate and C-reactive protein, despite their lack of specificity, may be useful in assessing the extent of inflammation. An elevated uric acid level could be a clue to unapparent gout as a cause of the FUO.[6]

Microbiological studies can be used to detect the presence of occult infection. Blood cultures can be very useful in detecting persistent or transient bacteremias caused by endocarditis, occult abscesses, and osteomyelitis. The highest sensitivity is obtained from three sets of blood cultures. Every effort should be made to obtain cultures with the patient off antibiotics.[8] Blood cultures utilizing lysis-centrifugation systems can be used to detect more fastidious organisms such as mycobacteria, endemic mycoses, *Bartonella* species, and *Brucella* species. A sputum Gram stain, acid-fast smear for mycobacteria, and routine and mycobacterial cultures can have utility if pulmonary disease is suspected. The tuberculin skin test may prompt consideration of mycobacterial disease. A urine culture can assist in diagnosing infections of the urinary tract and, if positive, may prompt a more thorough search for disease in this region. Finally, stool cultures for bacterial pathogens should be considered when gastrointestinal disease is suspected. Serologic studies may also be useful in the course of the diagnostic evaluation. Antibody testing for the human immunodeficiency virus may be warranted even if only risk factors are present.[10] In addition, rapid plasma reagent testing should also be performed if syphilis is under consideration.

Imaging Studies

Diagnostic imaging has in many ways revolutionized the evaluation of FUO. Abdominal and pelvic computed tomography (CT) may be of great utility in the course of the work-up of an undiagnosed fever. These aid in determining invasive diagnostic testing, which can be carried out via radiologically guided biopsies and aspirations or by surgery, when necessary. Direct communication of the patient's history with the evaluating radiologist is helpful in ensuring proper understanding of potential abnormalities. One drawback to CT scanning is that it may be too sensitive and may identify abnormalities that are unrelated to the cause of fever and that lead the further diagnostic work-up astray.

Ultrasonography in the form of echocardiography has a well-established and useful role.[9] Ultrasonography of the right upper quadrant can occasionally give better biliary tract detail than an abdominal CT scan. Ultrasonography of the lower extremities may be useful in establishing the diagnosis of occult deep venous thromboses as a cause of fever in a few patients.

Given its utility in diagnosing many different causes of fever, echocardiography is also useful in the evaluation of an FUO. An initial transthoracic echocardiogram may identify valvular vegetations or thrombi. When a transthoracic echocardiogram is unrevealing, a transesophageal echocardiogram (TEE) is recommended. TEE has superior ability to visualize cardiac valvular abnormalities as well as to detect the presence of a pericardial effusion.

Nuclear medicine modalities have several roles in localizing disease, and their role continues to evolve.[11] These studies are most useful in further elucidating potential infectious or inflammatory foci. Different radiopharmaceuticals are used to localize sites of inflammation via different mechanisms. Indium-111-labeled autologous leukocytes have been considered the nuclear medicine gold standard for identifying inflammation and infection because of their specificity. There is high uptake in any predominantly neutrophilic infiltrates, and lesions can be apparent early in their evolution.[11] The gallium-67 scan is sometimes considered a better initial test because it has greater sensitivity in imaging acute, chronic, granulomatous inflammation and malignancy as well.[12] Gallium binds to transferrin in blood and extravasates at sites of inflammation and infection.[11]

More recently, it has been shown that positron emission tomography may have even greater utility in localizing different causes of an FUO. The positron emitting tracer, ^{18}F-deoxyglucose, is taken up in metabolically active cells. Increased ^{18}F-deoxyglucose uptake has been reported in many neoplastic and infectious diseases as well as vasculitides and granulomatous diseases.[13] Positron emission tomography scanning may become an effective modality in the evaluation of FUO as its benefits and limitations continue to be defined.[13]

Reevaluation

After the initial evaluation, it is often necessary to reassess the patient to ascertain the evolution of the fever and the emergence of new symptoms or physical signs. Additional laboratory tests should be performed. The clinician should give consideration to thyroid function testing. Other endocrinologic causes of fever, including adrenal insufficiency and pheochromocytoma, should be sought out if the history, vital signs, or serum electrolytes are suggestive. Multiple myeloma can manifest subtly with fever, and serum protein and urine protein electrophoresis might be worthwhile. Tooth abscesses can be occult, and teeth radiographs may be revealing. If TEE has not been performed, it should be considered. Additionally, if cross-sectional imaging has already been performed and found to be unrevealing, one should consider performing a nuclear medicine study in an attempt to locate a region of inflammation. This may be useful early in the course of work-up. Lower extremity ultrasonography to examine the deep leg veins is revealing in some cases.

Both rheumatologic and infectious serologies can occasionally be illuminating. DeKleijn et al[10] found diagnostic utility in determining serum mixed cryoglobulins during the reevaluation for an FUO. Other tests may provide additional clues to rheumatologic diseases, such as systemic lupus erythematosus and vasculitis. These include the anti-neutrophil cytoplasmic antibody, serum complements (C_3, C_4, and CH_{50}), anti-double-stranded DNA. Additional serologic testing to evaluate for infectious causes might include hepatitis antibodies, antistreptolysin O antibody, and antibodies against *Coxiella burnettii* and *Brucella, Borrelia,* or *Bartonella* species.[8] *Mycoplasma* species and *Chlamydia psittaci* rarely cause a culture-negative endocarditis, and serologic studies for these organisms may be helpful.[10]

Consideration should also be given to bone marrow biopsy. This could have significant utility in discovering occult malignancy or infection, and biopsy proves more useful than aspirate.[6] Cultures taken alone have little diagnostic yield.[14]

In the absence of additional clues, colonoscopy, liver biopsy, and, in patients older than 55 years of age, temporal artery biopsy may be helpful. Colonoscopy or sigmoidoscopy can provide biopsy samples for histology as well as bacterial, mycobacterial, and fungal cultures and can screen for occult colon malignancy. Since symptoms of temporal arteritis can be subtle, and the erythrocyte sedimentation rate need not be elevated, blind temporal biopsy has been shown to have diagnostic utility.[9]

Selected Causes

Many references have impressive lists of the causes of FUO, and these are both daunting and enlightening to peruse.[1–3,5,6,9] Some selected causes are discussed below.

Tuberculosis

For tuberculosis to cause an FUO, it must typically manifest as either disseminated or primarily extrapulmonary disease.[9] Approximately 25% of the time, a tuberculin skin test will be negative in this situation.[2] The diagnosis of extrapulmonary tuberculosis, in particular, can be challenging. A diagnosis may be achieved with a thoracoscopic lung biopsy or liver biopsy (manifesting as granulomatous hepatitis). Urinalysis may provide initial diagnostic clues to kidney involvement, and back pain may hint at spinal involvement. A bone marrow biopsy can be diagnostic.

Infective Endocarditis

Clinical history, physical examination, and blood cultures are chief aids in the diagnosis of endocarditis. Any evidence of microscopic hematuria, circulating immune complexes, and systemic signs of inflammation such as anemia or leukocytosis are also consistent. When endocarditis is suspected, and blood cultures are nondiagnostic, additional tests should be performed. Lysis-centrifugation system blood cultures and specific serologic analysis should be considered. Culture-negative pathogens are more easily diagnosed, owing to improved culturing techniques. However, *Bartonella, Brucella, Coxiella,* and the fastidious gram-negative HACEK organisms (*Haemophilus parainfluenzae, H. influenzae, H. aphrophilus, H. paraphrophilus, Actinobacillus actinomycetemcomitans, Cardiobacterium hominis, Eikenella corrodens,* and *Kingella* species) account for the majority of cases of culture-negative endocarditis and should be considered when clinically indicated.[8]

Cytomegalovirus

Cytomegalovirus is a common cause of a prolonged febrile illness. Cytomegalovirus often appears without the diagnostic clues of sore throat, lymphadenopathy, and splenomegaly that may be present in infection with Epstein-Barr virus. In most cases, atypical lymphocytosis is present on peripheral smear. Subtle abnormalities in liver-associated enzymes are potential diagnostic clues. Immunoglobulin M and G antibodies should be present and their levels elevated, and the serum cytomegalovirus antigen level should be high.[2]

Malignancy

Malignancies of all varieties have been reported to be associated with fever. In most series, hematologic malignancies account for a high percentage of cases of FUO. The most common causes are Hodgkin's and non-Hodgkin's lymphoma as well as leukemia.[2,3,6,9] Of the solid tumors, renal cell carcinoma and hepatocellular carcinoma are well established causes of fever.[6] Any patient with a prior history of malignancy should be investigated fully for recurrence of the malignancy or a secondary malignancy in the context of prior chemotherapy or radiation. A prior history of radiation therapy is also known to be associated with pneumonitis and pericarditis as a cause of fever.[9]

Collagen Vascular Diseases

Collagen vascular diseases are an important cause of FUO. Once life-threatening infectious and malignant causes of fever are ruled out, prolonged observation may be necessary before the diagnosis of one of these diseases becomes apparent.[6] Still's disease is an important consideration and is characterized by the presence of lymphadenopathy, polyarthritis, myalgias, splenomegaly, and serositis. An evanescent salmon-colored rash and a sore throat are usual findings. Fever can precede other symptoms by as long as 1 year, thus making the diagnosis difficult.[6] Laboratory abnormalities include highly elevated ferritin levels, leukocytosis, an elevated erythrocyte sedimentation rate, and mild abnormalities in liver-associated enzymes. Serologic markers for other rheumatologic diseases are negative. In elderly patients, polymyalgia rheumatica is another important consideration, particularly when stiffness or pain is present in the shoulder or hip girdles.

Drug Fever

All potential offending drugs should be stopped. Although some drugs are common causes of FUO, the list of etiologic agents causing drug fever is extensive. The drug may have been started many weeks before the fever began. There may be an associated rash or eosinophilia present. Typically, drug fever resolves within 48 hours of stopping the agent.

Factitious Fever

Factitious fever describes a fever that is simulated or induced.[15] Although some patients with factitious fever may be malingering, a factitious fever is often a sign of very serious mental illness. The classic patient is a young woman with some experience in health care, although this is certainly not always the case.[15] Clues that a fever is factitious can be gleaned from a constellation of symptoms that do not correlate with any known disease. Once the diagnosis is suspected, the patient should be handled with empathy, bearing in mind that this may be a presentation of major psychiatric pathology and instability. Given patient variability, it is difficult to formulate a standardized approach, and psychiatric consultation is recommended.

Hereditary Fever

Much progress has been made over the last two decades in elucidating the molecular mechanisms and pathogenesis of the hereditary fever syndromes. Patients with hereditary fever syndromes have recurrent febrile attacks that may be weeks, months, or years apart. The precipitants of these febrile episodes are not well characterized. There are three well-established periodic fever syndromes at this point.[7]

Familial Mediterranean Fever is an inherited autosomal recessive disease that is most common in people of eastern Mediterranean descent, such as Armenians, Sephardic Jews, Arabs, and Turks.[7] It usually manifests before the age of 20 years, and patients typically present with periodic attacks of fever and serositis (peritonitis, pleuritis, or arthritis) that last for several days. The symptoms of serositis often predominate. Diagnosis is based on molecular genetic analysis, and this is important to establish because treatment with colchicine decreases the incidence of subsequent amyloidosis in these patients.[7]

The hyper IgD syndrome is seen in western Europeans, most commonly the Dutch and French, and is also inherited in an autosomal recessive pattern.[7] During attacks, patients have chills and high fevers that typically last for 4 to 6 days. Cervical lymphadenopathy and abdominal pain with vomiting and diarrhea usually accompany attacks. In the large majority of patients, symptoms begin in the first year of life, although it is possible for a patient to evade diagnosis for many years. The serum IgD level is typically elevated in this syndrome and should be checked in a young person of European descent as part of a recurrent fever work-up. The genetic defect is in the mevalonate kinase enzyme of the cholesterol metabolism pathway.[16] During attacks, levels of this enzyme are elevated in the urine and can be determined to corroborate with the diagnosis.[16]

The tumor necrosis factor receptor-associated periodic syndrome was first known as Familial Hibernian Fever, after its initial description in a large Irish family. It has since been seen in a number of ethnic cohorts. The syndrome is inherited in an autosomal-dominant pattern and usually manifests before the age of 20 years.[7] Unlike the prior diseases, attacks can vary in length from 1 day to longer than 1 week. More than 80% of patients experience pain and tightness of local muscle groups.[7] Abdominal pain, gastrointestinal symptoms, a macular rash, and painful conjunctivitis are other prominent features. Genetic sequencing is the recommended method for definitive diagnosis.[7] The disease is steroid responsive,[7] but it is unclear whether treatment with etanercept, a tumor necrosis factor-α antagonist, will decrease the incidence of long-term complications.[16]

Prognosis

In a recent case series, the cause of an FUO was found to be undetermined in 10% to 25% of cases.[2,3,12] Close observation of the patient may be required to determine whether the fevers resolve or a disease becomes apparent. When a patient is clinically deteriorating, however, watchful waiting is not appropriate. In this situation, the clinician should consider empiric therapeutic trials in conjunction with consultation with an infectious disease physician, rheumatologist, or oncologist, if clues lead in one or more of these directions.

Knockaert et al[12] followed a group of 60 of these patients for 5 years to determine the prognoses of patients with undiagnosed FUO. Approximately 20% of patients had a diagnosis established and 50% had resolution of symptoms soon after their evaluation. Less than 10% had persistent symptoms.

The inability to make a diagnosis can be an anxiety-provoking prospect for a patient who has submitted to countless tests in the hopes of finding a diagnosis. In this situation, one should council the patient on the generally favorable prognosis in this situation, modifying the discussion for factors that might apply in relation to the diagnostic findings. The fever itself should be managed symptomatically. Nonsteroidal anti-inflammatory drugs are the first-line agents for this. Meanwhile, observation, with emphasis on a noninvasive approach, should continue.

Key Points: Fever of Unknown Origin

⊂⋗ An extensive history and physical examination often will establish potential clues for the diagnosis of FUO.

⊂⋗ Key elements of this history include establishing the fever itself, exposure history, prodromes, dietary history, travel history, military service, and detailed medical history including prior surgeries, implanted devices and transfusions, and all prescribed and over-the-counter medications and supplements.

⊂⋗ Symptoms may be subtly present. The review of symptoms should be detailed and should be taken on repeated occasions, as symptoms may change or the patient may note their presence only on repeated questioning.

⊂⋗ The initial panel of laboratory testing should be reviewed in detail, again looking for subtle clues that can guide further diagnostic work-up. A clinical microbiologist should be informed of infections you are searching for, so that special specimen collection or laboratory procedures can be employed. Radiologic imaging and nuclear medicine studies can have important roles in localizing pathology. Serologic testing has an important role in the diagnosis of both rheumatologic disorders and many infectious diseases with nonspecific symptomology.

⊂⋗ When a diagnosis is not established after exhaustive searches, specialists can help in suggesting further diagnoses or recommending whether therapeutic trials are appropriate.

References

1. Petersdorf RG, Beeson PB: Fever of unexplained origin: Report on 100 cases. Medicine (Baltimore) 40:1–30, 1961.
2. Mackowiak PA, Durack DT: Fever of unknown origin. In Mandell GL, Bennett JE, Dolin R, eds: Mandell, Douglas, and Bennett's Principles and Practice of Infectious Diseases, 5th ed. Philadelphia: Churchill Livingstone, 2000:959–974.
3. deKleijn EM, Vandenbroucke JP, van der Meer JW: Fever of unknown origin: 1. A prospective multicenter study of 167 patients with FUO, using fixed epidemiologic entry criteria. Medicine (Baltimore) 76:392–400, 1997.
4. Norman DC: Fever in the elderly. Clin Infect Dis 31:148–151, 2000.
5. Gelfand JA, Dinarello CA: Fever and hyperthermia. In Fauci AS, Braunwald E, Isselbacher KJ, et al, eds: Harrison's Principles of Internal Medicine, 14th ed. New York: McGraw Hill, 1998:84–90.
6. Arnow PM, Flaherty JP: Fever of unknown origin. Lancet 350:575–580, 1997.
7. Drenth JP, van der Meer JW: Hereditary periodic fever. N Engl J Med 345:1748–1757, 2001.
8. Brouqui P, Raoult D: Endocarditis due to rare and fastidious bacteria. Clin Microbiol Rev 14:177–207, 2001.

9. Hirschmann JV: Fever of unknown origin in adults. Clin Infect Dis 24:291–302, 1997.

10. DeKleijn EM, van Lier H, van der Meer JW: Fever of unknown origin: II. Diagnostic procedures in a prospective multicenter study of 167 patients. Medicine (Baltimore) 76:401–414, 1997.

11. Corstens F, van der Meer JW: Nuclear medicine's role in infection and inflammation. Lancet 354:765–770, 1999.

12. Knockaert DC, Dujardin KS, Bobbaers HJ: Long-term follow-up of patients with undiagnosed fever of unknown origin. Arch Intern Med 156:618–620, 1996.

13. Blockmans D, Knockaert D, Maes A, et al: Clinical value of ^{18}fluoro-deoxyglucose positron emission tomography for patients with fever of unknown origin. Clin Infect Dis 32:191–196, 2001.

14. Mourad O, Palda V, Detsky A: A comprehensive evidence-based approach to fever of unknown origin. Arch Intern Med 163: 545–551, 2003.

15. Wurtz R: Psychiatric diseases presenting as infectious diseases. Clin Infect Dis 26: 924–932, 1998.

16. Hull K, Kastner D, Baiow J, et al: Hereditary periodic fever [letter]. N Engl J Med 346:1415–1416, 2002.

Diagnosis and Treatment of Lyme Disease

chapter

24

Maureen Cassin, M.D.

Lyme disease is the most common vector-borne illness in the United States and is an important outpatient "hot topic" because its incidence is on the rise.[1] In fact, Healthy People 2010 lists reduction in the incidence of Lyme disease among its public health goals for the next decade.[2] Lyme disease is caused by the spirochete *Borrelia burgdorferi*. The organism is transmitted by tick vectors, which require host mammals and seasonal variation to complete the life cycle. Lyme disease remains most prevalent in areas that provide a hospitable environment for ticks and their hosts. Prompt diagnosis and treatment are vital to symptom resolution and prevention of long-term sequelae.

This chapter reviews the epidemiology of Lyme disease, discusses the tick life cycle, and provides an overview of the key features of diagnosis and management of the disease. Strategies for the prevention of tick bites are also addressed.

Epidemiology

The incidence of Lyme disease increased more than 30-fold from 1982 to 1996.[3] In 2000, 17,730 cases were reported, representing an 8% increase from 1999.[4] The incidence is highest in the Northeast (especially Connecticut, Rhode Island, New Jersey, New York, Delaware, Pennsylvania, Massachusetts, New Hampshire, and Vermont), the mid-Atlantic (particularly Maryland), and the Midwest (Wisconsin, Minnesota). Lyme disease has also been identified on the West Coast. There are endemic and hyperendemic counties within these states (Figure 1).

The distribution of Lyme disease is bimodal, typically occurring in children 5 to 9 years of age and adults 50 to 59 years of age, with a slightly higher number of males affected. The majority of cases occur in June, followed by July and August.[4] People who live and work in residential or wooded areas are at greatest risk. Lyme disease became re-

Figure 1. Number of cases of Lyme disease, by county—United States, 2000. (From Centers for Disease Control and Prevention: Lyme Disease. CDC division of vector-borne infectious diseases. *www.cdc.gov.ncidod/dvbid/lyme/index.htm*. Accesssed Sept 23, 2002.)

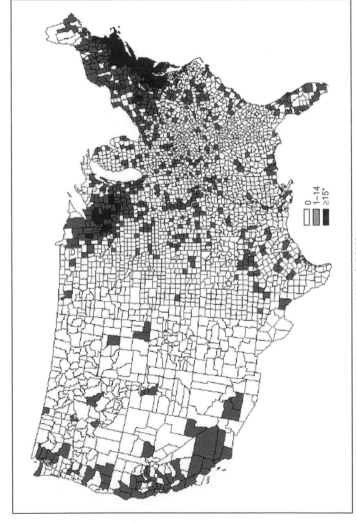

0
1–14
≥15*

*Total number of cases from these counties represented 90% of all 2000 cases.

portable to the Centers for Disease Control and Prevention (CDC) in 1991.

Life Cycle

Understanding the tick life cycle is an important step in assessing the risk of Lyme disease after a bite and developing strategies to prevent infection. Ticks from the genus *Ixodes*, typically *I. scapularis* in the northeastern United States and *I. pacificus* on the West Coast, are the vectors of Lyme disease. The species differ in animal host and vegetation preferences, factors governed by geographic availability. The life cycle of *Ixodes* takes 2 years to complete.

The ticks develop through larval, nymphal, and adult stages, each requiring a blood meal to advance to the next stage. Adult ticks lay eggs in early spring and the eggs hatch into larvae in the summer. Larvae feed on small mammals and birds into late summer and early fall before they molt into nymphs and become dormant.[5] In late spring, dormant nymphs emerge to feed on rodents, small mammals, and humans. After a blood meal, nymphs molt into adults in the fall. *B. burgdorferi* is transmitted during feeds. Large mammals, deer in particular, are the preferred hosts for adult ticks. Adults feed and mate on deer and then drop off to lay eggs in spring,[5] beginning the cycle again. Animal hosts are not harmed by infection.

Nymphs transmit the majority of *B. burgdorferi* infections to humans. They feed from late May into early September, when humans are most active and least covered. They typically occupy low-lying shrubs and grass, which allows them to crawl onto and attach to a host as it brushes past. The nymphs' tiny size helps them to escape detection long enough for successful attachment and feeding. Adults also transmit *B. burgdorferi*, but they are often discovered early and removed before attachment. Larvae do not carry *B. burgdorferi* when they first feed and are not important in human infections.

History

The patient history provides important clues in determining the likelihood of Lyme disease transmission.[6] Clinicians should focus on the following questions:

- Is Lyme disease endemic in the area in which the exposure occurred?
- During what season did the exposure occur? Was it a season in which nymphs feed? (Nymphs feed from late May into early September.)

- Was the tick attached? (The tick must be attached to take its blood meal and transmit disease.)
- How much time elapsed between high-risk exposure and discovery of a tick? (Ticks must be attached for 48 to 72 hours to transmit *B. burgdorferi.*)
- How long did it take for symptoms to develop? (Symptoms typically develop 7 to 14 days from tick exposure, but they may develop as early as 3 days or as late as 30 days after a bite.)

Clinical Signs and Symptoms

The CDC developed a case definition for Lyme disease for the purpose of surveillance in 1990, and this is reviewed in Table 1.[7] Clinical signs and symptoms of Lyme disease can be divided into three stages: early localized, early disseminated, and late or persistent infection (Table 2).

TABLE 1. CDC Case Definition of Lyme Disease[7]

Definition: Erythema migrans (EM) or at least one late manifestation and laboratory confirmation.

- **Erythema migrans** diagnosed by a physician. EM typically begins as a red macule or papule and expands over a period of days to weeks to form a large round lesion, often with partial central clearing. A solitary lesion must reach at least 5 cm in size. Lesions occurring within several hours of a tick bite represent hypersensitivity reactions and do not qualify as EM.

- **Late manifestations**
  Musculoskeletal: recurrent, brief attacks (weeks or months) of objective joint swelling in one or a few joints, sometimes followed by chronic arthritis in one or a few joints. Manifestations not considered as criteria for diagnosis include arthralgia, myalgia, fibromyalgia syndromes, chronic progressive arthritis not preceded by brief attacks, and chronic symmetrical polyarthritis.
  Neurologic: lymphocytic meningitis, cranial neuritis, particularly facial palsy (may be bilateral); radiculoneuropathy; encephalomyelitis, alone or in combination. Encephalomyelitis must be confirmed by showing a higher titer of antibody against *Borellia burgdorferi* in cerebrospinal fluid than in serum. Headache, fatigue, paresthesia, or mild stiff neck alone are not criteria for neurologic involvement.
  Cardiovascular: acute onset, high-grade (second- or third-degree) atrioventricular conduction defects that resolve in days to weeks, sometimes associated with myocarditis. Palpitations, bradycardia, bundle branch block, or myocarditis alone are not criteria for cardiovascular involvement.

- **Laboratory confirmation** of infection includes isolation of *B. burgdorferi* from tissue or body fluid, detection of diagnostic levels of immunoglobulin M or immunoglobulin G antibodies in serum or cerebrospinal fluid, or demonstration of a significant change in antibody levels in paired acute- and convalescent-phase serum samples. Syphilis and other causes of false-positive serologic test results should be excluded when diagnosis has been based on serologic testing alone.

TABLE 2. Clinical Manifestations of Lyme Disease
Early localized disease: local effects of *Borrelia burgdorferi*
General: fatigue, malaise, arthralgias, myalgias, headache, regional lymphadenopathy
Dermatologic: erythema migrans
Early disseminated disease: effects of spirochetemia and immune response
General: fatigue, malaise, generalized lymphadenopathy
Dermatologic: multiple annular lesions
Cardiac: varying degrees of atrioventricular block, myopericarditis, cardiomyopathy
Neurologic: aseptic meningitis, encephalitis, cranial nerve palsy, radiculopathy, peripheral neuropathy
Rheumatologic: migratory mono- or polyarthralgias/arthritis, myalgias
Late or persistent disease: effects of chronic infection and immune response
Dermatologic: acrodermatitis atrophicans
Neurologic: subtle cognitive disturbances, encephalitis, peripheral neuropathy, dementia
Rheumatologic: chronic migratory mono- or polyarthritis, synovitis

Early localized disease occurs a few days to a month after infection. It manifests as erythema migrans, a slowly spreading localized skin lesion at the site of the bite in about 80% of patients.[8] Although the classic erythema migrans lesion is described as a "bulls eye rash," the minority of patient actually develop this classic rash. The lesion begins as a red macule or papule at the location of the bite. The area of erythema gradually expands to a maximum median diameter of 15 cm (range, 3 68 cm) over 3 to 32 days (median, 7 days).[9] As the red rim expands, the center may become clear or even turn blue. In other cases, the center becomes necrotic, vesicular, or erythematous and indurated. An erythematous streak at the hairline may be the only clue to a bite on the head.[9]

Associated nonspecific symptoms include fatigue, myalgias, arthralgias, headache, malaise, and regional or generalized adenopathy. Patients may also report fever.

Early disseminated disease occurs days to months after tick bites. Carditis occurs in 5% to 10% of untreated patients and may include varied degrees of atrioventricular block and, less commonly, myopericarditis or cardiomyopathy. Dermatologic signs include multiple annular skin lesions away from the bite location. Neurologic manifestations occur in 10% to 15% of untreated patients and include cranial nerve palsies (usually facial nerve), aseptic meningitis, encephalitis, peripheral neuropathy, or radiculopathy. Rheumatologic complications such as polyathritis or arthralgias typically affect large weight-bearing joints, particularly the knees. Joints are involved in 50% to 60% of untreated patients.[8]

Late or chronic disease may be seen months to years after a tick bite. It typically affects joints, nervous system, and skin. Approximately 50% to 60% of untreated patients develop rheumatologic manifestations, including migrating polyarthritis, chronic monoarthritis, or synovitis. Neurologic signs and symptoms include encephalopathy (subtle cognitive dysfunction, sleep disturbances), peripheral neuropathy, or dementia.[8,10] Late dermatologic findings such as acrodermatitis chronica atrophicans, a chronic skin condition marked by telangiectasia, sclerosis, or atrophy, are more common in Europe.

Diagnosis

Who Should Be Tested?

The diagnosis of early Lyme disease is based on clinical evidence and a known exposure in an area with a high prevalence of Lyme disease (see Figure 1).[5] Current guidelines from Centers for Disease Control and Prevention and the American College of Physicians[5,11] support empiric therapy for patients with objective clinical signs of early disease and a high-risk exposure. Serologic testing is indicated in patients with clinical findings consistent with early disseminated or late disease.

Who Should Not Be Tested?

It is very important to consider pretest probability before testing for Lyme disease. In areas of low prevalence, false-positive findings outnumber true-positive findings.[11] Patients are needlessly subjected to the costs and complications of antibiotic therapy. Patients with nonspecific complaints such as myalgias, fatigue, headache, and fever in the absence of objective signs or exposures should not be tested.[11]

Serologic Testing

Serologic evidence supports the diagnosis in patients with clinical findings suggestive of early disseminated or late disease. For this group of patients, CDC guidelines recommend enzyme linked immunosorbent assay (ELISA) or indirect fluorescent antibody (IFA) test, two sensitive assays, for initial evaluation. If results are positive or equivocal, the more specific Western blot test should be used to verify or support ELISA or IFA results.[5] Western blot analysis detects immunoglobulin M (IgM) and immunoglobulin G (IgG) antibodies directed against B. burgdorferi proteins. If the ELISA or IFA results are negative, no further testing is necessary.

Western blot analysis findings are positive in the minority of patients during the first few weeks of infection. Positive results usually demonstrate IgM antibody. If suspicion of Lyme disease is high, and the early serologic testing result is negative, paired acute and convalescent samples obtained 2 to 4 weeks apart can be tested for IgM and IgG antibodies. Approximately 70% to 80% of convalescent serum samples will be positive, even after antibiotic therapy.[8] The IgG antibody isotype is more common in convalescent samples. A positive Western blot finding for IgM antibody after 1 month or more of illness is likely a false-positive finding and should be ignored.[8]

The presence of antibodies alone cannot make the diagnosis of Lyme disease. They may persist for years after appropriate therapy and resolution of infection. Polymerase chain reaction testing of skin, blood, cerebrospinal fluid, and synovial fluid has not been standardized and is not reliable. Urine antigen testing is also not useful.[8]

Treatment

Tables 3 and 4 summarize the treatment guidelines that follow.

Early Lyme Disease

Treatment of early Lyme disease is aimed at resolution of symptoms and prevention of late complications. For the treatment of early localized or early disseminated disease without third-degree heart block or neurologic complications in adults, current guidelines recommend doxycycline 100 mg orally twice daily or amoxicillin 500 mg orally three times daily for 14 to 21 days as first-line therapy. Cefuroxime axetil at 500 mg orally twice daily is a costly alternative for patients who

TABLE 3. Adult and Pediatric Dosages of Antibiotics Used in the Treatment of Lyme Disease		
Drug	Adult Dose	Pediatric Dose
Amoxicillin*	500 mg PO tid	50 mg/kg/day PO divided into three doses (maximum 500 mg/dose)
Doxycycline*	100 mg PO bid	1–2 mg/kg PO bid (maximum 100 mg/dose[†])
Cefuroxime axetil	500 mg PO bid	30 mg/kg/d PO divided into two doses (maximum 500 mg/dose)
Ceftriaxone*	2 g IV daily	75–100 mg/kg IV daily (maximum 2 g)
Cefotaxime	2 g IV tid	150–200 mg/kg/day IV divided into three or four doses (maximum 6 g daily)
Penicillin G	18–24 million units IV/day divided into q4-hr doses	200,000–400,000 units IV/kg/day divided into six doses (every 4 hours)

*Preferred therapy
[†]Age ≤ 8 years is a relative contraindication to doxycycline therapy.
Adapted from the Infectious Disease Society of America guidelines for the treatment of Lyme disease.[10]

TABLE 4. Route and Duration of Antibiotic Therapy for Lyme Disease*		
Manifestation	Route of Therapy	Duration
Erythema migrans	Oral	14–21 days
Early neurologic		
Meningitis, radiculopathy	Parenteral	14–28 days
Cranial nerve palsy	Oral	14–21 days
Cardiac		
First- or second-degree atrioventricular block	Oral	14–21 days
Third-degree atrioventricular block	Parenteral	14–21 days
Late rheumatologic		
Arthritis without neurologic disease	Oral	28 days
Recurrent arthritis after oral therapy	Oral	28 days
	Parenteral	14–28 days
Recurrent arthritis after 2 courses of treatment	No antibiotics	—
Central/peripheral nervous system disease	Parenteral	14–28 days

*Adapted from the Infectious Disease Society of American guidelines for the treatment of Lyme disease.[10]

cannot tolerate doxycycline or amoxicillin. Pregnancy and lactation are relative contraindications to doxycycline therapy.

Pediatric regimens include amoxicillin 50 mg/kg/day orally divided into three doses up to a maximum of 500 mg per dose or, for children 8 years or older, doxycycline 1 to 2 mg/kg/day divided into two doses up to a maximum of 100 mg per dose. Alternative therapy with cefuroxime axetil at 30 mg/kg/day divided into two doses up to a maximum of 500 mg per dose is recommended for children who cannot take amoxicillin or doxycycline. Age $\leq$ 8 years is a relative contraindication to doxycycline therapy.

Macrolides should be reserved for patients who cannot tolerate amoxicillin, doxycycline, or cefuroxime axetil. Adult regimens include azithromycin 500 mg orally daily for 7 to10 days or erythromycin 500 mg orally four times daily for 14 to 21 days, or clarithromycin 500 mg orally twice daily for 14 to 21 days. Pediatric macrolide regimens include azithromycin 10 mg/kg/day up to a maximum of 500 mg per dose or erythromycin 12.5 mg/kg four times daily up to 500 mg per dose, or clarithromycin 7.5 mg/kg twice daily up to 500 mg per dose.

Early Lyme Disease with Acute Neurologic Involvement

Acute neurologic involvement includes aseptic meningitis or radiculopathy. Parenteral therapy with ceftriaxone, penicillin G, or cefotaxime is recommended for both children and adults (see Tables 3 and 4 for dosages and duration of therapy). Oral or parenteral doxycycline can be used for patients over 8 years of age with intolerance of penicillins or cephalosporins.

Lumbar puncture may be reserved for patients with severe headache, nuchal rigidity, or other signs and symptoms of central nervous system involvement. If cerebrospinal fluid study findings are normal, an oral regimen is preferred. In cases of cranial nerve palsy, an oral regimen may be used to prevent further sequelae.

Cardiac Disease

For Lyme disease complicated by first- or second-degree atrioventricular block, oral therapy is adequate. In cases of third-degree atrioventricular block, current guidelines recommend parenteral antibiotics given in the hospital setting. Insertion of a temporary pacemaker may be necessary.

Late Disease

Arthritis without neurologic disease can be treated with a 28-day course of oral amoxicillin or doxycycline. However, some patients go on to develop signs of neuroborreliosis after treatment with an oral regimen, necessitating parenteral antibiotics anyway. Treatment of arthritis with neurologic involvement is the same as treatment of early Lyme disease with central nervous system involvement and includes parenteral ceftriaxone, penicillin G, or cefotaxime.

Recurrent or persistent arthritis can be treated with oral or parenteral therapy. It is important to wait for months between courses of treatment given the slow resolution of inflammation. If arthritis persists or recurs after two courses of oral therapy or one course of parenteral therapy, symptomatic treatment with nonsteroidal anti-inflammatory drugs may be effective. No further antibiotic therapy is recommended.

Late Neuroborreliosis

Current guidelines recommend 14 to 28 days of parenteral therapy with ceftriaxone, cefotaxime, or penicillin G for adults and children (see Tables 3 and 4). Repeat therapy is recommended only if relapse can be objectively demonstrated.

Chronic Lyme Disease

Despite appropriate treatment, some patients experience persistent fatigue, myalgias, arthralgias, neurocognitive dysfunction, and other subjective symptoms similar to those reported in cases of fibromyalgia or chronic fatigue syndrome. There is still debate over whether chronic Lyme disease represents a separate disease entity. Some experts believe that Lyme disease may trigger the onset of fibromyalgia. In a study by Kalish et al,[12] chronic subjective symptoms were reported to occur more commonly in patients who presented with early dissemination to the nervous system, especially if antibiotic therapy was delayed. In contrast, a recent longitudinal cohort study reports that symptoms consistent with chronic Lyme disease were just as common in age-matched, uninfected control subjects.[13] Prolonged or repeated courses of antibiotics have no demonstrated efficacy in these patients and should be avoided.[10]

Coinfection With Other Agents

Ixodes scapularis ticks also transmit *Ehrlichia* species and *Babesia microti,* the agents of human granulocytic ehrlichiosis (HGE) and babesiosis. Doxycycline therapy for Lyme disease also treats HGE. However, patients with persistent symptoms despite appropriate Lyme disease therapy may be coinfected with *Babesia.* Symptoms usually resolve with proper therapy directed against babesiosis, typically clindamycin and quinine.[14]

Monitoring for Complications of Therapy[6]

- Leukopenia has been associated with the use of beta-lactam antibiotics. Weekly complete blood cell counts should be performed.
- Biliary complications such as sludge formation may complicate ceftriaxone therapy. Weekly liver function testing is recommended, even in asymptomatic patients.
- Photosensitivity is a well-documented side effect of doxycycline therapy.
- *Clostridium difficile* colitis is a potential complication of antibiotic therapy.

Prophylaxis

Current guidelines do not recommend routine antimicrobial prophylaxis or serologic testing after a tick bite. Although several experts recommend prophylaxis after bites by engorged *I. scapularis* nymphs, it is very difficult to accurately identify the tick species and assess the degree of engorgement. Testing recovered ticks for *B. burgdorferi* is not recommended.[10]

People who have been bitten by a tick need close monitoring for development of skin lesions, temperature exceeding 38°C (suggestive of babesiosis or HGE), or other signs of illness for up to 1 month. If illness develops, patients should be evaluated for a tick-borne disease.

Prevention

Despite widespread awareness about Lyme disease, only 40% to 50% of adults take steps to prevent tick bites.[3] Effective strategies include wearing long pants and tucking pant legs into socks. Checking for ticks after time spent outdoors allows prompt detection (within 24–48 hours) and removal before attachment. Ticks are more easily seen on light-colored clothing. Bites typically occur in hidden, moist areas, such as the axilla, groin, or behind the knee and constricted areas such as waistbands. Unfortunately, only 30% of patients even recall a tick bite.[9] Nymphs often occupy the periphery of wooded areas, so following the middle of paths and trails helps minimize contact.

Avoidance of tick-infested areas is an effective but often impractical approach to Lyme disease prevention. Strategies to reduce tick population density include leaf removal and grass cutting. Because tick eggs are deposited on the ground in leaf litter, clearing this reduces the *Ixodes* population by 72% to 100%; however, the tick population returns within several months.[3] A Massachusetts study demonstrated that mowing grass reduced the tick population by 70%. Seventeen months later, the population remained 53% lower.[3] Large scale pesticide use is limited by toxicity to plants, birds, and animals.

The use of repellents and toxins is widely recommended. Repellents containing N,N-diethyl-3-methylbenzamide (DEET) are the most effective but must be reapplied often. Permethrin 0.5% fabric spray kills ticks, but skin contact should be avoided. Despite these shortcomings, the benefits of repellents and toxins likely outweigh the risks. The Lyme disease vaccine is no longer available.

Additional Information

For more information, visit the CDC website at *www.cdc.gov*. Click on "L" under "topics A-Z" for the link to the Lyme disease home page. The site contains information clearly presented in lay terms as well as excellent pictures, diagrams, and maps.

References

1. Orlowski KA, Hayes EB, Campbell GL, Dennis DT: Surveillance for Lyme disease—United States, 1992–1998. MMWR Morbid Mortal Wkly Rep 49:S1–11, 2000.
2. US Department of Health and Human Services: Healthy People 2010. Washington, DC: USDHHS, 2000.
3. Poland G: Prevention of Lyme disease: A review of the evidence. Mayo Clin Proc 76:713–724, 2001.

4. Centers for Disease Control and Prevention: Lyme disease—United States, 2000. MMWR Morbid Mortal Wkly Rep 51:29–31, 2000.
5. Centers for Disease Control and Prevention: Lyme Disease. CDC division of vector-borne infectious diseases. www.cdc.gov.ncidod/dvbid/lyme/index.htm. Accesssed Sept 23, 2002.
6. Sigal LH: Epidemiology and clinical manifestations of Lyme disease. UpToDate 2001; version 10.1. www.uptodate.com. Accessed Sept 23, 2002.
7. Centers for Disease Control and Prevention: Case definitions for public health surveillance. MMWR Morbid Mortal Wkly Rep 39:1–43, 1990.
8. Steere AC: Lyme disease. N Engl J Med 345:115–125, 2001.
9. Steere AC, Bartenhagen NH, Craft JE, et al: The early clinical manifestations of Lyme disease. Ann Intern Med 99:76–82, 1983.
10. Wormser GP, Nadelman RB, Dattwyler RJ, et al: IDSA practice guidelines for the treatment of Lyme disease. Clin Infect Dis 31:S1–S14, 2000.
11. Tugwell P, Dennis DT, Weinstein A, et al: Laboratory evaluation in the diagnosis of Lyme disease. Position paper: Clinical guideline. Ann Intern Med 127:1109–1123, 1997.
12. Kalish RA, Kaplan RF, Talor E, et al: Evaluation of study patients with Lyme disease, 10–20 year follow-up. J Infect Dis 183:453–460, 2001.
13. Seltzer EG, Gerber MA, Carter ML, et al: Long-term outcomes of persons with Lyme disease. JAMA 283:609–616, 2000.
14. Krause PJ, Spielman A, Telford SR, et al: Persistent parasitemia after acute babesiosis. N Engl J Med 339:160–165, 1998.
15. Centers for Disease Control and Prevention: Notice to readers: Recommendation for test performance and interpretation from the second national conference on serologic diagnosis of Lyme disease. MMWR Morbid Mortal Wkly Rep 44:590–591, 1995.
16. Nadelman RB, Nowakowski J, Forseter G, et al: The clinical spectrum of early Lyme borreliosis in patients with culture-confirmed erythema migrans. Am J Med 100:502–508, 1996.
17. Smith RP, Schoen RT, Rahn DW, et al: Clinical characteristics and treatment outcome of early Lyme disease in patients with microbiologically confirmed erythema migrans. Ann Intern Med 136:421–428, 2002.
18. Dinerman H, Steere AC: Lyme disease associated with fibromyalgia. Ann Intern Med 117:281–285, 1992.
19. Steere AC: Lyme disease. N Engl J Med 321:586–596, 1989.

Syphilis

Carolyn V. Gould, M.D., and
Harvey Rubin, M.D.

chapter
25

Syphilis is a worldwide chronic sexually transmitted disease caused by the spirochete *Treponema pallidum.* Notorious for its variable clinical manifestations, syphilis is often referred to as the "great imitator." Prior to World War II, syphilis was a common disease in the United States, with about 1 of every 13 Americans infected.[1] With the advent of penicillin in the 1940s, along with improved public health measures, disease rates declined markedly.[1-3] Syphilis became relatively rare in the United States, resulting in a lack of familiarity with the disease by most clinicians. In the late 1980s and early 1990s, syphilis made a resurgence, which was linked to the acquired immunodeficiency syndrome epidemic and later with epidemics of illegal drug use, especially crack cocaine.[2,3] Since then, syphilis rates have declined markedly, with an all-time low rate of 2.5 cases per 100,000 population in 1999, making future eradication of the disease a possibility.[4]

To continue this trend and prevent the potentially devastating sequelae of untreated syphilis, primary care physicians should be familiar with the diagnosis and management of syphilis. The most common clinical dilemmas that arise are how to interpret serologic findings, when to perform a lumbar puncture, and how to assess response to therapy.[5] This chapter reviews the transmission and clinical findings of syphilis in adults, discusses diagnostic testing, and outlines the latest recommendations for treatment and follow-up. Special considerations, including syphilis in patients with the human immunodeficiency virus (HIV) and syphilis in pregnancy, with regard to prevention of congenital syphilis, are also discussed.

Etiology

Syphilis is caused by *Treponema pallidum,* a slender, tightly coiled bacterium in the family Spirochaetaceae.[6] Too slender to be seen on direct microscopy, *T. pallidum* can be detected with darkfield microscopy and has a characteristic rotary movement with central flexion, which is diagnostic.[7] The organism cannot be cultured in vitro.

Transmission

In the vast majority of cases, syphilis is acquired by sexual intercourse with an infectious individual, during which *T. pallidum* gains access to the subcutaneous tissues through intact mucous membranes or microperforations in the skin.[6] Disease transmission is most likely during early (primary and secondary) syphilis, especially when active mucocutaneous lesions are present. An infectious syphilitic individual has about a 50% chance of transmitting the disease during a sexual encounter.[1] In general, patients can no longer transmit the disease by sexual contact 4 years after infection.[6]

Other means of transmission include close contact with an active lesion, passage through the placenta or during delivery (congenital syphilis), blood transfusion, and accidental direct inoculation, as in a needle stick injury. In developed countries, transfusion syphilis is extremely rare, owing to routine screening of donated blood for syphilis since the 1930s.[1]

Syphilis is most common among sexually active persons with multiple partners, making it is necessary to rule out other sexually transmitted diseases, especially HIV, when a diagnosis of syphilis is made and vice versa. Because of the high transmission rate of syphilis, empiric treatment of incubating syphilis in sexual contacts is warranted whenever possible.

Clinical Manifestations

Syphilis is divided into the following clinical stages: incubating, primary, secondary, latent, and late (tertiary) syphilis. The median incubation period after infection is 3 weeks but may range from 3 to 90 days, depending on the size of the inoculum.[6] Within hours to days after infection, *T. pallidum* disseminates throughout the body through lymphatics or blood and can invade any organ system, especially the central nervous system (CNS).

Primary Syphilis

Primary syphilis is characterized by the development of a *chancre,* a painless ulceration that usually begins as a papule at the site of inoculation. The ulcer has a smooth base and firm, raised borders with no exudate or inflammation. Spirochetes are present in the lesion, which is highly infectious. The chancre appears wherever the inoculum occurred; common sites include the external genitalia, cervix, mouth, perianal area, and anal canal. Lesions may become secondarily infected, especially in the oral and perianal region. Painless regional lymphadenopathy is often present.

Because of its painless nature, the chancre may go unnoticed, resulting in lack of diagnosis and continued transmission. Furthermore, lesions are frequently atypical or absent in primary syphilis, especially with a low inoculum, intercurrent antibiotics, or previous syphilis infection.[6] Multiple chancres may also occur, particularly in patients with HIV. Chancres typically heal within 2 to 8 weeks. In immunocompromised patients, such as those with HIV, however, chancres may take longer to heal and are often present when manifestations of secondary syphilis begin.[8]

The lesions of primary syphilis must be distinguished from genital ulcers caused by herpes simplex and *Haemophilis ducreyi* (chancroid), which are most often painful. Other potential mimickers of primary syphilis include lymphogranuloma venereum, granuloma inguinale, trauma, malignancies, and atypical nonvenereal infections such as tularemia.

Secondary (Disseminated) Syphilis

Secondary syphilis is a systemic illness that may develop 2 to 12 weeks (mean, 6 weeks) after resolution of the chancre and occurs in about 25% of patients with untreated syphilis.[9] During this stage, a high degree of spirochetemia occurs despite a vigorous immune response by the host. Constitutional symptoms are prominent during secondary syphilis, often with fever, malaise, anorexia, weight loss, and generalized lymphadenopathy. Involvement of epitrochlear lymph nodes is a classic finding.

A rash is the most typical manifestation of secondary syphilis. Lesions usually begin on the trunk and may become widely distributed, characteristically involving the palms and soles. Lesions can be macular, maculopapular, papular, or pustular, but are never vesicular (except in cases of congenital syphilis).

Other characteristic findings of secondary syphilis include *patchy alopecia* due to involvement of hair follicles (follicular syphilids), *condylomata lata*—broad, grayish-white to erythematous eroded papules that develop in warm, moist intertriginous areas—and *mucous patches*—silvery-gray erosions with a red border that develop on mucous membranes. Condylomata lata and mucous patches are highly infectious and teeming with spirochetes. They are painless unless secondarily infected.

Central nervous system involvement occurs in up to 40% of patients during this stage.[10] Cerebrospinal fluid (CSF) analysis often reveals elevated protein levels and a lymphocytosis. Symptoms may include headache, meningismus, and cranial nerve deficits, although only 1% to 2% of patients have symptoms of acute aseptic meningitis.[1] Eye involvement, particularly uveitis, is present in 5% to 10% of patients with secondary syphilis, especially in HIV-infected patients, and gets worse with steroids.[11]

Virtually any organ may be involved in secondary syphilis, with gastrointestinal, renal, and musculoskeletal disease reported. When untreated, patients spontaneously recover from secondary syphilis over the course of a few days to 10 weeks.

Latent Syphilis

Untreated secondary syphilis resolves spontaneously, leading to latent syphilis, an asymptomatic phase characterized only by a positive treponemal serology. Based on the likelihood of mucocutaneous relapse and therefore of "infectiousness," patients are classified as having *early latent syphilis* during the first year after infection, when 90% of relapses occur, and *late latent syphilis* beyond this time.[12] Although patients with late latent syphilis can no longer transmit the disease by sexual contact, transplacental or blood transmission is still possible.

Late (Tertiary) Syphilis

Late syphilis is a progressive inflammatory disease that may develop in 25% to 40% of patients with untreated syphilis, usually occurring 5 to 30 years after the initial infection.[13] This stage can be divided into late neurosyphilis, cardiovascular syphilis, and gummatous syphilis, depending on the organ system involved.

Late Neurosyphilis

Central nervous system invasion by *T. pallidum* often occurs in the earliest stages of infection, as noted, and can be symptomatic or asymptomatic. The majority of untreated patients recover spontaneously from this initial infection, but a subset of patients go on to develop chronic neurosyphilis. The persistence of CSF abnormalities for more than 5 years in the untreated patient is highly predictive of progression to clinical neurosyphilis.[13]

Late neurosyphilis may be asymptomatic or symptomatic. Symptomatic neurosyphilis can be categorized as either meningovascular or parenchymatous neurosyphilis, although patients usually have overlapping features.

Asymptomatic neurosyphilis, the most common presentation of chronic neurosyphilis, is diagnosed by the finding of at least one CSF abnormality: a pleocytosis, an elevated protein level, a decreased glucose concentration, or a positive nontreponemal or reaginic test (discussed on page 283). Meningovascular neurosyphilis, which occurs 4 to 7 years after infection, results from the pathologic finding of endarteritis obliterans of the small blood vessels of the brain, meninges, and spinal cord, which leads to multiple microscopic areas of infarction. Both stroke and progressive neurologic deficits may develop, causing hemiparesis, aphasia, and seizures.

Parenchymatous neurosyphilis typically occurs decades after infection and results from the destruction of nerve cells by direct invasion of spirochetes in the cerebral cortex, causing general paresis, and, in the spinal cord, causing tabes dorsalis. The result is a combination of psychiatric and neurologic manifestations. *General paresis* is a progressive dementing illness marked by changes in personality, affect, sensorium, and intellect. Speech may be slurred, reflexes are hyperactive, and the classic Argyll-Robertson pupils (small, irregular pupils that do not respond to light but accommodate to near vision) may be present.

In tabes dorsalis, there is demyelinization of the posterior column, dorsal roots, and dorsal root ganglia. This results in the characteristic ataxic, wide-based gait and footslap. Patients may have paresthesias, "lightning" (sudden, severe) pains in the extremities, and urinary and fecal incontinence. On examination, there is a loss of position and vibratory sense, deep pain and temperature sensation, and decreased ankle and knee reflexes. The Argyll-Robertson pupil is typical of tabes dorsalis, and the Romberg sign is a classic finding. Loss of sensation may result in Charcot's joints and traumatic sores on the feet and lower extremities.[6]

Ocular syphilis is common in CNS infection with syphilis, and usually manifests as anterior uveitis, although any inflammatory process of the eye can occur. Patients who are HIV-infected or are receiving steroids are most prone to uveitis. Optic atrophy occurs most often in patients with tabes dorsalis, resulting in "gunbarrel sight."[6]

Syphilitic otitis, causing asymmetric deafness and tinnitus, is a particular form of neurosyphilis that may occur at any stage of disease. Because the CSF profile is typically normal, it is difficult to diagnose. Therefore, any patient with unexplained hearing loss or other vestibular abnormality with a positive treponemal antibody test finding should be treated for syphilitic otitis.

Cardiovascular Syphilis

Now largely a historical curiosity, cardiovascular syphilis was once the leading cause of cardiovascular disease in middle-aged adults at the turn of the 20th century.[6] As in meningovascular neurosyphilis, the pathologic lesion in cardiovascular syphilis is endarteritis obliterans, in this case involving the vaso vasorum of the aorta. Medial necrosis causes aortitis with a predilection for the ascending aorta, causing aortic regurgitation, coronary artery stenosis, and saccular aneurysms, which rarely dissect. Linear calcifications of the ascending aorta on chest radiographs are a typical finding. In the past, symptomatic syphilitic aortitis occurred in 10% to 15% of untreated patients with syphilis, although up to 86% of untreated cases were found to have pathologic findings on postmortem examination.[2]

Gummatous (Late Benign) Syphilis

Gummatous syphilis is an indolent late manifestation of untreated syphilis, and in the post-antibiotic era tends to occur most commonly in HIV-infected patients.[13] Granulomatous-like lesions (gummas) can form in any organ but tend to develop in the skeletal system, skin, and mucocutaneous tissues. Clinical manifestations result from local tissue destruction. Gummatous hepatitis may be symptomatic and lead to eventual cirrhosis. Other causes of granulomatous disease must be distinguished from syphilis. Gummas generally heal rapidly with penicillin therapy.

Diagnosis

Primary and Secondary Syphilis

The most direct way to diagnose syphilis in the early stages is by darkfield examination or immunofluorescence staining of mucocutaneous lesions. The highest yield comes from examining serous transudate from moist lesions such as the primary chancre, condylomata latum, or mucous patches, which have the largest number of organisms.[7] Darkfield examination may not be able to distinguish nonpathogenic treponemes that reside in the mouth from *T. pallidum,* so specific direct fluorescent antibody staining should be done on oral specimens.[7]

For darkfield examination, lesions should be rinsed with nonbactericidal saline and lightly abraded with dry gauze so as not to induce bleeding. The resulting serous exudates can be squeezed onto a glass slide and covered with a cover slip to be examined. Under darkfield examination, a characteristic corkscrew appearance and spiraling movement with flexion about the center establishes the presence of *T. pallidum.* Darkfield examination must be done immediately after specimen collection so that the organisms remain viable; however, motility is not required for diagnosis by the direct fluorescent antibody test. In addition, because numerous organisms are required for visualization, a negative test finding does not rule out the diagnosis.

Biopsy specimens are sometimes useful to diagnose syphilis. Specific immunofluorescence or immunoperoxidase staining is preferred over silver staining for ease of diagnosis.

Polymerase chain reaction assays can detect *T. pallidum* in clinical specimens, but this is currently not available for routine use.[2]

Serology

Both nonspecific nontreponemal reaginic antibodies and specific antitreponemal antibodies are measured in the serologic testing for syphilis, and they are generally measured in tandem to confirm the diagnosis.

Nontreponemal Reaginic Tests. The nontreponemal antibody test is a rapid and inexpensive test used for screening large numbers of sera for syphilis and to monitor disease activity and response to treatment. Patients infected with *T. pallidum* generate immunoglobulin M and immunoglobulin G antibodies that cross-react with cardiolipin antigens that are used for testing. The standard nontreponemal test is the Venereal Disease Research Laboratory (VDRL) slide test, which utilizes a cardiolipin-cholesterol-lecithin antigen. A modified test used by most laboratories and blood banks is the rapid plasma reagin (RPR) card test.

Levels of nontreponemal antibody vary during the course of the disease, with the highest titer being in the secondary and early latent periods. In cases of primary syphilis, antibodies will not be present until 1 to 4 weeks after the chancre has formed.[7] In cases of later disease, antibody titers generally decline to less than 1:4, with about one quarter of untreated cases eventually developing negative titers.[3] It is important to remember that a prozone phenomenon may occur in 1% to 2% of patients with secondary syphilis, in which the spirochetal antigen load is the highest, and during pregnancy.[7] Therefore, appropriate dilutions should be done to rule out the diagnosis when there is a high clinical suspicion.

Because of the nonspecificity of the test, false-positive reactions are common, especially in conditions of immune upregulation, such as in cases of chronic infectious diseases (such as HIV), autoimmune disease, and intravenous drug use (Table 1).

Specific Treponemal Tests. The specific treponemal antibody tests are the fluorescent treponemal antibody, absorbed (FTA-ABS) test, and the *T. pallidum* hemagglutination assays (TPHA and MHA-TP). They are used primarily to verify a positive nontreponemal antibody test finding. The FTA-ABS is an indirect immunofluorescent antibody assay that tests the patient's serum against *T. pallidum* cultivated in rabbit testes. Once a patient has a positive treponemal antibody test finding, it usually remains positive for life, despite treatment, although reversion to a negative status may occur in some patients, especially if treated early. Spe-

TABLE 1. Possible Causes of False-Positive Serologic Tests for Syphilis

	Infectious	Noninfectious
Nontreponemal tests (RPR, VDRL)		
• Bacterial	Pneumonia	Pregnancy
	Pneumococcal	Chronic liver disease
	Mycoplasma	Advanced cancer
	Scarlet fever	Intravenous drug use
	Leprosy	Multiple myeloma
	Lymphogranuloma venereum	Advanced age
		Connective tissue disease
	Relapsing fever	
	Bacterial endocarditis	Multiple blood transfusions
	Psittacosis	
	Leptospirosis	
	Chancroid	
	Tuberculosis	
	Rickettsial disease	
• Viral	Vaccinia vaccination	
	Chickenpox	
	Human immunodeficiency virus	
	Measles	
	Infectious mononucleosis	
	Mumps	
	Viral hepatitis	
• Parasitic	Trypanosomiasis	
	Malaria	
Treponemal tests (FTA-ABS, MHA-TP)	Lyme disease	Systemic lupus erythe-
	Leprosy	matosus
	Malaria	
	Infectious mononucleosis	
	Relapsing fever	
	Leptospirosis	

FTA-ABS, fluorescent treponemal antibody, absorbed test; MHA-TP, microhemagglutination assay–*Treponema pallidum;* RPR, rapid plasma reagin; VDRL, Venereal Disease Research Laboratory.

Modified from Hook EW, Marra CM: Acquired syphilis in adults. N Engl J Med 326:1060–1068, 1992.

cific treponemal antibody tests are highly sensitive and specific, although false-positive results may occur in about 1% of the population in association with certain conditions, such as systemic lupus erythematosus (see Table 1).[7]

Diagnosis of Neurosyphilis

The diagnosis of neurosyphilis often poses a challenge, since there is no one test that is both sensitive and specific. The diagnosis is usually made based on a combination of reactive serologies, abnormalities of

CSF cell count and protein, or a reactive VDRL-CSF.[12] The VDRL-CSF is the standard serologic test for CSF and is diagnostic of neurosyphilis when reactive (except in cases of gross contamination of CSF with blood). However, it is an insensitive test, so a negative result does not rule out the diagnosis. An FTA-ABS test on CSF appears to be more sensitive than the VDRL but may lead to more false-positive results and currently still has investigational status. The high sensitivity of the FTA-ABS CSF test may make it most useful in ruling out the diagnosis of neurosyphilis.[7]

Typical abnormalities in the CSF profile in the setting of neurosyphilis include a mild mononuclear pleocytosis or an elevated protein level, or both, and these findings should be considered indicative of neurosyphilis in a patient with reactive serologic tests with or without clinical evidence of neurosyphilis.

Indications for Cerebrospinal Fluid Evaluation in Syphilis

Primary and Secondary Syphilis

• Neurologic or ophthalmic signs or symptoms
• Treatment failure

Although patients with primary and secondary syphilis often have early CNS invasion by spirochetes, the majority of these patients do not go on to develop clinical neurosyphilis when given the standard treatment regimens used for primary and secondary syphilis. Therefore, a CSF evaluation is not recommended in patients with primary and secondary syphilis in the absence of clinical manifestations of neurosyphilis.[12]

Latent Syphilis

• Neurologic or ophthalmic signs or symptoms
• Evidence of active tertiary syphilis (e.g., aortitis, gumma, iritis)
• Treatment failure
• HIV infection with late latent syphilis or syphilis of unknown duration

A common problem in the primary care setting is the elderly patient with some cognitive deficits who is found to have a reactive serologic test for syphilis with an unknown or remote history of treatment. While strict adherence to sexually transmitted disease treatment guidelines would dictate a CSF evaluation in these cases, the likelihood of having treatable disease in this population is small, and there are no recent data in favor or against this practice.[14]

Treatment

Penicillin G, administered parenterally, is the preferred treatment for all stages of syphilis in nonallergic patients (Table 2). The preparation, dose, and duration of treatment depend on the clinical stage of syphilis being treated.[12]

All patients with syphilis should be tested for HIV infection, and patients with primary syphilis should be retested for HIV after 3 months if the first test is negative.

TABLE 2. Recommended Treatment of Syphilis in Adults	
Type of Disease	**Treatment Regimen**
Primary, secondary, and early latent syphilis	Benzathine penicillin G, 2.4 million units intramuscularly in a single dose For patients allergic to penicillin: doxycycline, 100 mg orally bid or tetracycline, 500 mg orally qid for 14 days*
Late latent syphilis or syphilis of unknown duration	Benzathine penicillin G, 7.2 million units total, administered intramuscularly as 2.4 million units per week for 3 weeks For patients allergic to penicillin: doxycycline, 100 mg orally bid or tetracycline, 500 mg orally qid for 28 days*
Late syphilis	
Gummatous or cardiovascular	As for late latent disease, with appropriate management of complications
Neurosyphilis or ocular syphilis	Aqueous crystalline penicillin G, 18–24 million units per day intravenously (3–4 million units every 4 hours or continous infusion) for 10–14 days, or procaine penicillin G, 2.4 million units intramuscularly once daily plus probenecid, 500 mg orally qid for 10–14 days For patients allergic to penicillin: ceftriaxone 2 g daily, intravenously or intramuscularly, for 10–14 days†
Exposure	
Sexual contact of persons with infectious syphilis	As for early disease

*Data to support the use of alternatives to penicillin are limited and should be used only in conjunction with close serologic and clinical follow-up. The use of these alternative regimens in HIV-infected patients has not been studied and should be undertaken with caution. Alternative regimens to penicillin cannot be used in pregnant patients. Pregnant patients who are allergic to penicillin should be desensitized and treated with penicillin.

†Cross-reactivity may occur between ceftriaxone and penicillin. Patients with serious penicillin allergies (i.e., urticaria, angioedema, or anaphylaxis) should be densensitized and treated with penicillin.

Primary and Secondary Syphilis

Treatment. Benzathine penicillin G, 2.4 million units intramuscularly in a single dose, is recommended for both primary and secondary syphilis in adults.

Penicillin Allergy. For nonpregnant penicillin-allergic patients, either doxycycline (100 mg orally twice daily) or tetracycline (500 mg four times daily) for 14 days is considered an acceptable alternative. There are some data to support the use of azithromycin, as a single 1 or 2 g dose, as an acceptable alternative therapy for primary and secondary syphilis.[14]

Assessing Response to Therapy. Following treatment, patients should be reevaluated clinically and serologically at 6 months and 12 months. Nontreponemal test titers should decline fourfold (two dilutions) at 1 year following treatment. Treatment failure is probable if nontreponemal titers do not decline fourfold by 6 months. These patients should be retested for HIV infection. Some specialists recommend CSF examination in the case of an inadequate serologic response, as treatment failure may be a result of unrecognized CNS infection. The recommended retreatment regimen is benzathine penicillin G 2.4 million units by weekly intramuscular injections for 3 weeks, unless neurosyphilis is present.

Latent Syphilis

Treatment. For early latent syphilis (patients who acquired syphilis within the preceding year), benzathine penicillin G 2.4 million units IM in a single dose is recommended. Patients who have latent syphilis of unknown duration should be treated as having late latent syphilis. Treatment for late latent syphilis is benzathine penicillin G 7.2 million units total, given intramuscularly as three doses of 2.4 million units each at 1-week intervals.

Penicillin Allergy. In cases of penicillin allergy, nonpregnant patients with early latent syphilis can be treated with the same alternative regimens as those with primary and secondary syphilis. In cases of late latent syphilis or latent syphilis of unknown duration, acceptable regimens include doxycycline (100 mg orally twice daily) or tetracycline (500 mg orally four times daily) for 28 days. However, outcomes using these regimens have not been well documented, requiring close clinical and serologic follow-up.

Assessing Response to Therapy. Quantitative nontreponemal serologic tests should be repeated at 6, 12, and 24 months following treatment of latent syphilis. Retreatment for latent syphilis (with normal CSF examination) is indicated if (1) titers increase fourfold, (2) an initial high titer ($\geq$1:32) does not decline fourfold within 12 to 24 months of therapy, or (3) signs or symptoms of active syphilis develop.

Late (Tertiary) Syphilis

Treatment. Data regarding the clinical response of patients with late syphilis are lacking, and these patients should be managed in consultation with an infectious diseases specialist. Those with gummatous or cardiovascular syphilis with no evidence of neurosyphilis (CSF should be examined) can be treated with benzathine penicillin G 7.2 million units total, given intramuscularly as three doses of 2.4 million units each at 1-week intervals (same regimen as for late latent syphilis). However, some clinicians would treat patients with cardiovascular syphilis with a regimen for neurosyphilis.

Penicillin Allergy. Patients who are penicillin-allergic can be treated with the same regimens recommended for late latent syphilis.

Assessing Response to Therapy. There are no clear data concerning response to therapy and follow-up for cardiovascular and gummatous syphilis.

Neurosyphilis

Treatment. The main goal in treatment of symptomatic late neurosyphilis is to halt progression of the disease, since much of the damage to the CNS is irreversible.[3] Patients who have neurosyphilis or ocular syphilis should be treated with aqueous crystalline penicillin G, 18 to 24 million units per day, given as 3 to 4 million units intravenously every 4 hours or continuous infusion, for 10 to 14 days. An alternative regimen that requires strict assurance of compliance is procaine penicillin G, 2.4 million units IM once daily *plus* probenecid 500 mg orally four times daily, both for 10 to 14 days. Since the duration of therapy for neurosyphilis is shorter than the 3-week course recommended for latent syphilis, which theoretically may coexist, many specialists recommend an additional intramuscular dose of benzathine penicillin, 2.4 million units, after completion of the 2-week therapy for neurosyphilis to achieve at least 3 weeks of serum penicillin levels.[14]

Syphilitic otitis should be treated the same way as neurosyphilis, regardless of CSF results. Adjunctive systemic steroids are often used in this setting, but the benefit of such therapy has not been proven.

Penicillin Allergy. Ceftriaxone, 2 g IM or IV daily for 10 to 14 days, is an alternative regimen for patients with a penicillin allergy, although there is potential for cross-reactivity. No other regimen has been adequately evaluated for treatment of neurosyphilis. Therefore, if ceftriaxone is not considered a safe alternative, the patient should undergo skin testing to confirm the penicillin allergy and be desensitized if necessary.

Assessing Response to Therapy. Patients with elevated cell counts in the CSF prior to treatment should have repeated lumbar punctures every 6 months until the pleocytosis resolves. Changes in the VDRL-CSF and protein counts may take longer to occur, and persistent elevations may not be significant. As a general guideline, the cell count should decrease after 6 months and the CSF should normalize after 2 years; otherwise, retreatment should be considered.

Jarisch-Herxheimer Reaction

Following treatment of syphilis, the rapid death and release of lipopolysaccharide from circulating spirochetes may result in the Jarisch-Herxheimer reaction, an acute systemic reaction characterized by fever, chills, myalgias, headache, tachycardia, flushing, and mild hypotension. It typically occurs 1 to 2 hours following treatment and resolves within 24 to 48 hours.[6] The reaction is most likely to occur during treatment of secondary syphilis when spirochetemia is highest. Treatment with antipyretics or prednisone may ameliorate symptoms.[6]

Syphilis in HIV-Infected Patients

Syphilis and HIV are often found in association with one another, suggesting that syphilitic genital ulcers increase the risk of HIV transmission.[3] In addition, HIV-infected patients with syphilis seem to be at greater risk for florid clinical syphilis and may be more prone to treatment failure and development of neurologic complications than HIV-negative patients.[15,16] Recent studies in HIV-positive patients with syphilis have demonstrated no treatment failures, however, despite slower serologic responses with standard therapy.[14] Both nontreponemal and treponemal serologic tests for syphilis are generally reliable in most patients with HIV and can be used and interpreted in the usual way.[3]

The recommended treatment regimens for HIV-infected patients do not differ from those recommended for HIV-negative patients, although some experts advocate more vigorous and prolonged treatment in the setting of HIV coinfection to prevent neurologic complications.[1] In either case, more frequent follow-up to ensure treatment response is recommended. All patients with either late latent syphilis or syphilis of unknown duration should have a CSF examination before treatment.[12]

The efficacy of nonpenicillin regimens in HIV-infected patients has not been well studied, so penicillin is recommended for use whenever possible.[12]

Syphilis During Pregnancy

Prevention and detection of congenital syphilis depends on serologic screening of the mother during pregnancy. Women should be screened for syphilis with serologic testing at the first prenatal visit. Women at high risk for syphilis should be screened at 28 weeks' gestation and at delivery, in addition to the routine early testing.[12] Screening at delivery is also mandated in some states. In addition, a woman who delivers a stillborn infant after 20 weeks' gestation should be screened for syphilis. All pregnant women with syphilis should also be tested for HIV.[12]

Treatment during pregnancy with penicillin is effective in preventing maternal-fetal transmission and in treating an infected fetus. Pregnant women should receive the same penicillin regimens as nonpregnant patients, appropriate for the stage of syphilis, and the same serologic follow-up testing. No alternatives to penicillin have proven efficacy for syphilis in pregnancy. Erythromycin does not reliably cure syphilis in the fetus, and there are insufficient data for the use of ceftriaxone and azithromycin.[17] Tetracycline and doxycycline should not be used in pregnancy. Therefore, all pregnant patients with syphilis who have a history of a penicillin allergy should be desensitized and treated with penicillin, with or without the use of skin testing.[12]

The Jarisch-Herxheimer reaction develops in up to 45% of pregnant women treated with penicillin and may precipitate uterine contractions, preterm labor, and fetal heart-rate decelerations during the second half of pregnancy.[18] Routine hospitalization for fetal monitoring after treatment is not currently recommended, however, unless the fetus has evidence of fetal syphilis on ultrasonogram.[17] Women being treated in early pregnancy should be counseled to stay well hydrated and to take acetaminophen for uterine cramping, pain, or fever, whereas those at greater than 20 weeks' gestation should seek obstetric evaluation for fever, decreased fetal movement, or symptoms of labor.[17] Treatment is largely supportive and may require continuous fetal heart rate monitoring. There is not enough evidence to recommend prophylactic therapy to prevent this reaction.[17]

References

1. Tramont EC: Syphilis in adults: From Christopher Columbus to Sir Alexander Fleming to AIDS. Clin Infect Dis 21:1361–1371, 1995.
2. Singh AE, Romanowski B: Syphilis: Review and emphasis on clinical, epidemiologic, and some biologic features. Clin Microbiol Rev 12:187–209, 1999.
3. Hook EW, Marra CM: Acquired syphilis in adults. N Engl J Med 326:1060–1068, 1992.
4. Centers for Disease Control and Prevention: Primary and secondary syphilis— United States, 1999. MMWR Morbid Mortal Wkly Rep 50:113–117, 2001.

5. Birnbaum NR, Goldschmidt RH, Buffett WO: Resolving the common clinical dilemmas of syphilis. Am Fam Phys 59:2233–2240, 1999.
6. Tramont EC. *Treponema pallidum* (syphilis). In Mandell GL, Bennett JE, Dolin R, eds: Mandell, Douglas, and Bennett's Principles and Practice of Infectious Diseases, 5th ed. Philadelphia: Churchill Livingstone, 2000:2474–2489.
7. Larsen SA, Steiner BM, Rudolph AH: Laboratory diagnosis and interpretation of tests for syphilis. Clin Microbiol Rev 8:1–21, 1995.
8. Hutchinson CM, Hook EW, Shepherd M, et al: Altered clinical presentation of early syphilis in patients with human immunodeficiency virus infection. Ann Intern Med 121:94–99, 1994.
9. Clark EG, Danbolt N: The Oslo study of the natural course of untreated syphilis: An epidemiologic investigation based on a re-study of the Boeck-Bruusgaard material. Med Clin North Am 48:613–623, 1964.
10. Lukehart S, Hook E, Baker-Zander S, et al: Invasion of the central nervous system by *Treponema pallidum:* Implications for diagnosis and treatment. Ann Intern Med 109: 855–862, 1988.
11. Ross WH, Sutton HF: Acquired syphilitic uveitis. Arch Ophthalmol 98:496, 1980.
12. Centers for Disease Control and Prevention: Sexually transmitted diseases treatment guidelines 2002. MMWR Morbid Mortal Wkly Rep 51(RR-6):1, 2002.
13. Sparling PF, Hicks CB: Late syphilis. In UpToDate 2002. *www.uptodateonline.com* Accessed Dec. 2, 2002.
14. Augenbraun MH: Treatment of syphilis 2001: Nonpregnant adults. Clin Infect Dis 35(Suppl 2):S187–90, 2002.
15. Musher DM, Hamill RJ, Baughn RE: Effect of human immunodeficiency virus (HIV) infection on the course of syphilis and on the response to treatment. Ann Intern Med 113:872–881, 1990.
16. Gordon SM, Eaton ME, George R, et al: The response of symptomatic neurosyphilis to high-dose intravenous penicillin G in patients with human immunodeficiency virus infection. N Engl J Med 331:1469–1473, 1994.
17. Wendel GD Jr, Sheffield JS, Hollier LM, et al: Treatment of syphilis in pregnancy and prevention of congenital syphilis. Clin Infect Dis 35(Suppl 2):S200–209, 2002.
18. Klein VR, Cox SM, Mitchell MD, Wendel GD Jr: The Jarisch-Herxheimer reaction complicating syphilotherapy in pregnancy. Obstet Gynecol 75:375–380, 1990.

Approach to the Patient with Fever and Rash

*Vincent Lo Re III, M.D., and
Stephen J. Gluckman, M.D., FACP*

The evaluation of the patient who presents with fever and a rash is a challenging task for clinicians and remains one of the "hot topics" of internal medicine. The differential diagnosis of this syndrome is extensive and encompasses illnesses that range from trivial to life-threatening. Since a variety of infectious and noninfectious disease processes can manifest in this fashion, an organized approach to the diagnosis is necessary. A thorough history, particularly reviewing exposures as well as associated symptoms, can provide the initial clues to uncovering the diagnosis. The evolution and appearance of the rash are equally critical and can help further narrow the list of possible causes. Based on the history and physical examination, the clinician must decide whether hospitalization, isolation, or empiric antimicrobial therapy is warranted.

This chapter provides an organized approach to the patient with fever and rash. Essential questions that should be asked during the medical history are reviewed. Recognition of the key clinical features of a rash during physical examination is emphasized. Eruptions are characterized based on their clinical appearance, and a number of important infectious and noninfectious causes of fever and rash are reviewed to further assist the clinical diagnosis.

Patient History

The details of the medical history can provide the first clues to identifying the cause of fever and a rash. In particular, questions should focus on the following factors.

Drug Use. Prescription and nonprescription drugs are common causes of hypersensitivity reactions that manifest as fever and a rash, and those used within the past 30 days should be identified. Frequently implicated prescription medications include penicillins, sulfonamides, phenytoin, barbiturates, procainamide, quinidine, and allopurinol.[1] In addition, over-the-counter and alternative or complementary medications should also be determined, since these, too, may be involved. Illicit drug use, especially injection drug use, can expose individuals to a variety of bacterial and viral pathogens.[1] Injection drug use predisposes to cellulitis and infectious endocarditis and allows the transmission of hepatitis B, hepatitis C, and human immunodeficiency virus (HIV). Clinicians should also be alert for the possibility of necrotizing fasciitis in injection drug users.[2]

Diet. Food allergies may also cause hypersensitivity reactions, resulting in fever and a rash. Eggs, nuts, chocolates, and shellfish have been identified as common precipitants.[1] Exposure to undercooked or possibly contaminated foods can predispose unwary eaters to a number of infectious diseases that have cutaneous manifestations. For example, ingestion of raw seafood has been associated with *Vibrio vulnificus* infection, which can produce a severe hemorrhagic bullous eruption. Inadvertent consumption of fecally contaminated food or drink can expose a person to typhoid fever, which is associated with crops of small trunkal macules called *rose spots.*

Time of Year. The time of year in which the illness appears may be of importance, since a number of infections characterized by fever and rash have a distinct seasonal predisposition.

Ill Contacts. Exposure to sick persons within the recent past can result in the transmission of many infectious diseases that can cause cutaneous eruptions. Viral illnesses in particular can be acquired in this manner, and sexually transmitted diseases should also be considered.

Occupational Exposures. Although often overlooked, the occupation of an individual may be useful in determining the cause of fever and a rash. For example, florists and gardeners have a higher rate of exposure to the fungal pathogen *Sporothrix* because of their contact with spiny plants (especially roses) and soil.

Animal Exposures. A number of viral and bacterial pathogens are carried by vectors such as ticks, mosquitoes, mites, or lice. Exposure to any of these insects may provide a useful clue to the diagnosis. Exposure to domestic and wild animals can also predispose to various infections with cutaneous manifestations, and the degree of contact should be ascertained.

Travel. Travel to certain geographic regions in the United States or other parts of the world may expose individuals to infections that are uncommon in their home areas, and these can have various skin manifestations.[3] The epidemiology of diseases endemic in all travel destinations should be determined (see Chapters 28 and 29), and activities and exposures during travel should be assessed.

Sexual History. Sexual contact allows the transmission of several diseases with cutaneous manifestations, such as gonorrhea, syphilis, hepatitis B, and HIV. A sexual history should be taken, and it should include the number of partners, types of sexual activities, and protection used.

Past Medical History. Previous illnesses, including all prior medication allergies, can occasionally point toward the clinical diagnosis. The immunization history should also be sought, since inadequately immunized individuals may be more susceptible to infections. The presence of valvular heart disease should be determined, since this increases the risk of infective endocarditis. Patients with a prior history of a rheumatologic illness or inflammatory bowel disease may develop fever and skin manifestations associated with those underlying conditions.

Immune Status. The immune status of the host should also be assessed, since cutaneous eruptions occur frequently in immunosuppressed individuals. The use of corticosteroids, immunosuppressants, or chemotherapeutic agents and the possibility of immunosuppression from asplenia, malignancy, or HIV should be considered. Fever and rash can be quite prominent in patients with neutropenia and those with HIV infection.[1,4,5] Neutropenia predisposes to many bacterial (*Pseudomonas,* staphylococci, streptococci), viral (herpesviruses), and disseminated fungal infections (particularly *Candida* and *Aspergillus*). HIV is associated with numerous cutaneous diseases. Primary infection with HIV itself may cause a trunkal or facial rash approximately 2 to 6 weeks after acute HIV infection.[6,7] A number of other systemic bacterial, viral, and fungal infections with various cutaneous manifestations may occur with greater regularity in patients with chronic HIV infection and low CD4 counts.

Characteristics of the Rash. Clinicians should elicit specific details about the rash, including the site where it began, rate and direction of spread, its association with pruritus, and the timing of the onset of the rash in relation to the onset of fever.[1,4] Rashes that begin on the face or trunk and spread outward are termed *centrifugal,* whereas those that begin on the extremities and spread inward are termed *centripetal.*

Associated Symptoms. Clinicians should question the patient thoroughly about all associated symptoms and note the exact onset and progression of all complaints.

General Physical Examination

The recognition of associated physical findings can assist the clinician in determining the origin of a patient's rash. The general physical examination should focus on the following:

- **General appearance**—The physician should rapidly determine whether the patient with fever and a rash appears toxemic.

- **Vital signs**—Measurements of blood pressure, heart rate, and oxygen saturation will help further assess the level of toxicity present.
- **Eyes**—Diligent examination of the conjunctivae should be performed. Conjunctival petechiae may be found in cases of infective endocarditis. Conjunctivitis may be present in cases of leptospirosis and severe drug hypersensitivity reactions (Stevens-Johnson syndrome and toxic epidermal necrolysis). Fundoscopic examination may reveal Roth spots associated with endocarditis.
- **Mouth**—Many diseases that cause fever and a rash also involve the mucous membranes, particularly the mouth, and these are called *enanthems*. The presence of an enanthem can help narrow the differential diagnosis even further. Examples of enanthems include the following:
  Koplik's spots: Present in measles (rubeola) infections, Koplik's spots are fine blue-gray papules on an erythematous base found on the buccal mucosa opposite the second-molar teeth.
  Forscheimer spots: These are punctate soft palate macules that may be found in rubella infections.
  "Strawberry tongue": An intensely erythematous tongue with prominent papillations, the "strawberry tongue" suggest the possibility of scarlet fever, Kawasaki's disease, or streptococcal toxic shock syndrome.
  Palatal petechiae: Petechiae can be identified on both the hard and soft palate in up to 50% of patients with infectious mononucleosis.[1] Palatal petechiae may also be found with infective endocarditis and thrombocytopenia. Palatal petechiae may also be found with infective endocarditis as well as a wide variety of diseases associated with thrombocytopenia, including meningococcemia.
  Oral ulcers: These can be found in a variety of diseases such as hand-foot-and-mouth disease (due to coxsackievirus A16), inflammatory bowel disease, Behçet's disease, and severe drug hypersensitivity reactions (Stevens-Johnson syndrome or toxic epidermal necrolysis).
- **Lymph nodes**—Generalized lymphadenopathy should prompt consideration of secondary syphilis, sarcoidosis, and drug hypersensitivity reactions (particularly with phenytoin).
- **Lungs**—Pulmonary findings consistent with pneumonia in the presence of a fever and a rash should suggest infections such as Rocky Mountain spotted fever, *Mycoplasma* infection, severe bacteremia, or measles.
- **Heart**—A heart murmur in the presence of suggestive skin findings should prompt consideration of infective endocarditis and acute rheumatic fever.

- **Liver/spleen**—Hepatosplenomegaly may be found in cases of infective endocarditis, miliary tuberculosis, infectious mononucleosis, and disseminated histoplasmosis as well as in association with many hematologic malignancies.
- **Joints**—Any joint complaint should prompt the clinician to evaluate for the presence of warmth, tenderness, and effusions and assess complete range of motion.
- **Genitals**—The genital examination is often overlooked in patients with fever and a rash. The presence of genital ulcers or a penile or vaginal discharge might suggest a sexually transmitted disease as the cause of the fever and rash.
- **Central and peripheral nervous system**—A neurologic examination should be performed to determine global function. The presence of nuchal rigidity should also be assessed. Neurologic abnormalities can be found in meningococcemia, Rocky Mountain spotted fever, staphylococcal or streptococcal toxic shock syndromes, leptospirosis, acute HIV infection, and enteroviral infections.

Clinical Appearance of the Rash

The appearance and distribution of a rash frequently provides valuable information toward the diagnosis. The examination of any cutaneous eruption should be performed while wearing gloves, since some infections (notably syphilis, herpes simplex virus, and varicella-zoster virus) may be transmitted by direct skin contact.[4] The clinician should assess the overall distribution of the rash and note the types of primary lesions present. A list of dermatologic terms used to describe cutaneous lesions, as well as their definitions, is provided in Table 1.

Rashes can generally be divided into five groups: (1) maculopapular, (2) diffuse erythema, (3) vesiculobullous-pustular, (4) petechial, and (5)

TABLE 1.	Definitions of Dermatologic Terms Used To Describe Lesions and Rashes
Term	**Definition**
Macule	A circumscribed, nonpalpable area of perceptible change in normal skin color.
Papule	A circumscribed, solid, palpable lesion that is elevated above the skin surface and measures ≤1 cm in diameter.
Nodule	A palpable, deep-seated, rounded lesion <1.5 cm in diameter, usually involving the epidermal, dermal, and/or subcutaneous tissues.
Vesicle	A circumscribed, elevated, fluid-filled lesion measuring ≤1 cm in diameter.
Bulla	An elevated, fluid-filled lesion that measures >1 cm in diameter.
Pustule	A circumscribed, elevated lesion filled with purulent fluid.
Petechia	A nonblanching lesion caused by hemorrhage into the skin.
Ecchymosis	A nonblanching lesion caused by extensive hemorrhage into the skin.

nodular. This classification system can help narrow the list of diagnostic possibilities. However, it should be noted that many rashes have overlying features, and a number of infectious and noninfectious diseases can produce more than one type of rash.[1,4] Thus, determining the diagnosis of a rash based on morphology alone is a daunting challenge. To assist in this process, an algorithmic approach to determining the primary lesion of any rash is presented in Figure 1. Once the primary lesion is identified, the clinician can then consider a narrower list of dis-

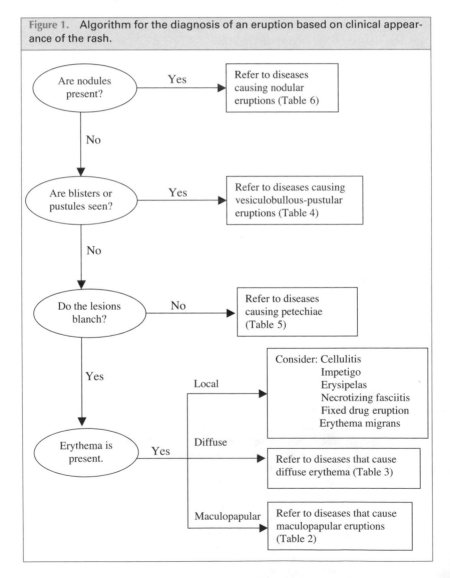

Figure 1. Algorithm for the diagnosis of an eruption based on clinical appearance of the rash.

eases. The important causes of rash and fever are listed by group in Tables 2 through 6, and selected diseases are also described in the following sections.

Maculopapular Rashes

Maculopapular rashes (Table 2) are the most common eruptions and are typically seen in patients with viral illnesses, most rickettsial illnesses, drug eruptions, and immune complex-mediated syndromes.[4,5] It

TABLE 2. Diseases Causing a Maculopapular Eruption		
Bacterial	**Viral**	**Noninfectious**
Centrally Distributed Eruptions		
Lyme disease (*Borrelia burgdorferi*)	Measles (rubeola)	Drug hypersensitivity
Typhoid fever (*Salmonella typhi*)	Rubella	Systemic lupus erythematosus
Acute rheumatic fever (group A streptococci)	Erythema infectiosum (parvovirus B19)	
Epidemic typhus (*Rickettsia prowazekii*)	Enteroviruses (coxsackievirus, echovirus)	
Endemic typhus (*Rickettsia typhi*)	Mononucleosis (Epstein-Barr virus) with ampicillin or amoxicillin	
Scrub typhus (*Rickettsia tsutsugamushi*)	Adenovirus	
Ehrlichiosis (*Ehrlichia* species)	Acute human immunodeficiency virus	
Bartonellosis (*Bartonella henselae, Bartonella quintana*)	Exanthem subitum (roseola, human herpesvirus 6)	
Leptospirosis (*Leptospira interrogans*)		
Peripherally Distributed Eruptions		
Secondary syphilis (*Treponema pallidum*)	Dengue fever	Drug hypersensitivity
Meningococcemia (*Neisseria meningitidis*)	Atypical measles (rubeola)	Pityriasis rubra pilaris
Rocky Mountain spotted fever (*Rickettsia rickettsii*)	Hand-foot-and-mouth disease (coxsackievirus A16)	Erythema multiforme*
Subacute bacterial endocarditis		
Bartonellosis (*Bartonella henselae, Bartonella quintana*)		
Disseminated gonococcal infection		

*Erythema multiforme may have underlying infectious causes.

TABLE 3. Disorders Causing Diffuse Erythema		
Bacterial	**Viral**	**Noninfectious**
Scarlet fever (group A streptococci)	Enteroviruses	Stevens-Johnson syndrome
Staphylococcal toxic shock syndrome		(drug hypersensitivity)
Streptococcal toxic shock syndrome		Toxic epidermal necrolysis
Staphylococcal scalded skin syndrome		(drug hypersensitivity)
		Kawasaki disease
		Exfoliative erythroderma
		Psoriasis
		Graft-versus-host disease
		Sézary syndrome

is useful to additionally categorize maculopapular eruptions as centrally (first appearing on the head or trunk) or peripherally distributed, since this can narrow the differential diagnosis further.[5,8]

Centrally Distributed Maculopapular Rashes

Measles (Rubeola). After approximately 4 days of fever and malaise, discrete maculopapular lesions appear on the face and spread downward, becoming confluent.[9] The rash last for 4 to 6 days, and the lesions gradually fade, leaving faint desquamation of the involved areas. Koplik's spots may also be identified in the mouth.

Rubella. This illness manifests likes measles, but its rash is quite pruritic and usually lasts for 2 to 3 days.[9] Forscheimer spots may be present on the soft palate.

Erythema Infectiosum. Caused by parvovirus B19, erythema infectiosum (also known as *fifth disease*) usually occurs in children, who present with fever, sore throat, and anorexia.[10] The fever then resolves, and a bright red facial rash ("slapped cheek") develops.[11] Several days

TABLE 4. Diseases Causing a Vesiculobullous-Pustular Eruption		
Bacterial	**Viral**	**Noninfectious**
Staphylococcal bacteremia	Varicella (chickenpox)	Stevens-Johnson syndrome
Disseminated gonococcal	Herpes zoster	(drug hypersensitivity)
bacteremia (*Neisseria*	Disseminated varicella	Toxic epidermal necrolysis
gonorhoeae)	Disseminated herpes	(drug hypersensitivity)
Rickettsial pox (*Rickettsia akari*)	zoster	Pemphigus vulgaris
Ecthyma gangrenosum		Bullous pemphigoid
(*Pseudomonas aeruginosa*)		
Vibrio vulnificus		
Necrotizing fasciitis		

TABLE 5.   Diseases Causing a Petechial Eruption

Bacterial	Viral	Noninfectious
Meningococcemia (*Neisseria meningitidis*) Rocky Mountain spotted fever (*Rickettsia rickettsii*) Bacteremia with/without disseminated intravascular coagulation Epidemic typhus (*Rickettsia prowazekii*) Subacute bacterial endocarditis	Enteroviruses (coxsackievirus A9, echovirus A9) Hepatitis B Dengue virus Viral hemorrhagic fevers Atypical measles (rubeola) Rubella	Thrombocytopeni Drug hypersensitivity Vasculitis Cryoglobulinemia Henoch-Schönlein purpura Systemic lupus erythematosus Thrombotic thrombocytopenic purpura

afterward, the rash progresses to a diffuse maculopapular eruption that may last for up to 8 weeks.

Erythema Migrans. The pathognomonic rash of Lyme disease, erythema migrans, consists of an enlarging, erythematous macule with central clearing, necrosis, or induration.[12] Smaller secondary lesions may develop and indicate early dissemination of the spirochete.

Drug Hypersensitivity. Allergic reactions to medications can manifest as any type of rash, but they most commonly occur as maculopapular eruptions.[13] The rash usually appears within the first week of drug use, but one may be at risk for up to 2 weeks after the medication is discontinued.

Peripherally Distributed Maculopapular Rashes

Erythema Multiforme Minor. The characteristic lesions of erythema multiforme minor are round macules or papules with a central area of erythema surrounded by a ring of normal-appearing skin and another

TABLE 6.   Diseases Causing Nodular Eruptions

Bacterial	Fungal	Noninfectious
Erythema induratum (mycobacteria) Pseudomonal bacteremia *Nocardia* species Bartonellosis (*Bartonella henselae, Bartonella bacilliformis, Bartonella quintana*)	Disseminated candidiasis Disseminated cryptococcosis Disseminated blastomycosis Disseminated histoplasmosis Disseminated coccidioidomycosis Disseminated sporotrichosis	Erythema nodosum Sweet's syndrome

ring of erythema ("target lesions").[4,5,14] They are usually distributed on the extensor surfaces of the extremities and, occasionally, on the trunk.[4,5,14] A number of conditions predisposes to erythema multiforme, but herpes simplex virus infection is a common precipitant.[4,5,14]

Secondary Syphilis. The lesions of secondary syphilis are commonly reddish-brown, scaly macules (occasionally papular or pustular) that are distributed diffusely and often include the palms and soles.[15] Ulcers and erosions can occur in the mouth or throat. The eruption may occur up to 10 weeks after the appearance of a chancre, but in some instances, the patient recalls no chancre. The lesions are highly infectious and can be acquired by contact. The rash of secondary syphilis may be accompanied by condyloma lata, which are pearly, papular lesions that arise in moist areas of the body, such as the anus, vulva, or scrotum.[15]

Diffuse Erythema

Scarlet Fever. This syndrome, typically caused by group A streptococci, produces a diffuse erythematous eruption, pharyngitis, and a strawberry tongue (Table 3). Petechiae may be identified in the skin folds of the antecubital areas and axillae ("Pastia's lines").[14]

Toxic Shock Syndromes. These may be caused by either staphylococci or group A streptococci and are usually characterized by fever, hypotension, diffuse erythema, and multiorgan system failure.[16] A staphylococcal infection is not required to produce toxic shock syndrome, and colonization by the bacteria in a wound or other areas of the body is sufficient.

Staphylococcal Scalded Skin Syndrome. This syndrome, caused by staphylococcal toxins (epidermolysins), usually occurs in infants and young children but may affect adults with immunosuppression, lymphoma, or renal failure.[4,5] The syndrome results in a diffusely tender erythroderma. Nikolsky's sign (shearing of the overlying skin with lateral pressure), though not specific for this condition, may be present.

Erythema Multiforme Major. Erythema multiforme major encompasses both Stevens-Johnson syndrome and toxic epidermal necrolysis. Both entities are associated with a prodrome of fever, malaise, and pharyngitis. Stevens-Johnson syndrome is characterized by the presence of mucosal ulcerations and generalized bullous lesions on or near large erythematous macules or plaques.[13] Toxic epidermal necrolysis is the most severe disorder of this entity. Generalized erythema, often with large bullae, may be seen on the trunk and proximal limbs. Epidermal detachment is common and often involves 30% or more of the body surface area.[13]

Vesiculobullous-Pustular Rashes

Varicella. After a mild prodrome of fever and malaise lasting 1 to 2 days, the rash of varicella (chickenpox), which is due to infection with varicella-zoster virus, begins on the face, scalp, or trunk and spreads to the extremities (Table 4).[5,14] The lesions first appear as erythematous macules, then evolve to form papules and umbilicated vesicles, and progress to pustules that ultimately crust over. The lesions are more prominent on the trunk than the extremities, and all stages of lesions may be present simultaneously. The cutaneous lesions of chickenpox can be difficult to distinguish from those of smallpox. One good clue is that in chickenpox, one can find lesions in all stages of development, while in smallpox, the lesions are all in the same stage.

Herpes Zoster. After primary varicella infection, varicella-zoster virus lies dormant in dorsal root ganglia but can reactivate at a later time. A prodrome of intense pain or numbness often precedes the rash by 2 to 3 days.[5] The characteristic vesicular eruption of herpes zoster usually affects a single dermatome, but in instances of immunosuppression, disseminated infection may develop.

Disseminated Gonococcal Infection. The characteristic rash of this infection is manifested by the presence of approximately 5 to 40 papules to pustules, which are often hemorrhagic in appearance.[17] Patients usually report arthralgias of the knees, ankles, elbows, or wrists, and physical examination may identify septic arthritis, tenosynovitis, or an overt genital infection.

Petechial Rashes

A petechial eruption often signals a life-threatening disease process (Table 5). When this is identified, the confirmation or elimination of one of the following disease processes is critical.

Meningococcemia. After a short prodrome of cough, headaches, sore throat, and nausea, infection due to *Neisseria meningitidis* causes a high fever and a petechial eruption, although the rash may occasionally be maculopapular in the early stages of the disease.[18] The petechial lesions often coalesce to form large areas of ecchymoses. Signs of meningeal irritation, including nuchal rigidity and confusion, may accompany the rash. The diagnosis is mainly confirmed by culture of the organism from the blood or cerebrospinal fluid. Patients with suspected meningococcemia must be isolated (droplet precautions), and empiric antibiotic therapy should be initiated. Consultation with an infectious diseases physician is recommended. The course of this disease is fulminant and can rapidly lead to death.

Rocky Mountain Spotted Fever. Infection with *Rickettsia rickettsii,* which is acquired by a tick bite, may also be life-threatening and have an equally fulminant course. The onset of symptoms is abrupt, and the key clinical features include fever, severe headaches, generalized myalgias, and photophobia. The rash usually begins as a pink macular eruption on the wrists, forearms, ankles, palms, and soles.[19] It spreads centripetally to the proximal extremities, trunk, and face. The lesions become petechial within 2 to 4 days of rash onset.[19] The diagnosis can be confirmed by serology or direct immunofluorescent examination of a skin biopsy sample for *R. rickettsii,* if available. Antimicrobial therapy, typically with doxycycline, should be initiated for suspected cases of Rocky Mountain spotted fever, and consultation with an infectious diseases physician is recommended. Isolation is unnecessary, since person-to-person transmission does not occur with this disease. About 10% of people with Rocky Mountain spotted fever do not have a rash.

Infective Endocarditis. A number of skin lesions are associated with bacterial endocarditis.[20] Petechiae may be found on the skin, conjunctivae, under the fingernail ("splinter hemorrhages"), and on the palate. Other cutaneous findings include Janeway lesions, which are erythematous macular lesions on the palms and soles, and Osler's nodes, painful papules on the finger and toe pads. Additional findings include a heart murmur and Roth spots, which are hemorrhagic lesions on the retina. Recognition of the manifestations of endocarditis should prompt the clinician to obtain three sets of blood cultures and consider empiric antimicrobial therapy.

Bacteremia. Severe bacteremia, often with shock and disseminated intravascular coagulation, can also cause petechiae, ecchymoses, and even peripheral gangrene.[4] Clinicians should obtain blood cultures and begin treatment with broad-spectrum antibiotics. The empiric antibiotic regimen may be narrowed once blood culture results become known.

Nodular Rashes

Erythema Nodosum. Erythema nodosum manifests as painful, erythematous nodules on the extensor surfaces of the lower extremities (Table 6). Both infectious and noninfectious causes are associated with this finding.[5] Histologic examination of these nodules reveals a septal panniculitis.

Disseminated Fungal Infections. A number of disseminated fungal infections, including blastomycosis, histoplasmosis, coccidioidomycosis, cryptococcosis, and candidiasis may present with subcutaneous nodules, usually in the immunocompromised host (see Table 6).

Laboratory Diagnosis

- **Aspirates/scrapings**—Lesions can be aspirated or scraped, and the material (fluid or tissue) can be Gram stained and cultured.[5] Vesicular lesions can be unroofed, and Tzanck smears or direct fluorescent antibody tests can be performed to evaluate for herpesvirus inclusions.
- **Skin biopsy**—A tissue biopsy should be considered for petechial, ecchymotic, and nodular lesions, as well as for ulcers. Diagnoses that can be confirmed histologically include Rocky Mountain spotted fever, disseminated fungal infections, herpesviruses, and vasculitides.[5,14]
- **Additional studies**—Blood cultures should be considered in all patients. In situations that are clinically relevant, cultures of the urethra, cervix, cerebrospinal fluid, and synovial fluid may be helpful. Other than testing for syphilis, serologic evaluation is of limited value in the acute setting but can offer confirmation of a diagnosis.

Infection Control

Some patients with fever and rash require immediate isolation. Patients with suspected meningococcemia should be placed on droplet precautions until appropriate antimicrobial therapy has been administered for 24 hours. Those with disseminated herpes zoster require both airborne and contact isolation, since the varicella-zoster virus can be spread in both manners.

References

1. Lindenauer PK, Sande MA: Fever and rash. In: Wilson WR, Sande MA, eds: Current diagnosis and treatment in infectious diseases. New York: McGraw Hill, 2001:247–254.
2. Chen JL, Fullerton KE, Flynn NM: Necrotizing fasciitis associated with injection drug use. Clin Infect Dis 33:6–15, 2001.
3. Kain KC: Skin lesions in returned travelers. Med Clin North Am 83:1077–1102, 1999.
4. Weber DJ, Cohen MS, Fine JD: The acutely ill patient with fever and rash. In Mandell GL, Bennett JE, Dolin R, eds: Mandell, Douglas, and Bennett's Principles and Practice of Infectious Diseases, 5th ed. Philadelphia: Churchill Livingstone, 2000: 633–650.
5. McKinnon HD: Evaluating the febrile patient with a rash. Am Fam Phys 62:804–816, 2000.
6. Kahn JO, Walker BD: Acute human immunodeficiency virus type 1 infection. N Engl J Med 339:33–39, 1998.
7. Perlmutter BL, Glaser JB, Oyugi SO: How to recognize and treat acute HIV syndrome. Am Fam Phys 60:535–542, 1999.

8. Kaye ET, Kaye KM: Fever and rash. In Fauci AS, Braunwald E, Isselbacher KJ, et al, eds: Harrison's Principles of Internal Medicine, 14th ed. New York: McGraw Hill, 1998:90–97.

9. Cherry JD: Contemporary infectious exanthems. Clin Infect Dis 16: 199–207, 1993.

10. Sabella C, Goldfrab J: Parvovirus B19 infections. Am Fam Phys 60:1455–1460, 1999.

11. Feder HM: Fifth disease. N Engl J Med 331:1062, 1994.

12. Steer AC: Lyme disease. N Engl J Med 345:115–124, 2001.

13. Roujeau JC, Stern RS: Severe adverse cutaneous reactions to drugs. N Engl J Med 331:1272–1285, 1994.

14. Schlossberg D: Fever and rash. Infect Dis Clin North Am 10:101–110, 1996.

15. Hook EW, Marra CM: Acquired syphilis in adults. N Engl J Med 362:1060–1069, 1992.

16. Stevens DL: The toxic shock syndromes. Infect Dis Clin North Am 10:727–746, 1996.

17. Sparling PF, Handsfield HH: Neisseria gonorrhoeae. In Mandell GL, Bennett JE, Dolin R, eds: Mandell, Douglas, and Bennett's Principles and Practice of Infectious Diseases, 5th ed. Philadelphia: Churchill Livingstone, 2000:2242–2258.

18. Rosenstein NE, Perkins BA, Stephens DS, et al: Meningococcal disease. N Engl J Med 344:1378–1388, 2001.

19. Spach DH, Liles WC, Campbell GL, et al: Tick-borne diseases in the United States. N Engl J Med 329:936–947, 1993.

20. Mylonakis E, Calderwood SB: Infective endocarditis in adults. N Engl J Med 345: 1318–1330, 2001.

Pre-Travel Immunizations

chapter
27

Vincent Lo Re III, M.D., and
Stephen J. Gluckman, M.D., FACP

With international travel to more exotic locations becoming increasingly popular, clinicians are finding it necessary to become familiar with current recommendations for travel health safety. Immunizations are a "hot topic" of pre-travel preparation discussions, and they offer one of the best ways to reduce the risks of infections in travelers. A wide spectrum of safe, efficacious vaccines is available, which can help international travelers prevent many of the serious diseases that are absent or uncommon in their home areas. Travel vaccines generally fall into three categories: (1) routine immunizations, which are typically administered during childhood but which may need to be updated; (2) required immunizations, which are necessary for entry into certain countries, and (3) recommended immunizations, which may be useful, depending on the risks of exposure at the travel destination.[1-3]

Advising travelers on vaccine preventable diseases is increasingly becoming the responsibility of the primary care physician. The approach to vaccine recommendations should be based on a thorough assessment of the risks for travel-related illnesses, the time available before trip departure, and current knowledge of the epidemiology of vaccine-preventable diseases. Practitioners should also take into account the adverse events and contraindications associated with each vaccine. This chapter reviews the overall approach to travel immunizations and provides an overview of the routine immunizations as well as those that are recommended or required for international travel.

Approach to Travel Immunizations

Risk Factors

Immunizations should be recommended according to the risk of travel-related diseases and not solely on geographic destination. However, determining vaccine recommendations based on health risk factors can be a major challenge for the health care practitioner. To properly assess a traveler's risk of illness, the health care provider must first consider the details of the planned journey.[4-6] Questions must be asked about the following:

- Exact itinerary, including all geographic destinations and possible stopovers
- Duration of stay in each location
- Style of travel (for example, business versus backpacking)
- Type of lodging (urban versus rural; hotel versus tent)
- Planned activities (possible animal contact, fresh water exposure, eating habits, and sexual activity)
- Purpose of the visit
- Time of year of the trip (seasonal risks)
- Level of anticipated contact with local residents (missionary, health care worker, Peace Corps volunteer)

Providers should then review the status of the traveler's general health, paying close attention to underlying diseases (particularly diabetes mellitus, transplantation, human immunodeficiency virus, chronic lung disease, renal insufficiency) that can have substantial implications for health during the trip and affect the immunogenicity of vaccines.[4] In some health conditions, such as pregnancy or a compromised immune system, live vaccines are relatively contraindicated. This may influence a traveler's plans.[4] Live viral vaccines include measles, mumps, rubella, yellow fever, oral polio, and varicella. The main live bacterial vaccine is the oral typhoid formulation. Past medical history, previous immunizations, allergies to medications and vaccine components (for example, eggs), and current medications should also be reviewed.[4-6] Special effort should be made to identify travelers who are at particularly high risk for travel-related illness (Table 1), since such travelers are more likely to acquire serious illnesses.[3,4] An overall approach to vaccination of travelers based on risk assessment is presented in Figure 1.

Time Before Departure

The time prior to the trip departure date determines whether the standard schedule for a primary immunization series can be used or whether

TABLE 1. Travelers at Particularly High Risk for Travel-Related Illnesses
Backpackers/trekkers
Elderly
Foreign-born persons visiting friends and relatives
Immunocompromised individuals*
Long-term travelers
* Patients with history of transplant, human immunodeficiency virus, or using immunosuppressive medications

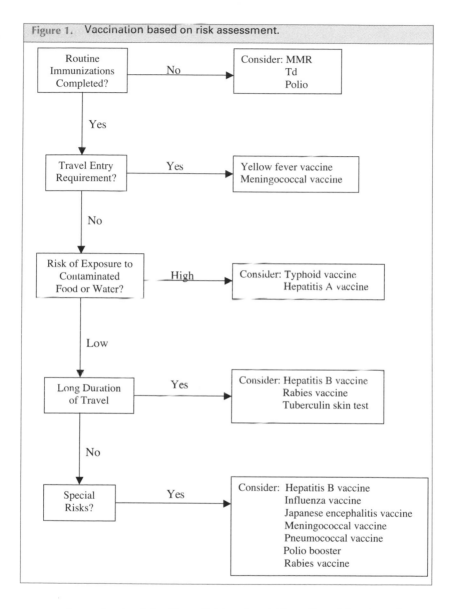

Figure 1. Vaccination based on risk assessment.

an accelerated schedule, if available, should be offered.[2] When departure is imminent and an accelerated vaccine schedule is used, vaccine efficacy may not be maximal by the time of departure, and this must be discussed with the vaccinee.[2] Furthermore, if multiple immunizations must be given concurrently, the health care provider should be aware of the vaccines and medications that may interfere with each other and limit the traveler's protection. In general, multiple vaccines can be given at the same time as long as different locations are used. The major exception is combining immunoglobulin with a live virus vaccine.

Epidemiology of Vaccine-Preventable Diseases

Practitioners who provide consultations to travelers should also base recommendations on the current epidemiology of vaccine-preventable diseases at each destination. The Centers for Disease Control and Prevention (CDC) publication, *Health Information for International Travel,* is one of the standard references for travel immunization recommendations and is updated regularly.[7] Additional information may be obtained from web page sites operated by the CDC (*www.cdc.gov/travel*) and the World Health Organization (WHO) (*www.who.int/ith*).

Routine Immunizations

Travel provides an opportunity to review and update routine vaccinations in adults.[1] Routine childhood vaccinations should be reviewed for all persons, and boosters should be administered as necessary.[4]

Tetanus and Diphtheria

Outbreaks of diphtheria have occurred throughout eastern Europe and the former Soviet Union during the past decade, and tetanus remains endemic throughout the world.[1] Previously immunized adults and children older than 7 years of age should receive a tetanus-diphtheria (Td, Aventis Pasteur) toxoid booster every 10 years.[8] Travelers to remote areas, where postexposure tetanus immunization might be unavailable, should consider receiving a booster dose prior to departure if 5 or more years have elapsed since their last vaccination.

Measles, Mumps, and Rubella

The measles-mumps-rubella vaccine (MMR, Merck) is a combined vaccine that is usually administered at 12 to 15 months of age.[9] Since up to 5% of vaccine recipients fail to respond to primary immunization, a second dose of MMR vaccine is given at the time of school entry.[9] Measles, in particular, is endemic in many developing nations, so immunity to the disease should be confirmed if a traveler's itinerary includes one or more of these countries. Rubella is primarily a concern for women of childbearing age without documented immunity. People can be considered immune to measles, mumps, or rubella if they were born before 1957 (exposure is assumed), have a documented history of these diseases, received two doses each of monovalent measles, mumps, and rubella vaccines or two doses of MMR vaccine, or have serum antibody titers against these diseases.[9] A booster of MMR vaccine is warranted for any person born after 1956 who does not have immunity. The vaccine rarely causes transient arthralgias, especially in nonimmune women of childbearing age.[1] Vaccination with this live attenuated viral vaccine is contraindicated in women who are pregnant or anticipate pregnancy within 2 to 3 months.[9]

Polio

Cases of poliomyelitis are still identified within developing countries of Africa, Asia, and eastern Europe. Wild-type poliomyelitis has been eliminated from the Western Hemisphere. However, there was a recent outbreak in the Dominican Republic and Haiti in 2000.[10] Travelers to Haiti, the Dominican Republic, Africa, Asia, and eastern Europe are advised to receive a single booster of inactivated polio vaccine (IPOL, Aventis Pasteur) if the primary series have already been administered.[7] For those with an incomplete primary immunization series, three doses of inactivated polio vaccine should be given prior to departure.

Varicella

Acute varicella (chickenpox) may be severe, particularly in adults, and can complicate travel and delay return home. Travelers may be exposed to this highly communicable virus (varicella-zoster virus) while traveling to their destination or through exposure to local populations after arrival.[1,7] The status of varicella immunity should be reviewed in long-term travelers as well as in those whose activities bring them into contact with children in schools, day care centers, refugee camps, or health care settings.[2] Adults who give no history of varicella or prior immunization should be tested for the presence of antibodies, since 71% to 93% of adults without a reliable history are actually immune.[7,11] Adults who grew up in tropical or subtropical countries are more likely to be at risk, since varicella infection is rare in childhood in these locations.[12] Children 1 to 12 years of age should receive a single dose of vaccine (Varivax, Merck), and those 13 years of age or older should receive two doses of vaccine 4 to 8 weeks apart.[7,11] Varicella vaccine may be administered concurrently (but at different sites) with any other vaccine.[7] Pregnant and immunocompromised individuals should not receive this live attenuated vaccine.[11] Immunization should occur prior to the initiation of antimalarial chemoprophylaxis, since these drugs will interfere the effectiveness of the vaccine.[7]

Pneumococcal

Pneumococcal vaccine should be a routine immunization for all adults over the age of 65 years and for younger adults with chronic cardiopulmonary disease, anatomic or functional asplenia, cirrhosis, and diabetes mellitus.[13] Since antibiotic-resistant strains of *Streptococcus pneumoniae* are being increasingly reported throughout the world and access to effective antibiotics may be limited while abroad, the pneumococcal vaccine should also be considered for travelers to developing countries.[7]

Influenza

In the United States, vaccination against influenza is routinely recommended for persons 65 years of age or older, for those with chronic cardiopulmonary conditions, and for persons who anticipate disease exposure. The influenza vaccine is also recommended for all international travelers during influenza season. While influenza typically occurs from November until March in the Northern Hemisphere, the incidence of the disease peaks from April until September in the Southern Hemisphere. Furthermore, influenza may occur at any time of year in the tropics. Practitioners should administer the most current vaccine available, since this is formulated on the recent epidemiology of the influenza virus.

Required Immunizations

Yellow Fever

Immunization against yellow fever is required by certain countries for entry, according to WHO regulations. Yellow fever is a rare but potentially fatal viral infection that is endemic in equatorial Africa and South America (Fig. 2a), where the virus is transmitted by day-biting mosquito vectors.[14] The clinical presentation of the disease ranges from a mild febrile illness to a life-threatening disease characterized by hepatitis, renal failure, hemorrhagic fever, and shock. Case-fatality rates range from 23% (sub-Saharan Africa) to 65% (South America).[7] The CDC and WHO regularly publish listings of areas with current yellow fever activity.

Yellow fever vaccination is required for entry by many countries within the areas of endemicity. Other countries may require proof of vaccination if one is traveling from an endemic area to prevent introduction of the disease. It is important to note that several countries within the yellow fever endemic zones do not require the immunization. Thus, immunization should be based on risk of exposure and not requirements. Practitioners can obtain country-specific requirements for yellow fever vaccination from the CDC's *Health Information for International Travel.* Yellow fever vaccine is recommended for persons older than 9 months of age who plan to live in or travel to areas where yellow fever is re-

Figure 2.   Yellow fever endemic zones, 2000. *A*, Africa (*figure continues on next page*).

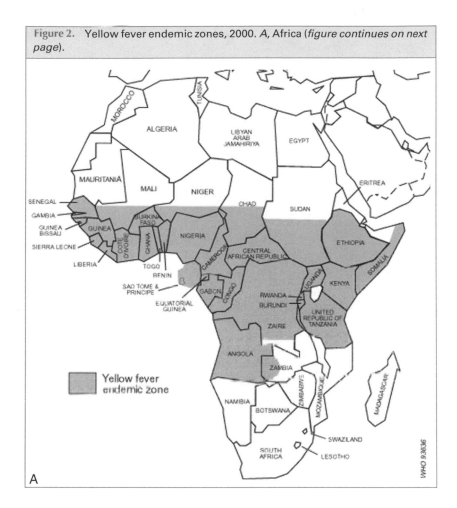

A

ported.[14] Vaccination is also recommended for travel in rural areas of countries that do not officially report yellow fever but that lie within the endemic zone.[14] For purposes of international travel, the vaccine must be administered at an approved yellow fever vaccination center. A list of these centers can be obtained from local or state departments of health. The vaccine is valid for 10 years and should be documented on the Official International Certificate of Vaccination Against Yellow Fever. The yellow fever vaccine (YF-VAX, Aventis Pasteur) is a live-attenuated virus preparation made from the 17D yellow fever strain grown in chick embryo cultures. It is delivered as a single subcutaneous inoculation of 0.5 mL and induces neutralizing antibodies in 99% of recipients within 30 days of receipt.[15] Immunity is likely lifelong, but, as mentioned, revaccination is required at 10-year intervals.[14]

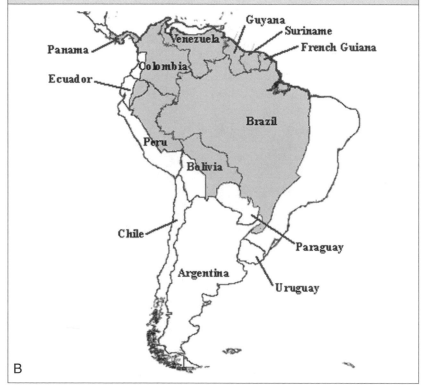

Figure 2. (*continued*) *B*, South America. (Reproduced from Centers for Disease Control and Prevention: Health Information for the International Traveler 2001–2002. Atlanta, U.S. Department of Health and Human Services, Public Health Service, 2001; www.cdc.gov/travel.)

Reactions to the yellow fever vaccine are generally mild and include headaches, myalgias, and low-grade fevers.[14] However, an analysis of yellow fever vaccine recipients in the United States from 1990 to 1998 found that persons 65 years of age or older were at an increased risk for neurologic or systemic reactions.[16] Thus, the vaccine's use should be considered carefully in this population and given only to those traveling to areas that report yellow fever. Yellow fever vaccination is not recommended in immunocompromised persons or in those with egg allergies. Vaccination should also be avoided in pregnancy, and nonimmune women should postpone travel to high-transmission areas until after delivery. If the travel itinerary of a pregnant woman does not present a substantial risk, and immunization is required only for entry, the pregnant traveler should be given a waiver letter from her physician.[7,14] Pregnant women who must travel to areas with active ongoing transmission should be vaccinated, since it is believed that the small risk to the mother and fetus from the vaccine is outweighed by the risk of yellow fever. Serologic response to yellow fever vaccine is not inhibited by administration of other vaccines, although if live virus vaccines (varicella, MMR) are not given concurrently, their administration should be separated by 1 month.[14]

Recommended Immunizations

Hepatitis A and Immunoglobulin

The risk of hepatitis A is present worldwide, particularly in areas where poor hygiene and sanitation allow fecal contamination of food or water.[2] Hepatitis A is the most frequently occurring vaccine-preventable disease among travelers.[17] The incidence of hepatitis A in nonimmune travelers to a developing country is 3 cases per 100 persons per month, and this rises to 20 cases per 1000 persons per month in those who travel to rural areas where poor hygienic conditions are present.[17]

The development of inactivated hepatitis A virus vaccines in the mid-1990s made long-term protection against this infection possible.[18] These vaccines are recommended for all international travelers except those going to destinations in North America (except Mexico), western Europe, Japan, Australia, and New Zealand.[7] There are two safe and highly efficacious inactivated hepatitis A virus vaccines available in the United States, Havrix (SmithKline Beecham) and VAQTA (Merck). The immunization schedule in adults for both formulations consists of a single 1.0 mL intramuscular dose. This is highly efficacious and lasts at least several years. For more sustained protection, one should get a single 1.0 mL booster 6 to 18 months later.[19] After both injections, a traveler has protective antibody levels for at least 10 years.[19] Travelers should preferably receive vaccination 4 weeks prior to departure to provide optimal immunity. Both vaccines provide protective antibody levels in 94% to 100% of patients within 4 weeks of vaccination, and they can be used interchangeably.[18,19] The main adverse effect is injection site soreness. The safety of the vaccine for pregnant women has not been determined. Simultaneous administration with other travel vaccines (at different sites) does not interfere with the immune response.[19]

Immunoglobulin protects travelers against hepatitis A virus infection through the passive transfer of preformed antibodies.[1,19] Active immunization is preferred, but the CDC recommends that travelers who are unable to receive hepatitis A vaccine at least 4 weeks prior to departure be given immunoglobulin at the time of hepatitis A immunization, since protection might not be completed until 4 weeks after vaccination.[7,19,20]

Immunoglobulin should also be offered to travelers who are allergic to the vaccine, younger than 2 years of age, or pregnant.[19] It is given by intramuscular injection and can provide protection for 3 to 5 months, depending on the dose used (0.02 mL/kg or 0.06 mL/kg). Immunoglobulin provides protection against hepatitis A infection in 85% to 90% of those inoculated.[19] Its major disadvantage is its limited time of protection (only 3 to 5 months). Adverse effects are very rare and consist mainly of local discomfort. Immunoglobulin has never been shown to transmit hepatitis B virus, hepatitis C virus, or human immunodeficiency virus.[7,19] Simultaneous administration of hepatitis A vaccine and immunoglobulin results in lower antibody titers than when only hepatitis A vaccine is given, but protective antibody levels exceed those achieved when immunoglobulin is given alone and persist for 6 months, at which time the booster dose is due.[2,21] The MMR and varicella vaccines should not be given concurrently with immunoglobulin.

Hepatitis B

Although childhood vaccination against hepatitis B is currently routine in the United States, many adult travelers have never been immunized. Hepatitis B is highly prevalent in parts of South America, Africa, Southeast Asia, and the South Pacific, and it is transmitted through unprotected sexual exposure and activities that involve contact with blood or blood-derived products.[7] The risk of hepatitis B infection for international travelers is generally low but increases the longer a person remains in an endemic area. The risk of infection may be associated with medical or dental care received abroad, exposure to blood products due to an accident or illness, and sexual or intravenous needle contact.[22]

Hepatitis B vaccination should be considered for the following people:
- Travelers who expect to have close contact with local populations that have high rates of hepatitis B transmission.
- Individuals who plan an extended stay (6 months or longer) in an area of hepatitis B endemicity.
- Persons who might have need for medical treatment while abroad.
- Travelers who anticipate sexual contact with local residents.
- Persons born overseas who travel back to their country of origin to visit family and friends.

Two hepatitis B vaccines are currently available in the United States, Recombivax-HB (Merck) and Engerix-B (GlaxoSmithKline).[23] The standard schedule with either formulation for adults 20 years of age and older calls for three doses of vaccine (each 1.0 mL) at 0, 1, and 6 months. For patients leaving immediately, an accelerated schedule with Engerix-B is available and consists of vaccination at 0, 1, and 2 months with a booster given 12 months after the first dose.[7,23] Serologic testing to assess immune response is not necessary in healthy hosts.[7] Pain at the injection site and occasional low-grade fever are the most common side effects among vaccines. The vaccine is not contraindicated in preganacy.[7]

Hepatitis A and B

A new combination hepatitis A and B vaccine (Twinrix, Glaxo-SmithKline) containing the same antigenic components as Engerix-B and pediatric Havrix was approved by the Food and Drug Administration in 2001 for use in adults older than 18 years, and this vaccine is as efficacious as each of the monovalent vaccines.[23,24] The indications for this vaccine are similar to those for hepatitis A and B vaccines in travelers. Primary immunization occurs at 0, 1, and 6 months. An accelerated schedule of 0, 1, and 3 weeks, with a fourth dose 12 months after the first dose, is as efficacious as with the standard schedule.[24] The main adverse effects are headache and nausea. Its safety in pregnancy has not been determined.

Japanese Encephalitis

Japanese encephalitis virus is an arboviral infection that is prevalent in the Indian subcontinent, China, Korea, Japan, and other Southeast Asian countries.[25] It is transmitted by day biting mosquitoes from May to October in endemic temperate areas and year-round in tropical regions.[7,25] The majority of human cases are asymptomatic, but in rare cases, the virus can cause severe encephalitis with residual neuropsychiatric sequelae. The case-fatality rate is 30%.[25]

Japanese encephalitis vaccine (JE-VAX, Aventis Pasteur) is not recommended for all travelers to Asia. The overall risk of Japanese encephalitis in areas where the virus is endemic is less than 1 case per million travelers.[25] However, this risk increases with travel to rural areas and a longer duration of stay. In general, the vaccination should be offered to individuals who plan to remain for 30 days or longer in endemic areas during the transmission season, especially if travel might include rural areas. Vaccination should also be considered for short-term travelers who may experience heavy exposure to mosquitoes, such as those who engage in extensive outdoor activities or visit areas of epidemic transmission.

Primary immunization in persons 3 years of age or older consists of three doses of 1.0 mL each given by subcutaneous injection on days 0, 7, and 30. An accelerated schedule, in which doses are given on days 0, 7, and 14, can be used when departure is imminent.[25] A single case-control study has measured the vaccine's efficacy to be 91% after two doses.[26] A booster dose may be given 3 years after the primary series if continued exposure in high-risk areas is expected.

The last dose of vaccine should be administered at least 10 days before trip departure to ensure an adequate immune response and to have ready access to medical care in the event of a delayed adverse reaction. Fevers, headaches, and myalgias are the most common adverse reactions reported by vaccinees.[25] However, generalized urticaria and angioedema of the face, lips, or oropharynx have occurred within minutes to as long as 2 weeks after immunization.[27] Patients with a history of allergic disorders (particularly to bee venoms and medications) appear to have a greater risk for developing adverse reactions to Japanese encephalitis vaccine.[27] The safety of the vaccine in pregnancy has not been determined. Pregnant women who must travel to an area where the risk of Japanese encephalitis is high should be vaccinated when it is felt that the risks of immunization are outweighed by the risk of infection to the mother and fetus.

Typhoid Fever

Typhoid fever is an acute, possibly life-threatening, febrile illness caused by *Salmonella typhi*. Typhoid fever immunization is recommended for travelers going to highly endemic areas in Central and South America, the Indian subcontinent, and Africa.[28] Typhoid vaccination is also recommended for travelers who will have prolonged exposure to potentially contaminated food and drink, such as individuals who visit friends and relatives in developing nations or those journeying beyond the usual tourist routes.[28]

Two types of typhoid vaccines are currently available in the United States:

- **Live-attenuated oral Ty21a vaccine** (Vivotif Berna, Berna Products) is made from a bacterial strain of *S. typhi* (Ty21a strain). Primary vaccination consists of one enteric-coated capsule taken on alternate days for four doses.[28] Vaccine-elicited immunity occurs 14 days after receipt of the last vaccine dose, and the overall efficacy is approximately 60% to 80%.[28] A booster dose is recommended every 5 years for those at continued risk and consists of the entire four-capsule regimen.[28] The most common adverse effect reported with this vaccine is mild gastrointestinal upset. The vaccine is contraindicated in pregnant women, children under the age of 6 years, and immunocompromised persons. Vaccination should be delayed at least 24 hours after the administration of antibiotics or mefloquine, since these can interfere with the antibody response.[7]

- **Capsular polysaccharide parenteral vaccine** (Typhim Vi, Aventis Pasteur) is composed of purified virulence ("Vi") antigen, the capsular polysaccharide elaborated by *S. typhi* isolated from blood cultures.[28] Primary immunization consists of a 0.5 mL dose given intramuscularly, and protective immunity is elicited 14 days after vaccine receipt.[28] The efficacy of this vaccine has been reported to be 50% to 80%.[7,28] A booster dose every 2 years is recommended for continued exposure. The main adverse effects reported include local pain, headaches, and low-grade fevers. The vaccine is not recommended for children younger than 2 years of age. No data have been reported regarding it use among pregnant women or immunocompromised hosts, although it theoretically is a safer alternative for these groups. It must be emphasized that current typhoid vaccines are only approximately 70% effective and cannot substitute for the careful selection of food and drink.

Meningococcal

Meningococcal vaccination may benefit travelers to areas where *Neisseria meningitidis* is endemic or where there is an outbreak, especially if extended contact with local persons is anticipated. Up to 10% of the population of countries with endemic meningococcal disease might be asymptomatic carriers.[7] In sub-Saharan Africa, epidemics of serogroups A or C meningococcal disease occur frequently during the dry season (December through June), particularly in the savannah areas extending from Senegal to Ethiopia in the so-called "meningitis belt" (Fig. 3).[29] Meningococcal vaccine is recommended for travel to this

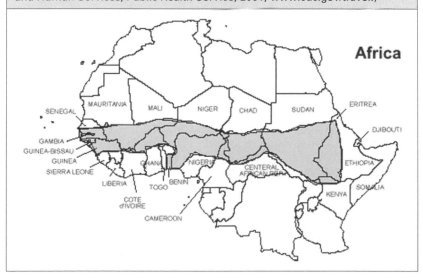

Figure 3. Endemic areas of meningococcal disease ("meningitis belt"). (Reproduced from Centers for Disease Control and Prevention: Health Information for the International Traveler 2001–2002. Atlanta, U.S. Department of Health and Human Services, Public Health Service, 2001; www.cdc.gov/travel.)

area. The vaccine is required for pilgrims entering Mecca, Saudi Arabia during the Hajj.[7] Epidemics of meningococcal disease have occasionally been reported in Kenya, Tanzania, Burundi, and Mongolia.[29] The CDC web site (www.cdc.gov/travel) can provide updated information about recent epidemics and review the geographic areas for which vaccine is recommended.

The currently available meningococcal vaccine (Menomune, Aventis Pasteur) is effective only against serogroups A, C, Y, and W-135.[23,29] Primary immunization in persons 2 years and older consists of a single 0.5 mL dose given by subcutaneous injection, and this confers immunity for at least 3 years.[29] Protective levels of antibody are achieved in 7 to 10 days.[7] Pain at the injection site is the most commonly reported adverse reaction. Vaccination is not contraindicated in pregnancy. Revaccination may be considered within 3 to 5 years for continued exposure.[29]

Rabies

International travelers are often unaware of the risk of rabies during their trip. Canine rabies remains endemic in the Indian subcontinent, China, Southeast Asia, the Philippines, parts of Indonesia, Latin America, Africa, and the former Soviet Union.[1,2] Globally, less than 10% of persons undergoing rabies postexposure prophylaxis for an animal bite receive appropriate therapy.[30] Preexposure rabies vaccination should, therefore, be considered in travelers who

- Plan a prolonged (more than 30 days) stay in a country where rabies is endemic.
- Travel in remote areas.
- Engage in activities that might involve working near animals or that could attract animals (e.g., cycling).
- Cannot report an exposure if bitten (young children).

In the United States, there are intramuscular formulations of the rabies vaccine adsorbed (BioRab, BioPort) and purified chick embryo cell vaccine (RabAvert, Chiron) and both intramuscular and intradermal formulations of the human diploid cell vaccine (Imovax, Aventis Pasteur). All three types of rabies vaccines are considered safe and efficacious. Preexposure rabies immunization consists of three 1.0 mL doses of one of the rabies vaccine formulations given on days 0, 7, and 21 or 28.[31] Adverse effects of the vaccine include headaches, myalgias, and localized lymphadenopathy. Travelers should be given basic information about what to do if they are bitten. After a high-risk bite, persons who underwent preexposure vaccination still require local wound care and two additional rabies vaccine doses (on the day of the bite and on day 3), but administration of rabies immunoglobulin is not necessary. Those who are bitten and who have not had prior rabies immunization must receive five doses of a rabies vaccine formulation on days 0, 3, 7, 14, and 28 as well as undergo inoculation with rabies immunoglobulin.

Cholera

Cholera is an acute intestinal infection caused by the toxigenic gram-negative bacillus *Vibrio cholerae* serogroup O1 or O139. Infection is typically acquired by ingesting contaminated food or water in endemic areas such as the Indian subcontinent, Africa, the Middle East, and Latin America.[7] The risk of cholera to travelers is so low (0.001% to 0.01%) and the protection of presently available vaccines is so poor that vaccination is believed to be of little benefit.[32] Furthermore, the only licensed cholera vaccine in the United States has been discontinued because of its frequent adverse effects and brief and unreliable immunogenicity.[7] Travelers to cholera-affected areas should be advised to avoid high-risk foods, especially poorly cooked or raw seafood.

References

1. Jong EC. Travel Immunizations. Med Clin North Am 83:903–922, 1999.
2. Jong EC: Immunizations for international travel. Infect Dis Clin North Am 12:49–66, 1998.
3. Ryan ET, Kain KC: Health advice and immunizations for international travelers. N Engl J Med 342:1716–1725, 2000.
4. Virk A: Medical advice for international travelers. Mayo Clin Proc 76:831–840, 2001.
5. Dick L: Travel medicine: Helping patients prepare for trips abroad. Am Fam Phys 58:383–398, 1998.
6. Gardner P: Immunizations, medications, and common sense for the international traveler. Infect Dis Clin North Am 4:179–197, 1990.
7. Centers for Disease Control and Prevention: Health Information for the International Traveler 2001–2002. Atlanta: U.S. Department of Health and Human Services, Public Health Service, 2001.
8. Centers for Disease Control and Prevention: Diptheria, tetanus, and pertussis: Recommendations for vaccine us and other measures. Recommendations of the Immunization Practices Advisory Committee (ACIP). MMWR Morbid Mortal Wkly Rep 40(RR-10):1–28, 1991.
9. Centers for Disease Control and Prevention: Measles, mumps, and rubella—vaccine use and strategies for elimination of measles, rubella, and congenital rubella syndrome, and control of mumps: Recommendations of the Advisory Committee on Immunization Practices (ACIP). MMWR Morbid Mortal Wkly Rep 47(RR-8):1–57, 1998.
10. Centers for Disease Control and Prevention: Poliomyelitis prevention in the United States: Updated recommendations of the Advisory Committee on Immunization Practices (ACIP). MMWR Morbid Mortal Wkly Rep 49(RR-5):1–22, 2000.
11. Centers for Disease Control and Prevention: Prevention of varicella: Updated recommendations of the Advisory Committee on Immunization Practices (ACIP). MMWR Morbid Mortal Wkly Rep 48(RR-6):1–5, 1999.
12. Wilson ME: Travel-related vaccines. Infect Dis Clin North Am 15:231–251, 2001.

13. Centers for Disease Control and Prevention: Prevention of pneumococcal disease: Recommendations of the Advisory Committee on Immunization Practices (ACIP). MMWR Morbid Mortal Wkly Rep 46(RR-8):1–24, 1997.
14. Centers for Disease Control and Prevention: Yellow fever vaccine: Recommendations of the Immunization Practices Advisory Committee (ACIP). MMWR Morbid Mortal Wkly Rep 39(RR-6):1–6, 1990.
15. Monath TP, Cetron MS: Prevention of yellow fever in persons traveling to the tropics. Clin Infect Dis 34:1369–1378, 2002.
16. Martin M. Weld LH, Tsai TF, et al: Advanced age a risk factor for illness temporally associated with yellow fever vaccination. Emerg Infect Dis 7:945–951, 2001.
17. Steffen R, Kane MA, Shapiro CN, et al: Epidemiology and prevention of hepatitis A in travelers. JAMA 272:885–889, 1994.
18. Werzberger A, Mensch B, Kuter B, et al: A controlled trial of a formalin-inactivated hepatitis A vaccine in healthy children. N Engl J Med 327:453–457, 1992.
19. Centers for Disease Control and Prevention: Prevention of hepatitis A through active or passive immunization: Recommendations of the Advisory Committee on Immunization Practices (ACIP). MMWR Morbid Mortal Wkly Rep 48(RR-12):1–37, 1999.
20. Wolfe MS: Protection of travelers. Clin Infect Dis 25:177–186, 1997.
21. Clemens R, Safary A, Hepburn A, et al: Clinical experience with an inactivated hepatitis A vaccine. J Infect Dis 171(Suppl 1):S44–49, 1995.
22. Centers for Disease Control and Prevention: Update: recommendations to prevent hepatitis B transmission—United States. MMWR Morbid Mortal Wkly Rep 48:33–34, 1999.
23. Advice for travelers. Med Lett Drugs Ther 44:33–38, 2002.
24. Steffen R: Immunization against hepatitis A and hepatitis B infections. J Travel Med 8(Suppl 1):S9–16, 2001.
25. Centers for Disease Control and Prevention: Inactivated Japanese encephalitis virus vaccine: Recommendations of the Advisory Committee on Immunization Practices (ACIP). MMWR Morbid Mortal Wkly Rep 42(RR-1):1–15, 1993.
26. Hoke CH, Nisalak A, Sangawhipa N, et al: Protection against Japanese encephalitis by inactivated vaccine. N Engl J Med 319:608–614, 1988.
27. Shlim DR, Solomon T: Japanese encephalitis vaccine for travelers: Exploring the limits of risk. Clin Infect Dis 35:183–188, 2002.
28. Centers for Disease Control and Prevention: Typhoid immunization: Recommendations of the Advisory Committee on Immunization Practices (ACIP). MMWR Morbid Mortal Wkly Rep 43(RR-14):1–7, 1994.
29. Centers for Disease Control and Prevention: Control and prevention of meningococcal disease: Recommendations of the Advisory Committee on Immunization Practices (ACIP). MMWR Morbid Mortal Wkly Rep 46(RR-5):1–10, 1997.
30. Dreesen DW: A global review of rabies vaccines for human use. Vaccine 15(Suppl):S2–6, 1997.
31. Centers for Disease Control and Prevention: Human rabies prevention—United States, 1999: Recommendations of the Advisory Committee on Immunization Practices (ACIP). MMWR Morbid Mortal Wkly Rep 48(RR-1):1–21, 1999.
32. Sanchez JL, Taylor DN: Cholera. Lancet 349:1825–1830, 1997.

Prevention of Malaria in Travelers

chapter

28

Vincent Lo Re III, M.D., and
Stephen J. Gluckman, M.D., FACP

The prevention of malaria has always been a "hot topic" among travelers to tropical locales. In 1998, the World Health Organization indicated that there were more than 270 million cases of malaria with more than one million deaths due to the disease.[1,2] In the United States, approximately 1400 cases are reported annually to the Centers for Disease Control and Prevention.[3] The evolving pattern of drug resistance by malaria parasites as well as the changes in the recommendations for chemoprophylaxis present a challenge to physicians who advise travelers on the prevention of this disease. Improving adherence to antimosquito measures and antimalarial medications could prevent many cases of malaria in travelers. This chapter provides an overall approach to malaria prevention in travelers. It reviews key risk factors for malaria acquisition, important measures to prevent mosquito bites, and drugs currently approved for chemoprophylaxis.

Life Cycle of *Plasmodium*

To better appreciate the methods of malaria prevention, it is necessary to understand the parasite's life cycle. Malaria is transmitted by the bite of an infected female *Anopheles* mosquito and is caused by infection with one of four species of the protozoa *Plasmodium* (*Plasmodium falciparum, Plasmodium vivax, Plasmodium malariae,* and *Plasmodium ovale*).[4,5] When an infected mosquito takes a blood meal during its feeding period between dusk and dawn, it injects sporozoites of *Plasmodium* from its salivary glands into the bloodstream of the host. The sporozoites circulate to the liver and invade hepatocytes, where they divide to form tissue schizonts and then merozoites, which escape into the bloodstream. Merozoites invade erythrocytes, they differentiate into trophozoites, and the trophozoites then divide to become blood schizonts. These then mature into merozoites, which, when released from red blood cells, can continue the cycle in the blood. A proportion of the sporozoites of *P. vivax* and *P. ovale* develop into dormant forms within the liver, called *hypnozoites,* that can activate months to years later to release more merozoites into the bloodstream, causing a symptomatic relapse. The life cycle is completed when merozoites differentiate into sexual forms called *gametocytes.* The female *Anopheles* mosquito ingests gametocytes during a blood meal, and sexual stages result in sporozoites that can be transmitted to the next susceptible human host.

Overall Approach to Malaria Prevention

The risk of malaria can be reduced by regular use of measures that limit contact with mosquitoes and by strict adherence to chemoprophylaxis.[6] To help travelers adhere to these recommendations, thorough pretravel advice must be provided by their health care providers. Even a brief exposure in an endemic area puts the unprotected traveler at risk. All travelers to endemic areas need to be aware of the threat of malaria in their destination and understand how to prevent it. Since no preventive regimen is completely effective, travelers should also know to seek medical attention urgently should they become febrile during or after their trip.

In summary, the overall approach to malaria prevention should consist of the following four principles:

1. Assess the risk of malaria infection on the basis of itinerary.
2. Discuss the available methods to reduce contact with *Anopheles* mosquitoes.
3. Identify the most appropriate antimalarials for chemoprophylaxis.
4. Alert the traveler to seek early diagnosis and treatment if fever develops during or after travel.

These principles provide a framework for the clinician to follow when counseling on malaria prevention during any pre-travel patient visit. Fig. 1 provides an algorithmic approach to the prevention of malaria in travelers.

Assessing the Risk of Malaria

Assessing malarial risk requires a detailed knowledge of a patient's travel itinerary and accommodations. The risk that a traveler will become infected depends on the overall rate of malaria transmission in the geographic area to be visited and on the extent of contact with infected mosquitoes.[7] Transmission rates may vary greatly from region to region, even within the same country. In countries where the overall risk is relatively low, there may be foci of intense transmission.

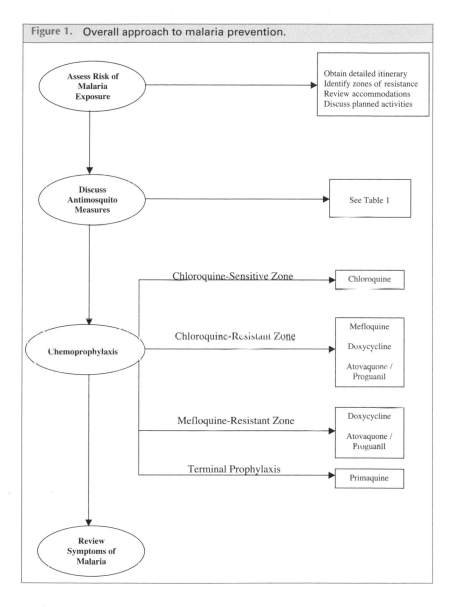

Figure 1.   Overall approach to malaria prevention.

The assessment of risk of malaria infection depends on several other considerations. Since malaria transmission often follows stringent seasonal patterns linked to rainfall, the timing of the trip may influence risk.[8] The elevation of the destination is important, because malaria transmission is rare above 2000 m altitude.[9] Finally, since the *Anopheles* mosquito feeds from dusk to dawn, the risk of transmission is influenced by a traveler's nighttime activities and accommodations.

Regular updated maps identifying malaria risk areas and times are available from several sources (Table 1) and can be valuable tools in counseling patients.[10] Details about risk within countries may be obtained from Web page sites operated by the Centers for Disease Control and Prevention (*www.cdc.gov/travel*) and the World Health Organization (*www.who.int/ith*).

Protection Against Mosquitoes

The most effective protection against malaria is to avoid exposure to the *Anopheles* mosquito that carries the disease.[6,8] All travelers to malaria-endemic areas need to be instructed on how best to avoid bites from these mosquitoes. A significant reduction in the risk of acquiring the disease can be achieved by simply limiting evening exposure to mosquitoes.

Travelers in endemic areas can substantially reduce the probability of infection with certain behavioral adaptations. Wearing clothes that minimize the amount of exposed skin is helpful. The use of insect repellent on exposed skin should also be encouraged. Repellents containing *N*, *N*-diethyl-3-methylbenzamide (DEET) in concentrations of approximately 30% are effective and safe.[11,12] DEET has been used safely by millions of people worldwide and is clearly superior to all alternative insect repellants.[13] It is generally well tolerated but has been noted to cause urticaria, irritation of the eyes, or headaches on rare occasion.[11] When in small, enclosed spaces such as a typical hotel room or tent, spraying with an ordinary household insecticide can "knock down" mosquitoes already in the room. Finally, since mosquitoes are not strong fliers, utilizing a fan can keep them out of the air.

Persons who will not be staying in rooms that are well screened or air-conditioned should consider sleeping under a mosquito bed net. The

TABLE 1.   Resources for Malaria Prevention
Centers for Disease Control and Prevention (CDC) Contacts
Voice Information Service: 1-888-232-3228
Fax Information Service: 1-888-232-3299
Malaria Hotline: 770-488-7788
Web Sites
CDC Traveler's Health Information, *http://www.cdc.gov/travel*
World Health Organization International Traveler's Health, *http://www.who.int/ith*
International Society of Travel Medicine, *http://www.istm.org*
American Society of Tropical Medicine and Hygiene, *http://www.astmh.org*
Malaria Foundation International, *http://www.malaria.org*

use of bed nets has been reported to reduce the mosquito attack rate by 97%.[14] Bed nets and sleeping bags impregnated with an insecticide such as permethrin are preferred, since they are effective barriers to vectors even when holes or tears are present.[6,15,16] Table 2 provides a summary of the protective measures against mosquitoes.

Chemoprophylaxis

A number of medications have been shown to have efficacy in preventing malaria infection. As with all treatments, the use of an antimalarial regimen should weigh the potential adverse effects against the risk of acquiring malaria.[8] The clinician must review the travel itinerary to assess the risk of malaria exposure and recognize areas of travel within drug-resistant zones. Contraindications to the use of specific antimalarials for that patient should be identified. Table 3 summarizes the current recommended chemoprophylactic agents.

Drug Resistance

Chloroquine-resistant *P. falciparum* exists throughout the entire malaria endemic world except for Mexico, Central America west of Panama, Argentina, the Caribbean, parts of China, and parts of the Middle East.[17] *P. falciparum* in any other part of the world must be assumed to be chloroquine-resistant. *P. falciparum* that is resistant to both mefloquine and chloroquine can be found in Southeast Asia along the Thailand-Myanmar (formerly Burma) and the Thailand-Cambodia borders.[17,18] Chloroquine-resistant *P. vivax* is also becoming an important problem, particularly in Papua New Guinea, Irian Jaya, Vanuatu, Myanmar, and Guyana.[19]

TABLE 2.   Personal Protective Measures Against Mosquito Bites
1. Minimize outdoor activities between dusk and dawn when *Anopheles* mosquitoes commonly bite.
2. Wear long-sleeved shirt and long trousers.
3. Apply insect repellent containing approximately 30% *N,N*-diethyl-3-methylbenzamide (DEET) to exposed skin at dusk. Repeated application may be required every 3 to 4 hours.
4. Stay in a building with air-conditioning or with screens over doors and windows. If no screens are available, windows and doors should be closed at sunset.
5. Use aerosolized insecticides in living or sleeping areas at dusk.
6. Utilize a strong fan to inhibit the flight of mosquitoes.
7. Use a mosquito bed net, preferably impregnated with permethrin, if accommodation allows entry of mosquitoes. Bed nets can be soaked in an insecticide solution and hung out to dry. They should be retreated every 6 months to maintain effectiveness.

TABLE 3. Drugs for Prophylaxis of Malaria				
Drug	**Usage**	**Adult Dosage**	**Wholesale Price**	**Comments**
Chloroquine (Aralen, Sanofi-Synthelabo)	In areas with chloroquine-sensitive *Plasmodium falciparum* Safe option in pregnancy	500 mg orally, once/week. Begin 2 weeks before exposure and continue 4 weeks after	$5.26/tablet	
Mefloquine (Lariam, Hoffman-LaRoche)	In areas with chloroquine-resistant *P. falciparum* Safe option in pregnancy	250 mg orally, once/week. Begin 2 weeks before exposure and continue 4 weeks after	$10.75/tablet	Not recommended in those with seizure disorders, cardiac conduction abnormalities, and psychosis.
Doxycycline (Vibramycin, Pfizer)	Alternative to mefloquine in areas with chloroquine-resistant *P. falciparum* Contraindicated in pregnancy	100 mg orally, daily. Begin 2 days before exposure and continue 4 weeks after	$5.80/tablet	Contraindicated in lactating women and children younger than 8 years of age. Should be taken with food.
Atovaquone/ Proguanil (Malarone, Glaxo SmithKline)	Alternative to mefloquine and doxycycline in areas with chloroquine-resistant *P. falciparum* Contraindicated in pregnancy	One adult tablet (250 mg atovaquone/100mg proguanil) orally, daily. Begin 1–2 days before exposure and continue 1 week after	$4.70/tablet	Contraindicated in severe renal failure (creatinine clearance < 30 ml/min) Should be taken with food.
Primaquine (base, Sanofi-Synthelabo)	For those with prolonged exposure to *P. vivax* and *P. ovale* or both. Contraindicated in pregnancy	26.3 mg orally, once/d for 14 days after departure from endemic area.	$0.90/tablet	Contraindicated in patients with glucose-6-phosphate-dehydrogenase deficiency For causal prophylaxis (not yet approved by Food and Drug Administration), take 2 tablets daily 1 day before exposure and continue for 7 days after.

Adapted from Centers for Disease Control and Prevention: Health Information for the International Traveler 2001–2002. Atlanta: U.S. Department of Health and Human Services, Public Health Service, 2001

Chloroquine

Because of the emergence of drug-resistant *P. falciparum* strains, chloroquine (Aralen, Sanofi-Synthelabo) is no longer the recommended chemoprophylaxis medication for most parts of the world. Chloroquine is still recommended for prophylaxis for travel to Central America west of the Panama Canal, Hispaniola (Haiti and the Dominican Republic), Argentina, parts of China, and parts of the Middle East (primarily Syria, Jordan, and Iraq).[17] The antimalarial dosage for a traveler to these areas is one 500 mg tablet (300 mg base) per week beginning 2 weeks before departure, one tablet weekly during exposure, and one tablet per week for 4 weeks after the trip. The most common side effect is dyspepsia, but it can also cause pruritus (especially in dark-skinned individuals), exacerbations of psoriasis, agranulocytosis, photosensitivity, and, rarely, neuropsychiatric disturbances such as vertigo or insomnia.[20,21] The drug is a safe option during pregnancy. Concurrent use of chloroquine interferes with antibody response to the intradermal administration of the human rabies vaccine.[9]

Mefloquine

Mefloquine (Lariam, Hoffman-LaRoche) is the drug of choice for most travelers to chloroquine-resistant regions.[9] The traveler takes a 250 mg tablet once a week for 2 weeks before departure, then takes a dose weekly during travel, followed by one dose per week for 4 weeks after returning home. In the past decade, many anecdotal reports of neuropsychological adverse effects have raised major concerns about this drug. However, adverse effects are similar in frequency and severity to those reported with weekly chloroquine use.[22] The most commonly reported side effects include nausea, dizziness, headaches, and vivid dreams. Mefloquine should be used with caution in patients with a history of psychosis, seizure disorder, or cardiac conduction defects. It is the most efficacious and safe option for the prevention of malaria in pregnant women traveling to areas with chloroquine-resistant *P. falciparum.*[17]

Doxycycline

Doxycycline (Vibramycin, Pfizer), a tetracycline, continues to be the preferred agent for persons unable to tolerate mefloquine or for those traveling to areas where mefloquine resistance is present.[1] The drug is taken in a dose of 100 mg daily during exposure and continued for 4 weeks after the traveler returns home. No loading dose is required. Doxycycline has been shown to have comparable prophylactic efficacy to mefloquine, but the need for daily dosing may reduce adherence and, therefore, the drug's effectiveness.[23] Side effects of doxycycline include gastrointestinal upset, esophagitis, and vaginal candidiasis. Furthermore, since the drug can be photosensitizing, its use requires adequate sunscreen protection. Doxycycline is contraindicated in pregnant or lactating women and in children younger than 8 years of age.[8] Long-term administration of tetracyclines has generally been well tolerated.[6]

Atovaquone/Proguanil

The U.S. Food and Drug Administration recently approved a fixed combination tablet of atovaquone and proguanil (Malarone, Glaxo Wellcome) for the chemoprophylaxis of malaria. Travelers need only take the medication during periods of exposure and for 1 week after departure.[24] This is an advantage over mefloquine and doxycycline, which need to be taken for 4 weeks following exposure. Atovaquone/proguanil has been found to be useful against strains of malaria that are resistant to other agents.[25,26] The adult dosing regimen for prophylaxis consists of one tablet (250 mg atovaquone/100 g proguanil) daily starting 2 days before travel, one tablet per day during travel, and one tablet daily for 7 days after leaving an endemic area. The most common adverse effects are abdominal pain, nausea, and headaches.[24] Since insufficient data exist on its safety in pregnancy, it should not be taken by pregnant or lactating women. Atovaquone/proguanil is also contraindicated in those with severe renal impairment. Overall, this combination is well tolerated and efficacious in the prevention of *P. falciparum*. More data are needed to confirm its efficacy against the other malaria species.

Primaquine

Primaquine (base, Sanofi-Synthelabo) has activity against both the blood and liver stages of malaria parasites.[1] In patients who have been infected with *P. vivax* or *P. ovale,* relapses can occur far after chemoprophylaxis is discontinued because the standard drugs fail to eliminate the liver hypnozoites. To prevent relapses, a course of primaquine may be given as terminal prophylaxis (to eliminate latent intrahepatic stages) at the conclusion of the standard post-travel chemoprophylaxis regimen. One 26.3 mg tablet is administered daily for 14 days after the trip. Terminal prophylaxis is generally indicated only for people who have a prolonged exposure in malaria endemic areas or who have visited areas of intense *P. vivax* transmission.[15] Primaquine causes acute intravascular hemolysis in those with an inborn deficiency of glucose-6-phosphate-dehydrogenase (G6PD).[21] The drug should not be prescribed without confirming a normal G6PD level. Primaquine should not be used in pregnant patients.

Future Options

Since primaquine is effective against the hypnozoites developing in the liver, it has recently been reconsidered for causal prophylaxis (to interfere with the early intrahepatic development) of malaria, particularly if the exposure is short. Travelers would need to take primaquine only during exposure and for 1 week after. Randomized controlled trials of the use of primaquine as a chemoprophylactic agent (30 mg base/day) have demonstrated protective efficacy against both *P. falciparum* and *P. vivax* infections, but at this time primaquine is not licensed for this indication.[27]

Tafenoquine is a long-acting primaquine analogue with the same mechanism of action, but this drug is not yet licensed in the United States. Like primaquine, it can be used for causal prophylaxis. It has a long elimination half-life (14–28 days for tafenoquine versus 4–6 hours for primaquine) that allows for infrequent dosing regimens. Preliminary reports indicate that a once-weekly dose is effective against *P. falciparum*, and a 3-day loading dose alone provides protection for several weeks.[27,28] Tafenoquine remains only a future option for the prevention of malaria, but it may improve medication compliance with malaria chemoprophylaxis.

Recognition of Illness

Travelers should be informed that although antimalarials can markedly decrease the risk for developing symptomatic malaria, none of the agents can guarantee complete protection.[9] Travelers should be told to seek medical attention immediately if fever develops during or after a visit to an endemic area. They should be warned that malaria is possible as early as 1 week after first exposure and as late as several months or even years (for *P. vivax*, *P. malariae*, and *P. ovale*) after returning from a trip. Symptoms of *P. falciparum* almost always begin within 2 months of departure from an endemic area, but only 50% of infected individuals with vivax malaria present in the first 2 months upon arrival home.[9]

Finally, travelers should be informed of the main symptoms of malaria. Fever, malaise, headaches, myalgias, arthralgias, chills, and sweats are seen in more than 80% of patients with malaria.[4] The typical cyclic fevers are often not seen in travelers returning to this country. Other symptoms include anorexia, nausea, vomiting, abdominal pain, and diarrhea.

References

1. Kain KC, Shanks GD, Keystone JS: Malaria chemoprophylaxis in the age of drug resistance. I. Currently recommended drug regimens. Clin Infect Dis 33:226–234, 2001.
2. Ryan ET, Kain KC: Health advice and immunizations for travelers. N Engl J Med 342:1716–1725, 2000.
3. Causer LM, Newman RD, Barber AM, et al: Malaria surveillance—United States, 2000. MMWR Morbid Mortal Wkly Rep 51(SS-05):9–21, 2002.
4. Krogstad DJ: *Plasmodium* species (malaria). In Mandell GL, Bennett JE, Dolin R, eds:

Mandell, Douglas, and Bennett's Principles and Practice of Infectious Diseases, 5th ed. Philadelphia: Churchill Livingstone, 2000:2817–2831.

5. Newton P, White N: Malaria: New developments in treatment and prevention. Annu Rev Med 50:179–192, 1999.

6. Lobel HO, Kozarsky PE: Update on prevention of malaria for travelers. JAMA 278: 1767–1771, 1997.

7. Wyler DJ: Malaria chemoprophylaxis for the traveler. N Engl J Med 329:31–37, 1993.

8. Baird JK, Hoffman SL: Prevention of malaria in travelers. Med Clin North Am 83: 923–944, 1999.

9. Kain KC, Keystone JS: Malaria in travelers: Epidemiology, disease, and prevention. Infect Dis Clin North Am 12:267–284, 1998.

10. Dick L: Travel medicine: Helping patients prepare for trips abroad. Am Fam Phys 58:383–398, 1998.

11. Fradin MS: Mosquitoes and mosquito repellents: A clinician's guide. Ann Intern Med 128:931–940, 1998.

12. Are insect repellents safe [editorial]? Lancet 2:610–611, 1998.

13. Fradin MS, Day JF: Comparative efficacy of insect repellants against mosquito bites. N Engl J Med 347:13–18, 2002.

14. Nevill CG, Watkins WM, Carter JY, Munafu CG: Comparison of mosquito nets, proguanil hydrochloride, and placebo to prevent malaria. BMJ 297:401–403, 1988.

15. Zucker JK, Campbell CC: Malaria: Principles of prevention and treatment. Infect Dis Clin North Am 7:547–567, 1993.

16. D'Alessandro U, Olaleye BO, McGuire W, et al: A comparison of the efficacy of insecticide-treated and untreated bed nets in preventing malaria in Gambian children. Trans R Soc Trop Med Hyg 89:596–598, 1995.

17. Centers for Disease Control and Prevention: Health Information for the International Traveler 2001–2002. Atlanta: U.S. Department of Health and Human Services, Public Health Service, 2001.

18. Nosten F, ter Kuile F, Chongsuphajaisiddhi T, et al: Mefloquine-resistant falciparum malaria on the Thai-Burmese border. Lancet 337:1140–1143, 1991.

19. Schwartz IK, Lackritz EM, Patchen LC: Chloroquine-resistant Plasmodium vivax from Indonesia. N Engl J Med 324:927, 1991.

20. Juckett G: Malaria prevention in travelers. Am Fam Phys 59:2523–2530, 1999.

21. White NJ: The treatment of malaria. N Engl J Med 335:800–806, 1996.

22. Lobel HO, Miani M, Eng T, et al: Long-term malaria prophylaxis with weekly mefloquine. Lancet 341:848–851, 1993.

23. Ohrt C, Richie TL, Widjaja H, et al: Mefloquine compared with doxycycline for the prophylaxis of malaria in Indonesian soldiers: A randomized, double-blind, placebo-controlled trial. Ann Intern Med 126:963–972, 1997.

24. Atovaquone/proguanil for malaria chemoprophylaxis. Med Lett 42:109–111, 2000.

25. Hogh B, Clarke PD, Camus D, et al: Atovaquone-proguanil versus chloroquine-proguanil for malaria prophylaxis in non-immune travelers: A randomized, double-blind study. Lancet 356:1888–1894, 2000.

26. Steffen R, Fuchs E, Schildknecht J, et al: Mefloquine compared with other malaria chemoprophylactic regimens in tourists visiting East Africa. Lancet 341:1299–1303, 1993.

27. Shanks GD, Kain KC, Keystone JC: Malaria chemoprophylaxis in the age of drug resistance. II. Drugs that may be available in the future. Clin Infect Dis 33:381–385, 2001.

28. Hale BR, Owusu-Agyei S, Fryauff DJ, et al: A randomized, double-blind, placebo-controlled, dose-ranging trial of twafenoquine for weekly prophylaxis against Plasmodium falciparum. Clin Infect Dis 36:541–549, 2003.

Fever in the Returned Traveler

chapter
29

Vincent Lo Re III, M.D., and
Stephen J. Gluckman, M.D., FACP

As the popularity of international travel, especially to exotic locations, continues to rise, physicians are increasingly encountering febrile patients who have recently visited tropical countries. It has been estimated that 15% to 37% of short-term travelers experience a health problem during international travel, and a febrile illness has been reported to occur in up to 11% of returned travelers.[1] There are many possible causes of fever in this population, and the clinician must search for clues during the evaluation to help make the correct diagnosis. In the majority of cases, the cause of the fever is a common illness such as a tracheobronchitis, pneumonia, or urinary tract infection. However, fever in the returned traveler should always raise suspicion of a severe or potentially life-threatening tropical infection. Malaria, in particular, must be considered if there was travel within an endemic area.

This chapter provides an overall approach to the evaluation of fever in the returned traveler. In addition, important tropical causes of fever are reviewed to familiarize clinicians with the key clinical features of these diseases.

Origin of Fever in the Returned Traveler

The majority of travelers with fever have infections that are common in nontravelers, such as upper respiratory tract infections, urinary tract infections, and community-acquired pneumonias.[2,3] Once routine infections have been considered, the differential diagnosis should be expanded to include travel-related infections. Malaria is the most important cause of fever in a returned traveler from the tropics.[2,3] *Plasmodium falciparum* malaria can be rapidly fatal but is curable with appropriate therapy, so this must be a key diagnostic consideration in such patients. Other important causes of fever in returned travelers include typhoidal and nontyphoidal salmonellosis, dengue fever, viral hepatitis, and rickettsial infections.[2,3] In rare instances, noninfectious diseases such as malignancies or collagen vascular diseases may appear coincidentally during travel and should be considered in the differential diagnosis.

Approach to the Diagnosis

A systematic approach to the evaluation of fever in the returned traveler is critical to obtaining a diagnosis. This evaluation should try to identify special risk factors, exposures, or physical findings that will help to focus the work-up. Consultation with an infectious diseases physician may be necessary to assist in arriving at a diagnosis.

Pre-Travel Preparation

Pre-travel immunizations and chemoprophylaxis taken during travel must be determined, since these will influence the probability of acquiring infections.[4,5] These interventions vary in efficacy. The proper administration of vaccines against hepatitis A, hepatitis B, and yellow fever effectively rules out each of these infections as a cause of a patient's illness.[6] However, vaccines against typhoid fever or use of immunoglobulin for the prevention of hepatitis A is only 70% to 80% effective, so these infections should still be considered among patients who have been immunized.[4] Childhood immunizations against diseases such as polio, diphtheria, and measles may not provide adequate protection in adults unless a booster has been administered or natural disease reported.[6] Immigrants from developing countries may not have received routine immunizations.

For travelers to malaria-endemic areas, the use of personal protective measures (insect repellents, bed nets) and chemoprophylaxis must be assessed.[4,6] Note that no antimalarial chemoprophylactic regimen is completely protective. Furthermore, poor compliance with antimalarials among travelers is a well-documented cause of failure.[4]

The health of the patient prior to travel is also of importance. The presence of underlying medical conditions (cardiopulmonary diseases, immunosuppression, asplenia) may increase susceptibility to various infections. Knowledge of the medications taken for treatment of a patient's illness prior to and during travel is also essential, since these may alter the presentation of certain diseases.

Travel History

Questions regarding the travel history should focus on the following factors.

Exact Travel Itinerary. The risk of acquiring a travel-related infection depends on the precise geographic location and length of stay in each destination.[4,5] Specific regions visited within each country should be determined, because some infections are focally transmitted, and risk is only present when traveling in endemic areas.[4,6] The Centers for Disease Control and Prevention publishes an excellent reference, *Health Information for the International Traveler,*[7] detailing specific infections that are found in different locations. Infections can be acquired en route, and layovers and intermediate stops should be identified. The type of transportation is also relevant, since outbreaks of many types of infections have been linked to airplanes, trains, and cruise ships.

Purpose of Travel. Determining the reason for travel can further assist in assessing the risk for certain infections.[8] Business travelers typically stay in modern accommodations in urban centers and have fewer disease exposures. Adventure travelers usually spend considerable periods of time in rural settings, where the possibility for disease exposure is greater.

Accommodations. Tourists who stay in modern hotels in major urban centers generally have fewer exposures than backpackers or volunteer workers who spend significant time in rural settings with the local population.[9] People who visit family and friends while abroad are also at increased risk for becoming ill during travel, since they often stay in local homes away from usual tourist routes.[10] These individuals also are more likely to forgo recommended vaccines and chemoprophylactic regimens.

Exposure History

The risk for acquiring a tropical infection is affected by the activities performed during travel.[11] Since many tropical illnesses have nonspecific symptoms and physical signs, identifying a unique exposure may provide the only clue to the correct diagnosis. Activities in remote areas, such as hiking or camping, increase the chance of exposure to insect vectors such as ticks, mosquitoes, and fleas as well as to fresh-water lakes and streams that may harbor schistosomes or leptospires.[5] Dietary indiscretions can place travelers at higher risk for foodborne illnesses.

Sexual contact with new partners is common during travel,[12] and this can result in exposure to sexually transmitted diseases. Although these patients usually present with genital lesions, occasionally only fever and nonspecific systemic symptoms are noted.[4,5] A sexual history should be taken and should include the number of partners, types of sexual activities, and protection used. Knowledge of illnesses among fellow travelers or exposures to sick contacts may also provide a diagnostic clue.[9] Specific exposures for a number of tropical infections are listed in Table 1.

Incubation Period

A precise travel and exposure history can allow the clinician to determine the approximate incubation period for the traveler's illness. This can help further narrow the differential diagnosis by prompting consideration or elimination of certain infections. Symptoms of dengue fever,

TABLE 1. Specific Exposures for Various Tropical Infectious Diseases	
Exposure	Specific Infections
Undercooked food	Cholera, nontyphoidal salmonellosis, trichinosis, typhoid fever
Untreated water/unpasteurized dairy products	Brucellosis, cholera, hepatitis A, nontyphoidal salmonellosis, typhoid fever, tuberculosis
Fresh water	Leptospirosis, schistosomiasis
Sexual contact	Chancroid, gonorrhea, hepatitis B, human immuno-deficiency virus, syphilis
Animals	Brucellosis, plague, Q fever, rabies, tularemia
Insects	
Mosquitoes	Dengue fever, malaria
Ticks	Rocky Mountain spotted fever, tularemia, typhus
Reduviid bugs	American trypanosomiasis
Tsetse flies	African trypanosomiasis
Sick contacts	Meningococcal disease, tuberculosis, viral hemorrhagic fevers

Adapted from Suh KN, Kozarsky PE, Keystone JE: Evaluation of fever in the returned traveler. Med Clin North Am 83:997–1017, 1999.

typhus, and viral hemorrhagic fever usually begin within 10 days of exposure, whereas fever appearing 3 weeks or more after return from an endemic area essentially rules out these diseases.[4,6] Typhoid fever may manifest up to 21 days after exposure to contaminated food or drink. The usual incubation period for *P. falciparum* malaria ranges from 8 to 40 days, but infection with the other three species of malaria (*Plasmodium vivax, Plasmodium ovale,* and *Plasmodium malariae*) may not become clinically apparent for several months to years after exposure. In addition, the usual incubation period of malaria can be lengthened by antimalarials taken by the traveler.[13] The incubation periods of various tropical diseases are listed in Table 2.

Symptoms and Physical Findings

Evaluation of the febrile traveler should include careful documentation of the associated symptoms and signs, since these can help guide the clinician toward the correct diagnosis. The mode of onset of the illness (acute versus gradual) and the precise sequence of symptoms should also be ascertained.

A thorough physical examination must also be performed to elicit additional clues.

Vitals Signs. Although rarely diagnostic, determination of a fever pattern may be helpful.[4–6,9] Several fever patterns have been identified (Table 3). However, it is logistically difficult to obtain accurately recorded temperatures, and the administration of antipyretics interferes

TABLE 2.   Typical Incubation Periods for Various Tropical Infectious Diseases

Less than 21 days	Greater than 21 days
East African trypanosomiasis	Acute human immunodeficiency virus
Dengue fever	Acute schistosomiasis (Katayama fever)
Leptospirosis	Amoebic liver abscess
Malaria	Leishmaniasis
Nontyphoidal salmonellosis	Malaria
Plague	Rabies
Typhoid fever	Viral hepatitis (A, B, C, D, E)
Typhus	West African trypanosomiasis
Viral hemorrhagic fevers	
Yellow fever	

Adapted from Suh KN, Kozarsky PE, Keystone JE: Evaluation of fever in the returned traveler. Med Clin North Am 83:997–1017, 1999.

with this task. In particular, although fevers every 48 to 72 hours are typical of malaria, these characteristic cyclical fevers are rarely seen in travelers, since they are much more likely to occur in a relapse of malaria rather than an initial infection. A pulse rate that is slow for the degree of fever (pulse-temperature dissociation) may suggest typhoid fever or rickettsial infections.

Skin. Many febrile patients have a rash that can assist in the diagnosis. A maculopapular rash may be seen with many travel-related infec-

TABLE 3.   Fever Patterns

Fever Pattern	Definition	Diseases Producing the Fever Pattern
Double quotidian fever	Two fever spikes within a 24-hour period	Gonococcal endocarditis, mixed malaria infections, visceral leishmaniasis
Dromedary fever (saddle-back or camelback fever)	Fever lasting several days, with a 1- to 4-day afebrile period, followed by a return of fever	Dengue fever, leptospirosis
Relapsing fever	Febrile episodes lasting a few days, separated by afebrile periods of about the same length	*Borrelia recurrentis*
Remittent fever	Persistent fever in which the temperature fluctuates but always remains above normal	African trypanosomiasis, bacterial septicemia, tuberculosis, typhoid fever
Intermittent fever	Fever in which the temperature fluctuates between febrile and afebrile levels every day	Miliary tuberculosis, pyogenic infections

Adapted from Saxe SE, Gardner P: The returning traveler with fever. Infect Dis Clin North Am 6:427–439, 1992.

tions, notably dengue fever, leptospirosis, and typhus, as well as with acute human immunodeficiency virus and acute hepatitis B.[4,6] A drug eruption should also be considered in the differential diagnosis of a maculopapular rash. Rose spots, crops of pink macules (2 to 3 mm in diameter) on the chest or abdomen, suggest typhoid fever. An eschar, a black necrotic ulcer with erythematous margins, may be found with many rickettsial diseases. Dengue fever, meningococcemia, Rocky Mountain spotted fever, and viral hemorrhagic fevers may present with petechiae, ecchymoses, or hemorrhagic lesions.

Eyes. The eyes should be examined for evidence of conjunctivitis (consider leptospirosis) or retinal hemorrhages (consider subacute bacterial endocarditis).

Sinuses, Ears, and Teeth. These are common sites of occult infection, and attention to these areas can help to avoid unnecessary testing for other causes of infections.[9]

Heart and Lungs. Auscultation of the lungs should focus on the detection of inspiratory crackles and wheezes, and auscultation of the heart is performed to evaluate for the presence of a murmur, since subacute bacterial endocarditis is always a major consideration.[5]

Abdomen. The presence of splenomegaly should be determined, since this is associated with a number of diseases, notably mononucleosis, malaria, visceral leishmaniasis, typhoid fever, and brucellosis.

Lymphadenopathy. Localized lymphadenopathy may be seen in many infections, and its presence is often less helpful than other signs. Generalized lymphadenopathy, however, has a more limited differential diagnosis, and this finding may be more useful.

Laboratory Investigation

The initial laboratory evaluation should focus on diseases that are life-threatening, and the chief considerations are falciparum malaria and typhoid fever.[9,10] Thick and thin blood films for malaria and blood cultures for typhoid fever are important initial diagnostic steps in the evaluation of febrile travelers. Thick smears for malaria are more sensitive, whereas thin smears are better for the determination of the malaria species. If the initial blood films are negative and malaria is still suspected, smears should be repeated every 8 to 12 hours, particularly during febrile episodes, for several days.[4–6,8,9,11] Blood cultures for typhoid fever, as well as other enteric infections, are usually positive within the first week of illness.[5]

Other useful screening tests include a complete blood cell count with a differential (paying close attention to eosinophilia), blood chemistries, liver-associated enzymes, and a urinalysis with urine culture. Since most viral and rickettsial infections are diagnosed by demonstrating an antibody response, storing a tube of acute serum when a patient is first evaluated may provide the diagnosis when accompanied with a convalescent sample at a later date.[4,5,9]

Major Tropical Causes of Fever in the Returned Traveler

Malaria

Malaria should be the first consideration in any febrile traveler returning from an endemic area. The disease is caused by a blood parasite that is transmitted by night-biting *Anopheles* mosquitoes. It is endemic throughout many tropical and subtropical areas of the world. Updated information on malarious areas is available in the Centers for Disease Control and Prevention's *Health Information for the International Traveler.*[7] It should be noted that even brief exposures in endemic areas can put travelers at risk for malaria, as in cases of runway or airport malaria.[14]

There are four species of malaria organisms that infect humans (*P. falciparum, P. vivax, P. ovale,* and *P. malariae*), but *P. falciparum* results in the most serious illnesses. Approximately 90% of cases of *P. falciparum* infection originate in Africa, and almost as many cases of *P. vivax* infection are acquired in Asia, particularly in India.[5] Up to 90% of travelers with *P. falciparum* infection become ill within 2 months of departure from a malarious area.[4] Symptoms resulting from infection with other species of malaria organisms may be delayed and can manifest months to years after international travel.[4]

The symptoms of malaria are nonspecific.[15,16] A typical presentation consists of the abrupt onset of rigors followed by high fevers and diaphoresis.[15] There may be profound malaise, severe headaches, myalgias, and vague abdominal pain.[15] Gastrointestinal symptoms of nausea, vomiting, and diarrhea may occur in up to 25% of cases and can potentially result in a delay in diagnosis. Jaundice and hepatosplenomegaly may be noted on physical examination. Anemia, thrombocytopenia, leukopenia, and abnormal liver-associated enzymes often accompany clinical illness.[15] Untreated *P. falciparum* can cause hypoglycemia, renal failure, pulmonary edema, and neurologic deterioration, leading to death.[4]

Clinicians must aggressively pursue the confirmation or exclusion of malaria by performing serial blood smears.[11] Three smears should be repeated every 8 to 12 hours, particularly during febrile episodes, as long as malaria is still considered a diagnostic possibility.[4,9,11] Any patient with falciparum malaria or in whom identification to the species level cannot be performed requires admission to the hospital. Consultation with an infectious diseases physician is recommended to ensure proper antimalarial treatment.

Enteric Fever

Enteric fever refers to a clinical syndrome caused by *Salmonella typhi* (typhoid fever) or, less commonly, *Salmonella paratyphi* (paratyphoid fever).[11,17] Disease may be acquired by either direct fecal-oral spread or through fecal contamination of food or water. Typhoid fever is common in many developing nations, and travel to Mexico, India, the Philippines, Pakistan, El Salvador, and Haiti accounts for the majority of cases.

Following an incubation period of 5 to 21 days, patients usually present with sustained fever, anorexia, malaise, and vague abdominal discomfort. Although diarrhea may occur early, it often resolves before fever develops, and constipation is the usual complaint on presentation.[4,17] A pulse-temperature dissociation may be noted on vital signs.[4] Rose spots are found in 30% to 50% of patients but are subtle and must be searched for carefully. Hepatosplenomegaly may also be identified. Laboratory findings are nonspecific, with anemia, leukopenia, and elevated transaminases common.

There are few distinctive clinical features, and the diagnosis should be considered in all febrile travelers, even those without gastrointestinal symptoms. Since current typhoid vaccines have an efficacy of approximately 70%, enteric fever is still a possibility in those who have been immunized.[18] Diagnosis is achieved by isolation of the organism in cultures of blood, stool, urine, bone marrow, and duodenal aspirates.[11] Prior or concurrent antibiotic use reduces the ability to isolate the bacterium. Fluoroquinolone antibiotics are the treatment of choice.[17]

Dengue Fever

Dengue fever is endemic in many tropical and subtropical countries.[19] The vector is the day-biting *Aedes* mosquito. Dengue is the most common arboviral cause of fever in the returned traveler,[2] and its area of endemicity has expanded considerably, particularly stretching into Mexico, the Caribbean, and Central and South America.[20,21] Infection may be caused by any of the four dengue virus serotypes (DEN 1, 2, 3, 4).[22] Subsequent infection with a different serotype may be more severe, resulting in dengue hemorrhagic fever or dengue shock syndrome.

After an incubation period of 3 to 10 days (range, 3–14 days), dengue fever typically manifests with the abrupt onset of fevers, frontal headaches, and severe myalgias.[19,22,23] Retro-orbital pain, exacerbated with movement of the eyes, is a usual complaint.[23] The typical rash associated with dengue fever is a macular or maculopapular erythroderma that blanches under light pressure.[11,22,23] A secondary centrifugal maculopapular rash may appear on the third or fourth day of illness.[23] Leukopenia and mild thrombocytopenia are frequent but nonspecific findings.[23] Rarely, travelers may develop dengue hemorrhagic fever, characterized by thrombocytopenia (platelet count <100,000/mm^3) and hemorrhagic manifestations (petechiae, purpura, gastrointestinal bleeding) or dengue shock syndrome, the hallmark of which is circulatory failure.[22] The diagnosis is made clinically and can be confirmed by noting a fourfold rise in antibody titer between acute and convalescent serum samples sent at least 4 weeks apart. Treatment is supportive.

Leptospirosis

Leptospirosis, caused mainly by the spirochete *Leptospira interrogans,* is a zoonosis that is common in tropical and subtropical climates. It infects wild and domestic animals, particularly rodents, and the organism is excreted in their urine.[24] Transmission to humans occurs when leptospires enter through abraded skin, mucous membranes, or conjunctiva following contact with urine-contaminated soil or water.[25] Exposure to the organism is either occupational (gardening, farming) or recreational (swimming, rafting, crossing streams).[24]

Leptospirosis may occur as two clinically distinguishable syndromes. The more common syndrome (85–90% of cases) is anicteric leptospirosis, which manifests as a biphasic illness.[25] After an incubation period of 7 to 12 days (range, 2–20 days), the initial septicemic phase is characterized by the abrupt onset of high fevers, headaches, and myalgias. Conjunctival suffusion, muscle tenderness, a maculopapular skin rash, and hepatosplenomegaly may also be noted. After 4 to 7 days, defervescence occurs. Two to 3 days later, during the secondary immune phase, leptospires disappear from the blood and cerebrospinal fluid, but circulating antibodies may cause immune-mediated aseptic menigitis, uveitis, or chorioretinitis.[25] Icteric leptospirosis, or Weil's syndrome, is less common (5–10%) and may be characterized by hepatic, renal, and vascular dysfunction. Fever, jaundice, and azotemia typically develop, and hypotension due to vascular collapse may ensue. The diagnosis is usually established retrospectively by serologic tests. Blood, urine, and cerebrospinal fluid can be obtained for culture. Empiric therapy with doxycycline or penicillin should be initiated if the diagnosis is considered.[24,25]

Rickettsial Infections

Rickettsial diseases are vector-borne illnesses usually carried by ticks, lice, fleas, or mites, and they are widely distributed throughout the world. Tick typhus (also known as *Mediterranean spotted fever* or *boutonneuse fever*) is the most common imported rickettsial disease in returning travelers.[26] It is endemic in southern Europe and the Middle East, where it is caused by *Rickettsia conorii,* and in southern Africa, where *Rickettsia africae* is the etiologic agent.[4,26] After a 5- to 7-day incubation period, fever, headaches, and myalgias may occur. A maculopapular rash involving the palms, soles, and face may accompany the illness. There is usually an eschar, called a *tâche noire* ("black spot") at the tick bite site.[4,11,26] The diagnosis is usually confirmed serologically. Doxycycline is the treatment of choice. Depending on the area visited, other rickettsial infections, such as Rocky Mountain spotted fever, epidemic typhus, endemic typhus, or scrub typhus, should be considered.

Approach to Fever in the Returned Traveler

The approach to the returning traveler with non-focal fevers can be summarized as follows:

1. Always consider nontravel-related causes.
2. Consider how long after return the fevers began:

Less than 21 days: The majority of patients will have malaria, typhoid fever, or dengue fever. Although very uncommon, consider meningococcemia and viral hemorrhagic fevers, since these diagnoses represent potential emergencies.

Greater than 21 days: The majority of patients have malaria or tuberculosis. If unimmunized, hepatitis A should be strongly considered.

3. If the diagnosis is still not established, consider uncommon diagnoses such as leptospirosis, rickettsial diseases, acute human immunodeficiency virus infection, and acute trypanosomiasis. An infectious diseases consultation is recommended.

References

1. Bruni M, Steffen R: Impact of travel-related health impairments. J Travel Med 4: 61–64, 1997.
2. O'Brien D, Tobin S, Brown GV, Torresi J: Fever in returned travelers: Review of hospital admissions for a 3-year period. Clin Infect Dis 33:603–609, 2001.
3. Doherty JF, Grant AD, Bryceson ADM: Fever as the presenting complaint of travellers returning from the tropics. Q J Med 88:277–281, 1995.
4. Suh KN, Kozarsky PE, Keystone JE: Evaluation of fever in the returned traveler. Med Clin North Am 83:997–1017, 1999.
5. Humar A, Keystone J: Evaluating fever in travellers returning from tropical countries. BMJ 312:953–956, 1996.
6. Strickland GT: Fever in the returned traveler. Med Clin North Am 76:1375–1392, 1992.
7. Centers for Disease Control and Prevention: Health Information for the International Traveler, 2001–2002. Atlanta: U.S. Department of Health and Human Services, Public Health Service, 2001.

8. Felton JM, Bryceson ADM: Fever in the returning traveller. Br J Hosp Med 55: 705–711, 1996.
9. Saxe SE, Gardner P: The returning traveler with fever. Infect Dis Clin North Am 6: 427–439, 1992.
10. Ryan ET, Wilson ME, Kain KC: Illness after international travel. N Engl J Med 347: 505–516, 2002.
11. Magill AJ: Fever in the returned traveler. Infect Dis Clin North Am 12:445–469, 1998.
12. Matteelli A, Coris G: Sexually transmitted diseases in travelers. Clin Infect Dis 32: 1063–1067, 2001.
13. Reyburn H, Behrens RH, Warhurst D, Bradley D: The effect of chemoprophylaxis on the timing of onset of falciparum malaria. Trop Med Int Health 3:281–285, 1998.
14. Conlon CP, Berendt AR, Dawson K, Peto TEA: Runway malaria. Lancet 335:472–473, 1990.
15. Svenson JE, MacLean JD, Gyorkos TW, Keystone J: Imported malaria: Clinical presentation and examination of symptomatic travelers. Arch Intern Med 155:861–868, 1995.
16. Dorsey G, Gandhi M, Oyugi JH, Rosenthal PJ: Difficulties in the prevention, diagnosis, and treatment of imported malaria. Arch Intern Med 160:2505–2510, 2000.
17. Mermin JH, Townes JM, Gerber M, et al: Typhoid fever in the United States, 1985–1994: Changing risks of international travel and increasing antimicrobial resistance. Arch Intern Med 158:633–638, 1998.
18. Centers for Disease Control and Prevention: Typhoid immunization: Recommendations of the Advisory Committee on Immunization Practices (ACIP). MMWR Morbid Mortal Wkly Rep 43(RR-14):1–7, 1994.
19. Jelinek T: Dengue fever in international travel. Clin Infect Dis 31:144–147, 2000.
20. Jelinek T, Dobler G, Holscher M, et al: Prevalence of infection with dengue virus among international travelers. Arch Intern Med 157:2367–2370, 1997.
21. Gubler DJ, Clark GG: Dengue/dengue hemorrhagic fever: The emergence of a global health problem. Emerg Infect Dis 1:55–57, 1995.
22. Rigau-Perez JG, Clark GG, Gubler DJ, et al: Dengue and dengue hemorrhagic fever. Lancet 352:971–977, 1998.
23. Schwartz E, Mendelson E, Sidi Y: Dengue fever among travelers. Am J Med 101: 516–520, 1996.
24. van Crevel R, Speelman P, Gravekamp C, Terpstra WJ: Leptospirosis in travelers. Clin Infect Dis 19:132–134, 1994.
25. Farr RW: Leptospirosis. Clin Infect Dis 21:1–8, 1995.
26. MacDonald JC, MacLean JD, McDade JE: Imported rickettsial disease: Clinical and epidemiological features. Am J Med 85:799–805, 1988.

Principal Agents of Bioterrorism

Vincent Lo Re III, M.D., and Kelly J. Henning, M.D.

chapter

30

The threat of bioterrorism, long ignored and denied, has heightened. The recent anthrax attacks in the fall of 2001 have forced the public health and medical community to face the very real possibility of future bioterrorist events. Bioterrorism is the use of biological agents to intimidate governments or societies on behalf of an ideological cause.[1] These agents are capable of causing large numbers of casualties with relatively minimal cost, technological expertise, and logistical requirements. Biological weapons have been used throughout the history of armed conflict (Table 1).[2,3]

Physicians need to be familiar with the effects of biological agents and the treatments associated with each disease. Health care professionals constitute the first line of defense against bioterrorism. The rapidity with which doctors reach a proper diagnosis and the speed with which they apply preventive and therapeutic measures could potentially save thousands of lives. Thus, physicians need to be alert to any constellation of symptoms that might be the harbinger of new outbreaks.

In 1999, the Centers for Disease Control and Prevention (CDC) identified several biological agents that would have significant impact on U.S. health and security if released into the population, and these were designated Category A agents.[4] This chapter provides a general overview of the pathophysiology, clinical presentation, diagnosis, and management of patients exposed to or infected with these Category A agents, which include anthrax, smallpox, plague, botulinum toxin, tularemia, and the hemorrhagic fever viruses.

Anthrax

Anthrax is caused by *Bacillus anthracis,* a spore-forming gram-positive rod. Naturally acquired infection results from contact with contaminated animals. No human-to-human transmission of the disease has ever been confirmed.

346 Principal Agents of Bioterrorism

TABLE 1. History of Biological Warfare and Bioterrorism
1347: Tartars hurl plague-infected bodies into Kaffa.
1754: Sir Jeffrey Amherst gives American Indians blankets and handkerchiefs containing smallpox.
1917: Germany attempts to infect livestock destined for shipments to the United States and Russia with anthrax and glanders.
1925: Geneva Protocols prohibit the use of biological agents.
1932: Japan creates Unit 731, a biological warfare research facility under the direction of Dr. Shiro Ishii.
1942: Britain tests strategic amounts of anthrax on Gruinard Island, near the coast of Scotland.
1942: U.S. creates Camp Detrick in Maryland for research in biological weapons.
1946: U.S. has strategic amounts of botulinum toxin and anthrax.
1972: Biological Warfare Convention is created and signed by more than 100 nations, prohibiting the development and possession of biological weapons.
1979: Outbreak of inhalational anthrax in Sverdlovsk, Russia (downwind from major Soviet microbiology facility); 79 cases identified, 68 deaths.
1984: Rajneeshee cult intentionally contaminates salad bars in 10 Oregon restaurants with *Salmonella*.
1995: Iraq admits to possession of anthrax, botulinum toxin, and rotavirus.
1995: Japanese cult Aum Shinrikyo releases sarin nerve gas into Tokyo subway. Police seize cult's arsenal of botulinum toxin and anthrax.
2001: U.S. anthrax bioterrorist attacks occur.

Pathogenesis

The virulence of *B. anthracis* is dependent on its capsule and the two toxins it produces.[5] The poly-D-glutamic acid capsule is antiphagocytic and prevents bacterial lysis of the organism by host proteins.[5,6] The anthrax toxins have been shown to be composed of three entities that act synergistically to produce the clinical effects of anthrax:

- *Protective antigen* (so named because it is the main protective constituent of the anthrax vaccine) binds to target cell receptors and then cleaves off a portion of its protein, which allows attachment by either edema or lethal factor.
- *Edema factor* can bind to the exposed region on protective factor and form edema toxin, which can disrupt cellular water balance, causing intracellular edema.
- *Lethal factor,* a metalloprotease, can bind to the exposed domain on protective antigen and form lethal toxin, which at sufficient concentrations inhibits neutrophil function and can destroy cellular tissues. Lethal toxin also stimulates macrophages to release tumor necrosis factor and interleukin-1, which contribute to sudden death in cases of systemic anthrax.[6]

Clinical disease can occur when endospores of *B. anthracis* are introduced into the body by abrasion, inhalation, or ingestion. These spores are ingested by local macrophages and transported to regional lymph nodes, where germination to form vegetative bacilli may occur up to 60 days later.[6,8] These bacteria release themselves from macrophages and multiply within the lymphatic system, elaborating toxins that overwhelm the clearance ability of regional lymph nodes. Bacteremia and the systemic production of toxins can then ensue.

Clinical Manifestations

There are three main types of anthrax infection:

Cutaneous anthrax results from direct contact with the microbe on the skin or mucous membranes. More than 95% of naturally occurring anthrax is the cutaneous form.[9] Approximately 1 to 7 days after anthrax endospores are introduced into the skin at a site of a previous cut or abrasion, a painless, pruritic macule or papule appears. Within 24 to 36 hours, the lesion forms a vesicle filled with clear or serosanguinous fluid containing numerous organisms that can be seen with Gram stain. The lesion undergoes necrosis, forming a painless ulcer covered by a characteristic central black eschar.[10,11] There is accompanying nonpitting edema, which may be extensive, and multiple bullae may occasionally develop. Low-grade fever and malaise may be present, and painful regional lymphadenopathy can occur. Incision and débridement of early lesions should be avoided, since this may increase the chance of bacteremia.[9] The eschar dries and falls off in 1 to 2 weeks, often with no residual scarring. The administration of antibiotics does not change the course of eschar formation but does decrease the likelihood of systemic disease. Although bacteremia is rare, the mortality rate has been reported to be as high as 20% without antibiotics but is less than 1% with them.[7]

Inhalational anthrax follows deposition of endospores into the alveolar spaces and may be a biphasic illness. The minimum infectious inhaled dose has not been precisely determined. Symptoms can develop 2 to 60 days after the inhalation of spores but usually develop after 6 days of incubation. The early phase is characterized by the insidious onset of fever, malaise, nonproductive cough, and dyspnea.[7,9,12–14] Nausea, vomiting, and abdominal pain may also be present. Pleuritic chest pain and drenching sweats were prominent features in the 2001 U.S. anthrax outbreak.[13,14] This stage of illness lasts from hours to a few days. Some patients may experience a brief period of apparent recovery. However, a second phase begins abruptly with spiking fevers, worsening dyspnea, and hypotension. A widened mediastinum due to massive mediastinal lymphadenopathy may be identified on chest radiograph. Pleural effusions may also be evident. These enlarged nodes can lead to partial tracheal compression and stridor.[15] Up to one half of patients develop hemorrhagic meningitis with subsequent coma. Death can occur within hours. The mortality rate was previously reported to approach 90%, but in the recent U.S. anthrax bioterrorist cases, lower mortality rates (approximately 40%) were observed.[14]

Gastrointestinal anthrax can occur following the deposition of endospores in the upper or lower gastrointestinal tract. It is presumed that endospores inoculate areas of mucosal breakdown. This form of anthrax has never been reported in the United States. Symptoms can appear 2 to 5 days after the ingestion of endospore-contaminated meat. If spores are deposited in the oropharyngeal region, clinical findings typically include oral or esophageal ulceration accompanied by cervical edema and lymphadenopathy. Patients may complain of dysphagia, nausea, vomiting, fever, and even respiratory difficulty. Lesions have the appearance of pseudomembranous ulceration.[6] If endospores are deposited in the lower gastrointestinal tract, patients may present with nausea, abdominal pain, fever, and bloody diarrhea. Hemorrhagic mesenteric lymphadenitis and massive ascites can also occur.[9] Death occurs from intestinal perforation and anthrax toxemia. The case-fatality rate of gastrointestinal anthrax ranges from 12% to 50%.[16]

Diagnosis

Clinical diagnosis of anthrax requires a high index of suspicion. During the recent postal-related outbreak of anthrax in the United States, the CDC used surveillance case definitions, which established a *confirmed case* of anthrax as a patient with a compatible clinical illness combined with either isolation of *B. anthracis* from a culture or laboratory evidence of infection based on at least two supportive tests (polymerase chain reaction [PCR], immunohistochemistry, or serology).[17] A *suspected case* was defined as a patient with a compatible clinical illness combined with either a single nonculture laboratory test or epidemiologic linkage to a source.

Gram stain and culture of *B. anthracis* can be obtained from blood, cerebrospinal fluid, vesicular fluid, and biopsy material from a cutaneous specimen. Growth of the bacillus is usually noted within 6 to 24 hours, and it is nonmotile and nonhemolytic and demonstrates spores in nutritionally deficient media.[6] Serologic testing requires the acquisition of acute and convalescent specimens and is not commercially available. Confirmation of identification can also occur with PCR, direct fluorescent antibody analysis, or immunohistochemical testing, which are generally available only through public health laboratories. Nasal swabs have been used in epidemiologic outbreak investigations but have no clinical utility in making treatment decisions. Although community laboratories can provide presumptive identification, confirmatory testing is available only through state health department laboratories.

Treatment and Postexposure Prophylaxis

The currently recommended therapies for adults and children with clinically evident gastrointestinal or inhalational anthrax are summarized in Table 2.[18] During the anthrax attacks of 2001, persons with inhalational anthrax treated with two or more antibiotics active against B. anthracis had a greater chance of survival.[14] Thus, two or three antibiotics in combination are recommended for treatment of persons with inhalational anthrax, and these should ultimately be based on susceptibility testing.[18] Treatment should continue for 60 days, since this has been the maximum time required for germination of spores acquired through inhalational exposure.[8] A switch from intravenous to oral formulations can occur once clinical improvement is demonstrated.

Adult patients with cutaneous anthrax can be treated with oral ciprofloxacin (500 mg twice daily).[10] If the strain is susceptible, oral doxycycline (100 mg twice daily) or amoxicillin (500 mg three times daily) may also be used.[18] When cutaneous anthrax occurs in the setting of a bioterrorist event, treatment should continue for 60 days (because of the risk of inhalational exposure) as opposed to 7 to 10 days for naturally acquired disease.

TABLE 2. Treatment of Gastrointestinal or Inhalational Anthrax in Adults			
Antimicrobial Agent*	Adult Dose	Pediatric Dose	Duration
Ciprofloxacin *or*	400 mg IV twice daily	10–15 mg/kg IV twice daily, not to exceed 1 g daily‡	60 days
Doxycycline *plus*	100 mg IV twice daily 100 mg IV twice daily‡	If weight is ≥ 45 kg, give 100 mg IV twice daily‡ If weight is < 45 kg, give 2.2 mg/kg IV twice daily‡	60 days
One or two additional antibiotics†			

*A switch to the oral formulations of these antimicrobial agents can be made once clinical improvement is demonstrated to complete 60 days of therapy.
†These include penicillin, ampicillin, imipenem, vancomycin, rifampin, chloramphenicol, clindamycin, and clarithromycin. Chloramphenicol is especially recommended for anthrax meningitis. Penicillin and ampicillin should not be used alone because of possible resistance by B. anthracis.
‡Although fluoroquinolones and tetracyclines have known adverse effects in children, these risks must be balanced against the risks of anthrax.
Adapted from Inglesby TV, O'Toole T, Henderson DA, et al: Anthrax as a biological weapon, 2002: Updated recommendations for management. JAMA 287;2236–2252, 2002.

An anthrax vaccine (BioThrax, BioPort), consisting of a noninfectious sterile filtrate from the culture of an attenuated strain of *B. anthracis,* has been approved for preexposure prophylaxis.[19] The Food and Drug Administration has recently approved the release of the vaccine by the manufacturer's (BioPort) newly renovated facility. Vaccination consists of six 0.5 mL subcutaneous doses given at 0, 2, and 4 weeks and then 6, 12, and 18 months after exposure. Annual boosters are recommended for continued immunity. Mainly minor adverse effects (local erythema and tenderness, fever, myalgias) related to its use have been reported.[20] Currently, routine preexposure vaccination is limited to military personnel. Postexposure prophylaxis with the anthrax vaccine has not yet been approved by the Food and Drug Administration but is under investigation.

If public health officials have determined that there is evident risk of exposure to anthrax, postexposure prophylaxis is necessary to prevent clinical disease. Recommended options are listed in Table 3.[18] A total of 60 days of therapy is recommended for postexposure prophylaxis.[18] However, owing to the unusually high potency of anthrax spores used in the bioterrorist attacks of 2001 and the theoretical possibility that weaponized spores might cause illness up to 100 days after exposure, the CDC has asked that clinicians caring for patients exposed to anthrax consider these additional recommendations: (1) an additional 40 days of antimicrobial prophylaxis (for a total of 100 days) and (2) administration of three doses of anthrax vaccine on days 0, 14, and 28.[21]

TABLE 3.	Recommendations for Postexposure Prophylaxis of Anthrax in Adults		
Antimicrobial Agent	Adult Dose	Pediatric Dose	Duration
Ciprofloxacin	500 mg PO twice daily	20–30 mg/kg/day PO in two daily doses, not to exceed 1 g daily[†]	60–100 days
Doxycycline	100 mg PO twice daily	If weight is ≥45 kg, give 100 mg PO twice daily[†] If weight is <45 kg, give 2.5 mg/kg PO twice daily[†]	60–100 days
Amoxicillin*	500 mg PO three times daily	If weight is ≥20 kg, give 500 mg three times daily If weight is <20 kg, give 40 mg/kg PO in three doses every 8 hours	60–100 days

*Amoxicillin should only be used after 10–14 days of ciprofloxacin or doxycycline *and* if a contraindication to continuing one of these therapies exists (pregnancy, lactation, age <18, intolerance).
[†]Although fluoroquinolones and tetracyclines have known adverse effects in children, these risks must be balanced against the risks of anthrax.
Adapted from Inglesby TV, O'Toole T, Henderson DA, et al: Anthrax as a biological weapon, 2002: Updated recommendations for management. JAMA 287:2236–2252, 2002.

Infection Control

No person-to-person transmission of the disease has been reported, although the risk of secondary transmission related to weaponized forms of anthrax is not fully defined.[22] Hospital personnel should use standard precautions when treating patients, but contact precautions should be established for patients who have draining cutaneous lesions.[9]

Smallpox

A global scourge for generations, the last case of endemic smallpox was identified in Somalia in 1977, and the global eradication of the disease was declared in 1980, marking one of the greatest achievements in modern medicine. In the wake of the 2001 anthrax bioterrorist attacks, there is heightened concern that smallpox might be used as a biological weapon.[23,24] This apprehension stems from its contagious nature, high rates of morbidity and mortality, and unknown existing human immunity to the virus.

The causative agent of smallpox is the variola virus, an orthopoxvirus within the Poxviridae family. Smallpox is a contagious disease characterized by fever and a vesicular and pustular rash.

Pathogenesis

Smallpox is readily transmitted from person to person via droplet nuclei, aerosols, or direct contact with contaminated fomites. Transmission generally occurs after the onset of the rash.[25] Infection begins once the virus implants onto the oropharyngeal or respiratory mucosa. It passes rapidly into local lymph nodes and multiplies. An asymptomatic viremia ensues, followed by multiplication of the virus in the reticuloendothelial system. The virus then localizes in the oropharyngeal mucosa and dermal blood vessels.

Clinical Manifestations

After the usual 12- to 14-day incubation period (range, 7–17 days), the patient typically presents with high fever, malaise, headache, and backache. Severe abdominal pain may also be present.[25] The characteristic rash usually begins 2 to 3 days after symptom onset. The rash is maculopapular and appears on the oropharyngeal mucosa, face, and forearms. It then spreads to the trunk and legs. Within 2 days, the rash becomes vesicular then pustular. Scabs usually appear on the eighth or ninth day of the rash, and pitted scarring develops. There may be a second, less pronounced temperature spike 5 to 8 days after the onset of the rash, particularly if there is secondary bacterial infection.[26]

The World Health Organization has described five types of smallpox:
- **Variola major**—The mortality rate in this most common form of smallpox is 30%.[25,26]
- **Variola minor**—The disease is milder, and the mortality rate is less than 1%.[26]
- **Hemorrhagic smallpox**—Frank bleeding can be seen in the skin and mucous membranes. This form of smallpox, which occurs in less than 3% of cases, is fatal within 6 days of appearance of the rash. Pregnant women are unusually susceptible.[25]
- **Malignant smallpox**—Confluent, flat, velvety lesions (no pustules) are seen in this variant of smallpox, and the case fatality rate exceeds 95%.[26]
- **Variola sine eruptione**—This form of smallpox, which occurs in previously vaccinated contacts, results in mild symptoms such as low-grade fever, headache, or malaise.

Diagnosis

Smallpox is primarily a clinical diagnosis and must be differentiated from other eruptive illnesses, particularly chickenpox. The distinguishing features between smallpox and chickenpox are listed in Table 4. A suspected case of smallpox is a public health emergency and requires immediate contact with local public health authorities.

Microbiological diagnosis can be achieved by PCR or growth of the virus in cell culture. Both of these techniques must be performed in specialized containment (Biosafety Level 4) laboratories available only at the CDC or United States Army Medical Research Institute for Infectious Diseases.

Treatment and Postexposure Prophylaxis

There is no treatment approved by the FDA for smallpox infection. Supportive care is the primary intervention. Any individual exposed to a patient with smallpox should be immunized immediately and placed on a fever watch for a period of 17 days.[25] If performed within 3 to 4 days of exposure, vaccination with vaccinia virus can attenuate or possibly prevent the clinical manifestations of smallpox.[25,26] Vaccine is administered with the use of a bifurcated needle, which is inserted into a bottle of reconstituted vaccine. The needle is held at right angles to the skin, and 15 perpendicular strokes into the dermis of the upper deltoid are given in an area of about 0.5 cm in diameter.[25,26] A trace amount of blood should appear at the vaccination site after 15 to 30 seconds. After vaccination, excess vaccine should be removed from the site, and a loose bandage placed to prevent inadvertent spread of the virus to other parts of the body.[26] Adverse reactions to the vaccine have included ur-

TABLE 4. Distinguishing Features of Smallpox and Chickenpox		
Feature	Smallpox (Variola Major)*	Chickenpox
Prodrome	Lasts 2–4 days, with high fever, headache, backache, severe prostration; vomiting and abdominal pain possible	Prodrome often absent; if present, mild and brief (1 day)
Distribution of rash	Begins on oral mucosa, spreads to face, then expands in centrifugal pattern (most dense on face and distal extremities)	Begins on trunk and expands in centripetal pattern (most dense on trunk)
Lesions on palms and soles	Common	Almost never
Timing for occurrence of lesions	Generally emerge over 1–2 days and then progress at same rate	Occur in different stages of maturation at any given point in time
Evolution of lesions	Progress from macules (day 1) to papules (day 2) to vesicles (days 3–7) to pustules (days 7–14) to scabs (days 14–20)	Progress quickly over ~24 hours from macules to papules to vesicles then to crusted lesions
Sensation associated with lesions	May be painful and only become pruritic during scabbing stage	Often intensely pruritic and not usually painful (unless bacterial superinfection occurs)
Depth of lesions	Extend deep into dermis and often cause pitted scarring	Superficial and generally do not cause scarring
Duration of illness	14–21 days	4–7 days
Severity	Patients often appear toxic; case-fatality rate is 30%	Patients often do not appear severely ill; disease is rarely fatal
Epidemiology	Cases can be expected to occur in all age groups	Most cases occur in children; adults likely to be immune

*Illness may be milder in patients with partial immunity (fever may be less common and fewer lesions may occur, with more rapid healing).
Adapted from Infectious Diseases Society of America: Distinguishing features between smallpox and chickenpox (http://www.idsociety.org).

ticarial rash, postvaccinial encephalitis, eczema vaccinatum, generalized vaccinia, and autoinoculation.[23,25] Vaccinia immunoglobulin (0.6 ml/kg intramuscularly in divided doses over 24 hours) can be used to treat the complications and adverse effects of vaccinia immunization, but its availability is severely limited.[25]

Infection Control

All patients with suspected cases of smallpox should be isolated in negative-pressure rooms. Airborne and contact precautions should remain in effect until all lesions have scabbed and separated.

Plague

Plague is caused by *Yersinia pestis,* a gram-negative coccobacillus. It is a zoonotic disease, and rodents, prairie dogs, and squirrels are the primary reservoirs.[23] In a bioterrorist event, intentional dissemination of plague would most likely be delivered as an aerosol of *Y. pestis,* resulting in cases of primary pneumonic plague.[27]

Pathogenesis

Plague is usually transmitted to humans by the bites of infected fleas.[27] This results in inoculation of thousands of *Y. pestis* organisms into a patient's skin. The bacteria migrate to regional lymph nodes and multiply, causing destruction of lymph node architecture and subsequent bacteremia.

Human infection can also be acquired by inhalation of plague bacilli via droplet nuclei.[27,28] After inhalation, the bacteria migrate to mediastinal lymph nodes, multiply, and subsequently disseminate into the bloodstream. Plague rarely occurs after ingestion of infected meat or handling of contaminated tissue.

Clinical Manifestations

There are three clinical syndromes of plague infection:

Bubonic plague typically occurs 2 to 8 days after a flea bite. It is characterized by the sudden onset of fever, chills, and fatigue. This is followed by the development of a bubo, an acutely warm, tender, swollen regional lymph node (usually in the groin, axilla, or cervical region). Buboes are nonfluctuant and often associated with considerable edema. Despite treatment, bubonic plague carries a 14% case-fatality rate.[27]

Septicemic plague develops in a small fraction of people infected by fleas. Buboes may or may not be present. Septicemic plague may lead to disseminated intravascular coagulation, plague meningitis, or gangrene of the digits or nose (thus the name "Black Death"). It carries a case-fatality rate of approximately 22% despite therapy.[27]

Pneumonic plague may be primary or secondary. Secondary pneumonic plague develops via hematogenous spread in a small number of patients with bubonic or septicemic plague. Patients experience dyspnea, chest pain, and hemoptysis. Primary plague pneumonia is most likely in the event of a bioterrorist attack. It occurs 2 to 4 days after an exposure and manifests with symptoms similar to those of secondary pneumonic plague. Abdominal pain, nausea, and vomiting are also prominent.[28] This syndrome rapidly progresses to sepsis and respiratory failure and is invariably fatal if therapy is delayed for more than 24 hours.

Diagnosis

The diagnosis of plague requires a high index of suspicion. Fever, cough, dyspnea, chest discomfort, and a fulminant course should immediately suggest the possibility of pneumonic plague or inhalational anthrax. The presence of hemoptysis in this setting suggests plague.

A Gram stain of infected blood or sputum may reveal safety pin-like gram-negative bacilli or coccobacilli. Cultures of sputum, blood, or lymph node aspirates are important in the diagnosis of the disease. Rapid diagnostic tests are not widely available. Direct antigen detection in urine, serologic tests, immunohistochemical staining of tissue, and PCR are available but usually are performed only in reference laboratories.[23]

Treatment and Postexposure Prophylaxis

Current recommendations for the treatment of plague are listed in Table 5. Postexposure prophylaxis for asymptomatic close contacts (less than 2 m) of patients with pneumonia consist of either oral doxycycline (100 mg twice daily) or ciprofloxacin (500 mg twice daily) for a total of 7 days.[27] Fever or cough in a close contact warrants immediate isolation.

Infection Control

All patients with suspected pneumonic plague should be isolated to avoid person-to-person spread, and droplet precautions should be

TABLE 5. Treatment of Patients with Plague			
Antimicrobial Agent	Adult Dose	Pediatric Dose	Duration
Streptomycin*	1 g IM twice daily	15 mg/kg IM twice daily	10 days
Gentamicin*	5 mg/kg IV or IM daily	2.5 mg/kg IV or IM three times daily	10 days
Ciprofloxacin	400 mg IV twice daily	15 mg/kg IV twice daily, not to exceed 1 g daily‡	10 days
	500 mg PO twice daily		
Doxycycline	100 mg IV twice daily	If weight is ≥45 kg, give 100 mg IV twice daily‡ If weight is <45 kg, give 2.2 mg/kg IV twice daily‡	10 days
Chloramphenicol†	25 mg/kg IV four times daily	25 mg/kg IV four times daily	10 days

*Preferred choice.
†Especially recommended for meningitis.
‡Although fluoroquinolones and tetracyclines have known adverse effects in children, these risks must be balanced against the risks of plague.
Adapted from Inglesby TV, Dennis DT, Henderson DA, et al: Plague as a biological weapon: Medical and public health management. JAMA 283:2281–2290, 2000.

maintained during the first 48 hours of antibiotic treatment. Persons living or working in close contact with patients with confirmed or suspected pneumonic plague should use surgical masks to prevent disease transmission.

Botulinum Toxin

Botulinum toxin is produced primarily by *Clostridium botulinum*, a spore-forming obligate anaerobe. The toxin targets neurons and mainly causes a flaccid muscle paralysis. The use of botulinum toxin as a biological weapon would most likely take the form of aerosolization or food contamination. This concern has heightened since Iraq's acknowledgement in 1995 of the production of 19,000 L of botulinum toxin, three times the amount needed to annihilate the entire human population.[29]

Pathogenesis

Botulinum toxin is a zinc-dependent metalloprotease that exists in seven distinct antigenic types (A through G).[30,31] Only types A, B, E, and F cause human disease.[30] These four types act by a similar mechanism and produce similar clinical manifestations when either inhaled or ingested.[31] Botulinum toxin can be inactivated by heat ($\geq$85°C for at least 5 minutes).[30]

Clostridium botulinum has three modes of entry into the human body: wound contamination, foodborne, and inhalation.[23] After toxin is absorbed, it enters the bloodstream and travels to peripheral cholinergic synapses, primarily the neuromuscular junction. Once at these sites, botulinum toxin is internalized and enzymatically prevents the release of acteylcholine. Recovery of neuromuscular function requires new synapses to form.[30] Symptoms of botulism typically develop 12 to 72 hours after exposure. This incubation period depends on the amount of toxin absorbed and the rate of absorption.[30] Person-to-person transmission of botulism does not occur.

Clinical Manifestations

Botulism is an acute symmetrical descending flaccid paralysis that often begins in the bulbar musculature. Prominent bulbar palsies typically include diplopia, dysarthria, dysphonia, and dysphagia (the so-called 4 Ds). Pupillary dilatation and subsequent blurry vision may also be present. The symmetric descending paralysis usually begins in the upper extremities and then progresses down the trunk and to the lower extremities, highlighted by the loss of deep tendon reflexes. Finally, respiratory muscle paralysis occurs.

Features that discriminate botulism from other paralyses include the following:
- Patients are afebrile
- Mental status remains clear
- Sensory deficits are not observed
- Neurologic findings are symmetric

Diagnosis

The diagnosis of botulism requires recognition of the key clinical features. Clinical samples used for naturally occurring disease include direct detection of botulinum toxin and identification of *C. botulinum* by culture of serum ($\geq$30 ml of blood in a red-top tube), stool, gastric aspirate, vomitus, and suspected food.[23,30] In a bioterrorism aerosol release, serology would be the primary method of diagnosis. Toxins produced by cultured isolates are confirmed by a mouse bioassay.

Treatment and Postexposure Prophylaxis

Treatment consists of supportive care and passive immunization with a trivalent equine antitoxin. Supportive care may include enteral nutrition, ventilatory support, and treatment of secondary infections. The reverse Trendelenburg position is recommended for nonventilated patients to prevent aspiration of secretions. Administration of the trivalent (containing types A, B, and E) equine antitoxin, available only through the CDC, should occur immediately after a clinical diagnosis is made and should not await laboratory confirmation. This can minimize subsequent nerve damage and reduce the severity of disease but does not reverse existent paralysis. The dose of licensed botulinum antitoxin is a single 10 ml vial per patient, diluted 1:10 in a 0.9% saline solution, and administered by slow intravenous infusion.[30] Since hypersensitivity reactions are common with the antitoxin, skin testing is usually performed as a screening tool.[30] If hypersensitivity is identified, patients can be desensitized before additional antitoxin is given.

It is unclear how best to care for patients who may have been exposed to botulinum toxin but who are not yet ill. The use of the trivalent equine antitoxin is limited by it scarcity and risk of hypersensitivity. An investigational pentavalent (ABCDE) botulinum toxoid is used by CDC laboratory workers at high risk and by the military for protection of troops against attack.[30] A recombinant vaccine is also in development.

Infection Control

Since person-to-person spread of botulism does not occur, no isolation is necessary. Physicians should use standard precautions when caring for patients with botulism.

Tularemia

Francisella tularensis, the causative agent of tularemia, is an aerobic, gram-negative coccobacillus. Tularemia is a zoonotic disease that humans may acquire through diverse environmental exposures and can develop into a severe and sometimes fatal illness. Voles, mice, squirrels, rabbits, and hares are natural reservoirs of infection.[31] Humans may acquire infection in various ways:
- Bite from an infected arthropod (tick, deerfly, mosquito)
- Handling infectious animal tissues
- Ingestion of contaminated foods or liquids
- Inhalation of infected aerosols

Transmission from person to person has not been documented.[32,33] An aerosol release would be the most likely route used in a bioterrorist event.

Pathogenesis

After *F. tularensis* is inoculated into the skin, mucous membranes, gastrointestinal tract, or lungs, the organisms are taken up by macrophages, where they multiply and spread to regional lymph nodes.[32] The bacteria can then disseminate to organs throughout the body, particularly targeting the lymph nodes, spleen, liver, lungs, and kidneys. Bacteremia may be present during dissemination. *F. tularensis* can remain viable in the environment for weeks and is able to resist temperatures below freezing.[33] However, it is easily killed by heat and disinfectants.

Clinical Presentation

Clinical illness due to tularemia occurs after an incubation period of 1 to 21 days (average, 3 to 5 days), and as few as 10 to 50 organisms may cause disease.[33] The onset of tularemia is abrupt and is characterized by fever, headaches, rigors, and generalized body aches (especially low back). Patients occasionally complain of abdominal pain, diarrhea, and vomiting. Pulmonary symptoms include a dry or slightly productive cough, substernal chest discomfort, dyspnea, and pleurisy. A pulse-temperature deficit is found in less than half of patients.[32] The overall case-fatality rate is approximately 2%.[32,33]

Tularemia can appear in one of six forms in humans, depending on the route of inoculation:

Ulceroglandular tularemia usually occurs following an infected arthropod bite but may also be acquired after the inoculation of skin with infected blood or body fluids. A papule usually appears at the inoculation site, becomes pustular, and then ulcerates.[32] Fever, chills, headaches, and malaise accompany the cutaneous findings. Regional lymphadenitis occurs within days of the appearance of the papule.

Oculoglandular tularemia follows inoculation of the conjunctiva by contaminated hands, infected tissue fluids, or infectious aerosols. Patients have painful, purulent conjunctivitis with preauricular or cervical lymphadenopathy. Fever, chemosis, periorbital edema, and pinpoint conjunctival ulcers may also be noted.

Glandular tularemia is characterized by fever and tender lymphadenopathy, without ulceration.

Oropharyngeal tularemia may be acquired by ingesting contaminated foods or liquids or by inhaling infectious aerosols. Patients typically develop an acute exudative pharyngotonsillitis with cervical or retropharyngeal lymphadenopathy.[33]

Typhoidal tularemia occurs mainly after inhalation of infectious aerosols but can occur after intradermal or gastrointestinal inoculation.[33] This is a systemic illness characterized by fever, headaches, weight loss, and malaise without lymphadenopathy. Abdominal tenderness and hepatosplenomegaly may be present on physical examination. Patients may develop shock, delirium, or coma.[33]

Pneumonic tularemia may occur after the inhalation of organisms (primary disease) or following the hematogenous spread of any form of tularemia to the lungs (secondary disease).[34-36] Disease onset is abrupt, with high fevers, dyspnea, nonproductive cough, and pleuritic chest pain. Patients may rarely develop mucopurulent sputum or hemoptysis.[34] On examination, inspiratory crackles may be heard in the involved areas of the lungs, and pleural friction rubs are common.[34]

Diagnosis

The clinical presentation and laboratory features of tularemia are generally nonspecific. Radiographic findings include lobar consolidations, miliary infiltrates, hilar or mediastinal lymphadenopathy, or pleural effusions, but these, too, are nonspecific. As with the other diseases caused by the agents of bioterrorism, clinical suspicion is necessary for diagnosis.[36] Physicians who suspect this disease should alert local or state public health authorities so that the appropriate epidemiologic and environmental investigations can be begun. The clinical microbiology laboratory should also be warned of the diagnosis, since isolation of the organism represents a clear hazard to laboratory personnel.

Francisella tularensis may be directly identified in human tissues or body fluids using antigen detection assays (direct fluorescent antibodies or immunohistochemical stains). A diagnosis can also be made by recovery of the organism from cultures of blood, ulcers, conjunctival exudates, sputum, gastric aspirates, and pharyngeal washings, although these should only be attempted in Biosafety Level 3 containment facilities.[32-34] The organism is quite fastidious, and growth may be delayed, so cultures should be held for 10 days before discarding. Culture may still be possible after the initiation of appropriate antimicrobial therapy.[33] Most diagnoses of tularemia are made serologically, and a fourfold change in titer between acute and convalescent serum specimens or a single titer of at least 1:160 is diagnostic for infection.[32,33,36] Serum titers usually do not reach diagnostic levels until 10 or more days after the onset of illness.

Treatment and Postexposure Prophylaxis

Streptomycin has historically been the drug of choice for tularemia, but alternative therapies should be considered, since this antibiotic is not readily available (Table 6). Gentamicin is an acceptable alternative, and treatment should be continued for 10 days.[32] Ciprofloxacin, which has intracellular activity, has been used successfully to treat tularemia after 10 days of therapy.[33] Doxycycline and chloramphenicol can also be used, but since these drugs are bacteriostatic, therapy should be continued for at least 14 days to reduce the risk of treatment failure and relapses.[32]

In a bioterrorist release, exposed persons should be prophylactically treated with a 2-week course of either oral ciprofloxacin (500 mg twice daily) or doxycycline (100 mg twice daily).[32] These individuals should be instructed to begin a fever watch. Those who develop fever or clinical symptoms should begin parenteral therapy as outlined in Table 6.

Infection Control

Isolation is not necessary for patients with tularemia, since person-to-person transmission has not been documented. Physicians should use standard precautions when caring for patients with tularemia.

TABLE 6. Antimicrobial Treatment of Tularemia			
Antimicrobial Agent	Adult Dose	Pediatric Dose	Duration
Streptomycin	1 g IM twice daily	15 mg/kg IM twice daily	10 days
Gentamicin	5 mg/kg IV or IM daily	2.5 mg/kg IV or IM daily	10 days
Ciprofloxacin	400 mg IV twice daily	15 mg/kg IV twice daily, not to exceed 1 g daily*	10 days
Doxycycline	100 mg IV twice daily	If weight is ≥45 kg, give 100 mg IV twice daily* If weight is <45 kg, give 2.2 mg/kg IV twice daily*	14 days
Chloramphenicol	15 mg/kg IV four times daily	15 mg/kg IV four times daily	14 days

*Although fluoroquinolones and tetracyclines have known adverse effects in children, these risks must be balanced against the risks of tularemia.
Adapted from Dennis DT, Inglesby TV, Henderson DA, et al: Tularemia as a biological weapon: Medical and public health management. JAMA 285:2763–2773, 2001.

Viral Hemorrhagic Fevers

The term *viral hemorrhagic fever* refers to a clinical illness associated with fever and a bleeding diathesis caused by a diverse group of RNA viruses in four separate families: filoviruses, arenaviruses, bunyaviruses, and flaviviruses.[37] These agents have limited geographic ranges, may be highly infectious by aerosol route, and are believed to have natural animal reservoirs and arthropod vectors.[33] Humans are incidental hosts, acquiring disease by direct contact with infected animal tissue, through inhalation of infectious aerosols, or by the bite of an infected arthropod. Person-to-person transmission may be possible, allowing infected individuals to spread the disease to close contacts. The flaviviruses (yellow fever, dengue virus) are not considered significant biological warfare threats.[33]

Pathogenesis

Infection with one of the hemorrhagic fever viruses leads to reduced levels of circulating platelets and coagulation factors due to a combination of disseminated intravascular coagulation and hepatic dysfunction. The filoviruses, Ebola and Marburg viruses, can directly damage the cells of hemostasis (platelets and endothelial cells), while the arenaviruses, Lassa fever virus and the New World arenaviruses (Argentine, Bolivian, Brazilian, and Venezuealan hemorrhagic fever viruses), produce inhibitors of platelet aggregation.[37] The pathogenesis of bunyavirus infections (most importantly Rift Valley fever) remains poorly understood, but a combination of hepatic necrosis and vasculitis has been hypothesized.[37]

Clinical Manifestations

A variety of clinical findings are possible following infection with a hemorrhagic fever virus. The incubation period for these viruses ranges from 2 to 21 days.[38] Patients initially develop a nonspecific prodrome that usually lasts for 1 week. Symptoms may include malaise, headaches, arthralgias, myalgias, abdominal pain, and nausea.[33,37,38] Early signs may include high fever, tachycardia, pharyngitis, and a skin rash.[33,37,38] Patients may progress to a hemorrhagic diathesis with circulatory shock, central nervous system dysfunction, multiorgan system failure, and death. Reported clinical sequelae in those who survive infection include hearing or vision loss and impaired motor coordination.[37] The clinical findings characteristic of the key hemorrhagic fever viruses are listed in Table 7.

Diagnosis

The variable clinical presentation of the hemorrhagic fever viruses presents a major diagnostic challenge, and a high index of suspicion is necessary. Common laboratory abnormalities include thrombocytopenia, co-

TABLE 7. Clinical Findings Characteristic of Key Hemorrhagic Fever Viruses

Family	Virus	Characteristic Clinical Findings
Filo-viruses	Ebola and Marburg viruses	Fever, prostration, myalgias Nausea, vomiting, diarrhea, pharyngitis Diffuse nonprurutic maculopapular rash after ~5 days of illness No transmission of disease before clinical symptoms and signs appear
Arena-viruses	Lassa fever	Cough, chest pain, abdominal pain Up to 20% may develop ulceration of buccal mucosa Exudative pharyngitis Cervical lymphadenopathy (may progress to severe swelling of the neck) Pleuropericardial effusions Survivors often develop deafness No transmission of disease before clinical symptoms and signs appear
	Argentine, Bolivian, Brazilian, Venezuelan hemorrhagic fevers (New World arena-viruses)	Generalized lymphadenopathy Retro-orbital pain, conjunctival injection Central nervous system dysfunction (tremors, myoclonic movements, gait disturbances) Generalized seizures No transmission of disease before clinical symptoms and signs appear
Bunya-viruses	Rift Valley fever	Retro-orbital pain, photophobia Jaundice Keratitis in 10% No reported cases of person-to-person transmission

agulation abnormalities, decreased fibrinogen, increased fibrin split products, elevated liver enzymes, and azotemia.[38] All suspected cases of viral hemorrhagic fever should be immediately reported to local and state health departments. Public health authorities will provide assistance in the processing and transport of laboratory specimens for the diagnosis of these diseases. Specific disease identification can only occur at special Biosafety Level-4 laboratories, and methods of diagnosis include antigen-capture enzyme-linked immunosorbent assay, immunoglobulin M antibody-capture enzyme-linked immunosorbent assay, PCR, and viral isolation.[33,38] Visualization by electron microscopy is also available.[33]

Treatment and Postexposure Prophylaxis

All therapy for viral hemorrhagic fevers is supportive, with careful attention to fluid and electrolyte balance and blood pressure control. Mechanical ventilation, renal dialysis, and antiseizure medication may be necessary. Intramuscular injections, nonsteroidal anti-inflammatory drugs, and anticoagulation therapies should all be avoided, since they may exacerbate bleeding. Ribavirin, a nucleotide analogue, has shown some activity against arenaviruses and bunyaviruses (though none against filoviruses) and is currently under investigation as a possible therapy.[37]

No available antiviral agents are effective for postexposure prophylaxis. Persons who have been exposed should be placed on a fever watch for a period of 21 days from the time of contact.

Infection Control

Since the hemorrhagic fever viruses can be transmitted from person to person by direct contact of infected body fluids or possibly through aerosol exposure, strict barrier and airborne precautions should be instituted for any person suspected of having clinical illness. Barrier precautions consist of the use of an impermeable gown, face shield, eye protection, shoe coverage, and double gloves. The patient should be placed in a negative-pressure room, and clinicians should not enter unless N-95 masks or powered air-purifying respirators are worn.

Key Points: Principal Agents of Bioterrorism

- To minimize the effects of a bioterrorist attack, physicians must have an increased index of suspicion that such an attack can occur.
- Physicians are at the frontline in this new form of warfare.
- An understanding of the clinical presentation of the principal agents that can be weaponized is crucial.
- By close attention to disease patterns, physicians can become aware of a potential problem in time to institute actions that may save numerous lives and decrease the impact of the disease.
- Additional resources for information on the Category A agents are listed in Table 8.

TABLE 8.   Additional Resources on Category A Agents of Bioterrorism

Web Sites
  www.bt.cdc.gov
  www.hopkins-biodefense.org
  www.usamriid.army.mil/education/bluebook.html
  www.idsociety.org/BT/ToC.htm
  www.acponline.org/bioterro/?hp
Books
  Alibek K: Biohazard. Random House, 1999.
  Department of Defense: 21st Century Bioterrorism and Germ Weapons—U.S. Army Field Manual for the Treatment of Biological Warfare Agent Casualties. Progressive Management, 2001.
  Miller J, Engelberg S, Broad WJ: Germs: Biological Weapons and America's Secret War. Simon & Schuster, 2001.
  Tucker, J. Scourge—The Once and Future Threat of Smallpox. Grove Press, 2001.

References

1. Huxsoll DL, Parrott CD, Patrick WC III: Medicine in defense against biological warfare. JAMA 262:677–679, 1989.
2. Christopher GW, Cieslak TJ, Pavlin JA, Eitzen EM: Biological warfare: A historical perspective. JAMA 278:412–417, 1997.
3. Lesho E, Dorsey D, Bunner D: Feces, dead horses, and fleas: Evolution of the hostile use of biological agents. West J Med 168:512–516, 1998.
4. Centers for Disease Control and Prevention: Biological and chemical terrorism: Strategic plan for preparedness and response. Recommendations of the CDC Strategic Planning Workgroup. MMWR Morbid Mortal Wkly Rep 49(RR-4):1–4, 2000.
5. Pile JC, Malone JD, Eitzen EM, Friedlander AM: Anthrax as a potential biological warfare agent. Arch Intern Med 158:429–434, 1998.
6. Dixon TC, Meselson M, Guillemin J, Hanna PC: Anthrax. N Engl J Med 341:815–826, 1999.
7. Inglesby TV, Henderson DA, Bartlett JG, et al: Anthrax as a biological weapon: Medical and public health management. JAMA 281:1735–1745, 1999.
8. Friedlander AM, Welkos SL, Pitt MLM, et al: Postexposure prophylaxis against experimental inhalational anthrax. J Infect Dis 167:1239–1242, 1993.
9. Swartz MN: Recognition and management of anthrax—an update. N Engl J Med 345:1621–1626, 2001.
10. Gallagher TC, Strober BE: Cutaneous *Bacillus anthracis* infection. N Engl J Med 345:1646–1647, 2001.
11. Roche KJ, Chang MW, Lazarus H: Cutaneous anthrax infection. N Engl J Med 345:1611, 2001.
12. Bush LM, Abrams BH, Beall A, Johnson CC: Index case of fatal inhalational anthrax due to bioterrorism in the United States. N Engl J Med 345:1607–1610, 2001.
13. Mayer TM, Bersoff-Matcha S, Murphy C, et al: Clinical presentation of inhalational anthrax following bioterrorism exposure: Report of 2 survivors. JAMA 286:2549–2553, 2001.
14. Jernigan JA, Stephens DS, Ashford DA, et al: Bioterrorism-related inhalational anthrax: The first 10 cases reported in the United States. Emerg Infect Dis 7:933–944,2001.
15. Shafazand S, Doyle R, Ruoss S, et al: Inhalational anthrax: Epidemiology, diagnosis, and management. Chest 116:1369–1376, 1999.
16. Sirisanthana T, Brown AE: Anthrax of the gastrointestinal tract. Emerg Infect Dis 8:649–651, 2002.
17. Centers for Disease Control and Prevention: Investigation of anthrax associated with inhalational exposure and interim public health guidelines, October 2001. MMWR Morbid Mortal Wkly Rep 50:889–893, 2001.
18. Inglesby TV, O'Toole T, Henderson DA, et al: Anthrax as a biological weapon, 2002: Updated recommendations for management. JAMA 287:2236–2252, 2002.
19. Friedlander AM, Pittman PR, Parker GW: Anthrax vaccine: Evidence for safety and efficacy against inhalational anthrax. JAMA 282:2104–2106, 1999.
20. Centers for Disease Control and Prevention: Surveillance for adverse events associated with anthrax vaccination. MMWR Morbid Mortal Wkly Rep 49;341–345, 2000.
21. Centers for Disease Control and Prevention: Additional options for preventive treatment for persons exposed to inhalational anthrax. MMWR Morbid Mortal Wkly Rep 50:1142, 1151, 2001.
22. Lo Re V III, Fishman NO: Recognition and management of anthrax [letter]. N Engl J Med 346:943–944, 2002.
23. Varkey P, Poland GA, Cockerill FR III, et al: Confronting bioterrorism: Physicians on the front line. Mayo Clin Proc 77:661–672, 2002.

24. Henderson DA: Smallpox: Clinical and epidemiological features. Emerg Infect Dis 5: 537–539, 1999.
25. Henderson DA, Inglesby TV, Bartlett JG, et al: Smallpox as a biological weapon: Medical and public health management. JAMA 281:2127–2137, 1999.
26. Breman JG, Henderson DA: Diagnosis and management of smallpox. N Engl J Med 346:1300–1308, 2002.
27. Inglesby TV, Dennis, DT, Henderson DA, et al: Plague as a biological weapon: Medical and public health management. JAMA 283:2281–2290, 2000.
28. Crook LD, Tempest B: Plague. A clinical review of 27 cases. Arch Intern Med 152:1253–1256, 1992.
29. Zilinskas RA: Iraq's biological weapons: The past as future? JAMA 278:431–432, 1997.
30. Arnon SS, Schechter R, Inglesby TV, et al: Botulinum toxin as a biological weapon: Medical and public health management. JAMA 285:1059–1070, 2001.
31. Franz DR, Jahrling PB, Friedlander AM, et al: Clinical recognition and management of patients exposed to biological warfare agents. JAMA 278:399–411, 1997.
32. Dennis DT, Inglesby TV, Henderson DA, et al: Tularemia as a biological weapon: Medical and public health management. JAMA 285:2763–2773, 2001.
33. Darling RG, Catlett, Huebner KD, Jarrett DG: Threats in bioterrorism I: CDC category A agents. Emerg Med Clin North Am 20:273–309, 2002.
34. Gill V, Cunha BA: Tularemia pneumonia. Sem Resp Infect 12:61–67, 1997.
35. Feldman KA, Enscore RE, Lathrop SL, et al: An outbreak of pneumonic tularemia on Martha's Vineyard. N Engl J Med 345:1601–1606, 2001.
36. Hornick R: Tularemia revisited [editorial]. N Engl J Med 345:1637–9, 2001.
37. Borio L, Inglesby TV, Peters CJ, et al: Hemorrhagic fever viruses as biological weapons: Medical and public health management. JAMA 287:2391–2405, 2002.
38. Isaäcson M: Viral hemorrhagic fever hazards for travelers in Africa. Clin Infect Dis 33:1707–1712, 2001.

Index

Page numbers in **boldface** type indicate complete chapters.

Candidiasis (*Cont.*)
as nodular eruption cause, 301, 304
as osteomyelitis cause, 186
as peritonitis cause, 133, 135, 136
as splenic abscess cause, 140
as urinary tract infection cause, 227
vulvovaginal, 217, 240, 242–243
Capnocytophaga canimorsus, 3, 177–178
Carbuncles, 162
Carbunculosis, 170
Cardiac examination, for fever of unknown origin evaluation, 255
Cardiomyopathy
hypertrophic obstructive, 74
Lyme disease-related, 269
Cat bites, 3, 178
CD4 cell count, in HIV infection, 212, 213
Cefadroxil, as cellulitis treatment, 156
Cefazolin, as infectious arthritis treatment, 198, 199
in prosthetic joint infections, 200
Cefdinir
as bacterial sinusitis treatment, 47
as pharyngitis treatment, 49
Cefditoren, as pharyngitis treatment, 49
Cefepime
as bacterial meningitis treatment, 10
as infectious arthritis treatment, 198
Cefixime
as infectious arthritis treatment, 198, 199
as urethritis treatment, 237
Cefotaxime
as bacterial meningitis treatment, 6, 9, 10
as Lyme disease treatment, 271, 273
as peritonitis treatment, 132

Cefotetan
as pelvic inflammatory disease treatment, 233, 234
as peritonitis treatment, 136
Cefoxitin
as pelvic inflammatory disease treatment, 233, 234, 235
as peritonitis treatment, 136
Cefprozil, as pharyngitis treatment, 49
Ceftriaxone
as bacterial meningitis treatment, 6, 8, 9, 10
as chancroid treatment, 248
as conjunctivitis treatment, 40, 41
as infectious arthritis treatment, 198, 199
as Lyme disease treatment, 271, 273
as neurosyphilis treatment, 288
as pelvic inflammatory disease treatment, 235
as peritonitis treatment, 132
as syphilis treatment, 286
as urethritis treatment, 237
Cefuroxime axetil
as bacterial sinusitis treatment, 47
as Lyme disease treatment, 271–272
as pharyngitis treatment, 49
Cell subset analysis, for HIV infection diagnosis, 213
Cellulitis, 155–156, 169
anaerobic, 169, 170
bite wound-related, 183
clostridial, 169
erysipelas variant of, 157
gangrenous, 169, 170
nonclostridial, 169
orbital, 36
perianal, 157
Pseudomonas-related, 157–158
Central nervous system, tuberculosis of, 95–96
Central nervous system tumors, as meningitis cause, 19

Dermatologic examination, for fever of unknown origin evaluation, 254–255
Dermatologic infections. *See* Skin infections
Dermatophyte infections, 160–161, 162–163
Desenex, 164
Dexamethasone, as bacterial meningitis treatment, 10
Dextromethorpan, as bronchitis treatment, 58
Diabetes mellitus
  foot osteomyelitis in, 187
  as infective endocarditis risk factor, 76
  urinary tract infections in, 227
Dialysis, peritoneal, as peritonitis cause, 135–137
Diarrhea
  acute infectious, **103–116**
  inflammatory, 104, 105
  noninflammatory, 104–105
  stool testing for, 103, 104–105, 106–108, 111, 112–113, 114
  treatment for, 114–115
  antibiotic-associated, 112
  definition of, 104
  persistent, 106
  traveler's, 106, 107, 114
Dicloxacillin
  as cellulitis treatment, 156
  as impetigo treatment, 159
N,N-Diethyl-3-methylbenzamide (DEET), 275, 326, 327
Diphtheria, 50
Diphtheria immunization, in travelers, 310, 334
Directly observed therapy, for tuberculosis, 98, 100–101
Diverticulitis, 142
Dog bites, 3, 177–178
Double quotidian fever, 337
Doxycycline
  as acute infectious diarrhea treatment, 107

Doxycycline (*Cont.*)
  as anthrax treatment, 349, 350
  as bite-wound infection treatment, 179, 182
  as community-acquired pneumonia treatment, 69
  as conjunctivitis treatment, 40, 41
  contraindications to, 272, 273, 290
  as infectious arthritis treatment, 198, 199
  as Lyme disease treatment, 271–272
  as malaria prophylaxis, 325, 327, 328, 329–330
  as pelvic inflammatory disease treatment, 233, 234, 235
  as plague treatment, 355
  as prostatitis treatment, 226
  side effects of, 274, 329–330
  as syphilis treatment, 286, 287
  as tularemia treatment, 360
  as urethritis treatment, 238
Dromedary fever, 337
Drugs. *See also* names of specific drugs
  as aseptic meningitis cause, 13, 15, 18–19, 20
  as fever and rash cause, 293–294
  as fever of unknown origin cause, 260–261
  hypersensitivity reactions to, 293–294, 296, 299, 300, 301
Dry eye syndrome, 39
Dysentery, 106, 115
Dysuria
  cystitis-related, 216
  differential diagnosis of, 217–218
  urethritis-related, 235

E
Eastern equine encephalitis virus, 24, 25, 28
Ebola virus, 361, 362
Ecchymosis, 297
Echinacea, as common cold treatment, 44

392 Index